The Good Housekeeping Illustrated Guide to Women's Health

The Good Housekeeping Illustrated Guide to Women's Health

Comprehensive Information and Advice About
Medical and Life-style Issues Facing Women Today

Kathryn A. Cox, M.D.
Medical Editor

Genell J. Subak-Sharpe, M.S.
Editorial Director

Diane M. Goetz
Managing Editor

Briar Lee Mitchell, M.A.
Illustrator

HEARST BOOKS
NEW YORK

Library of Congress Cataloging-in-Publication Data
The Good housekeeping illustrated guide to women's health / editors,
  Kathryn Cox, Genell J. Subak-Sharpe, Diane M. Goetz ;
  Briar Lee Mitchell, illustrator.
     p. cm.
  Includes index.
  ISBN 0-688-12116-0
  1. Women – Health and hygiene. I. Cox, Kathryn.
II. Subak-Sharpe, Genell J. III. Goetz, Diane M.
RA778.G688 1995
613'.04244 – dc20   94-9284
                                                                  CIP

Printed in the United States of America

First Edition

1 2 3 4 5 6 7 8 9 10

BOOK DESIGN BY CHARLES KRELOFF

GOOD HOUSEKEEPING

Editor-in-Chief: *John Mack Carter*
Executive Editor: *Mina Mulvey*
Good Housekeeping Medical Editor: *Madonna Behen*

EDITORS

Kathryn Cox, M.D.
Assistant Clinical Instructor in Obstetrics/Gynecology
The New York Hospital–Cornell Medical Center
Medical Editor

Genell J. Subak-Sharpe, M.S.
Editorial Director

Diane M. Goetz
Managing Editor

Briar Lee Mitchell, M.A.
Illustrator

MEDICAL ADVISORY BOARD

Psychiatry

Francine Cournos, M.D., Associate Clinical
Professor of Psychiatry, Columbia University
College of Physicians and Surgeons, New York

Breast Surgery

Alisan Goldfarb, M.D., Assistant Clinical Professor
of Surgery, Mt. Sinai Medical School, New York

Nutrition

Delia Hammock, M.S., R.D., Associate Director,
The Good Housekeeping Institute, New York

Endocrinology

Lois Jovanovic-Peterson, M.D., Clinical Professor of
Medicine, University of Southern California, Los
Angeles, and Senior Scientist, Sansun Medical
Research Foundation

Rheumatology

Steven K. Magid, M.D., Associate Professor of
Clinical Medicine, Cornell University Medical
College, New York

Exercise Physiology

William McArdle, Ph.D., Professor of Health and
Physical Education, Queens College, New York

Internal Medicine/Endocrinology

JoAnn E. Manson, M.D., Dr. P.H., Associate
Professor of Medicine, Harvard Medical School,
Boston

Plastic and Reconstructive Surgery

Richard A. Skolnik, M.D., Assistant Clinical
Professor of Surgery, Mt. Sinai Medical School,
New York

Preventive Medicine

Valerie Ulene, M.D., M.P.H., The New York
Hospital–Cornell Medical Center, New York

Occupational Medicine

Michael Wilkes, M.D., Ph.D., Assistant Professor of
Medicine and Health Services Research,
University of California, Los Angeles

Foreword

History is a profound teacher, one that reveals the attitudes, mores, and culture of a society. According to Eileen Power in *Medieval Women*, the position of women is often considered a test by which the civilization of a country is judged. The position of women is one thing in theory, another in legal position, yet another in "everyday life."[1] If Power is correct, then the twentieth century can be judged to have been a successful, if tumultuous, century for women, at least women of the industrialized world. The advancements realized by and for women have been far reaching and have occurred in a relatively short period of time.

Women now not only cast their ballots but they are those for whom ballots are also cast. Women who once ran homes now run corporations. Women who defended their homes now defend their countries. Few professions or activities are barred from women today who have the skill and ability to succeed. And women still retain the role of homemaker, caretaker, and nurturer. Health has been enhanced such that women, on average, live to 78 years of age. Many diseases have been eradicated and others have been brought under control.

Health is a constant theme throughout the study of civilizations, and history is a profound teacher especially as it concerns women. For centuries women's health has been misunderstood or neglected due to superstition and fear. Cyclical flow of blood, procre- ation and bearing of children, menopause, and other manifestations of womanhood have puzzled humans since recorded time. Michel Rouche, examining life in the early Middle Ages, comments that "for many men, women remained a mystery, sometimes good, some- times evil, a source of happiness, now of sorrow, at once terrifyingly pure and destructively impure."[2] This view, sometimes held by some women as well, has persisted for many centuries and has influenced the study of women's health. Indeed, it has been difficult to construct an accurate history of women's health as it has frequently been ignored or misrepresented in historical accounts of daily life and medicine.

This is no longer the case. As women have emerged on the public and professional scene in this century, so has the study of women's health and dis- ease. The focus on women's health has expanded from a concentration on reproductive organs to the "whole" woman. Increasingly, women recogize that heart disease is the leading cause of death among women as it is among men. And such conditions as alcoholism, drug abuse, and sexually transmitted dis- eases, which have for too long been stigmatized, are now receiving long overdue attention among women. Lung cancer, a disease of men until the middle of the twentieth century, especially among those who smoked, has now become the leading cause of cancer death among women since they have adopted for- merly male behaviors such as cigarette smoking.

---

[1]Power, E. *Medieval Women*. New York: Cambridge University Press, 1975, p. 9.

[2]Rouche, M. The early and middle ages in the west. *A History of Private Life*. Philippe Aries and Georges Duby (general editors), Cambridge, Massachusetts: Belknap Press of Harvard University Press, 1987, p. 482.

The focus on women's health, both in research and treatment, has come about late in the twentieth century, resulting from escalating demands from the scientific community, women's advocates, and from legislators intent upon equity.

One of the most important events in women's health came about when the National Institutes of Health, the premier federal biomedical research institution, created the Office of Research of Women's Health in 1990 with the resources to assure action. The creation of this office and legislation by the 103rd Congress mandating it and the inclusion of women in studies of diseases, disorders, and conditions that effect them meant that women's health and attendant research could no longer be ignored. Additional legislation also underscores that action should be undertaken to recruit and advance women in biomedical careers. Other agencies within the federal government's Department of Health and Human Services have underscored this focus on women's health with offices of their own: the Food and Drug Administration, the Health Resources and Services Administration, the Substance Abuse and Mental Health Administration, the Agency for Health Care Policy and Research, the Centers for Disease Control and Prevention, and Public Health Service's Office of Women's Health. Similar efforts are emerging in state and local governments, in private organizations and corporations, and in many health centers.

One of the most exciting aspects of women's health resulting from all of these actions is the necessary attention to the health of all of America's women—of all racial and ethnic groups and sexual orientation, across the life-span, wherever they reside. In the future, scientists and health care providers will know better whether a medication is as effective in Asian women as in African-American women; whether the dosage must be reduced in women compared to men; or whether the treatment is as effective in older women as in younger women.

These changes and advancements are exciting and hold great promise. Yet, we already possess considerable knowledge that will benefit women, that will prevent disease or identify and treat it early, thus enhancing quality of life. Unfortunately, too many women remain unaware of that knowledge. A 1993 survey of 2,500 women, conducted by the Commonwealth Fund, indicated that 44 percent of those questioned had not had a mammogram and 35 percent had not undergone a Pap smear. While heart disease, cancer, and stroke are the leading cause of death among women, most surveyed did not know how to take preventive action.

Today, each woman must take control of her health by becoming informed and acting upon that information. It is never too early to begin and never too late. Young women should never begin smoking cigarettes; older women should not fail to quit. This book will help you take control by providing a broad-based focus on women's health and well-being. It gives you information you need about your body and its functions—from your reproductive organs to your cardiovascular system. It addresses topical issues such as occupational health and domestic violence. It addresses prevention—eating right, exercising, managing stress, and avoiding such harmful habits as alcohol abuse and smoking.

As health care professionals and scientists, we know that our best chance for success is a partnership based on mutual understanding, information, and trust. If you understand your body and know what questions to ask, we will be prepared to guide and care for you. This book should be a useful supplement to that professional guidance. Join with us as we make history and enhance our health and well-being together.

Judith H. LaRosa, Ph.D., R.N.
Deputy Director
Vivian W. Pinn, M.D.
Director

Office of Research on Women's Health
Office of the Director
National Institutes of Health
Bethesda, Maryland
August 1994

Acknowledgments

In the more than two years it has taken to put this book together, dozens of people have provided invaluable expertise, guidance, and insight to make it a comprehensive reference. Although it is impossible to name all of them here, some must be acknowledged for their outstanding contributions.

We want first to acknowledge the expertise and dedication of our medical advisors—Francine Cournos, M.D., Alisan Goldfarb, M.D., Delia Hammock, M.S., R.D., Lois Jovanovic-Peterson, M.D., Steven Magid, M.D., JoAnn E. Manson, M.D., Dr. P. H. William McArdle, Ph.D., Richard A. Skolnik, M.D., Valerie Ulene, M.D., M.P.H., and Michael Wilkes, M.D., Ph.D.—who managed to review the manuscript while working full time at writing, editing, teaching, conducting research, and practicing medicine and surgery.

A bevy of expert consultants lent their skills and knowledge to the project. Our thanks to James B. Bakalar, J.D., Gayle S. Sanders, J.D., Meg Kaplan, Ph.D., Claudia B. Scalzi, M.P.S., Joyce Zeitz of the American Fertility Society, and, from *Good Housekeeping Magazine*, John Mack Carter and Madonna Behen.

A skilled team of medical writers and editors brought their talen to bear on these pages. They include: Brenda Becker, Diana Benzaia, Cathy Caruthers, Diana Debrovner, Stephanie Denmark, Nancy Gagliardi, Rachel Hager, Andrea Kott, Ricki Lewis, Helene MacLean, Linda Murray, Emily Paulsen, Roberta Chopp Rothschild, Caroline Tapley, Luba Vikhanski, Eileen Wallen, and Judith Weinstein.

Our talented illustrator, Briar Lee Mitchell, deserves special thanks for her extraordinary patience and diligence. So does Barbara Gold, who made it all seem so easy as she executed the interior layout and gave new life to the book.

We want to pay tribute to our editors at Hearst Books for their guidance and support. We are grateful to Ann Bramson, for having a special vision about this book; Sonia Greenbaum, for combing the manuscript for inconsistencies and smoothing out its style with her straightforward prose; Ann Cahn, whose expertise and experience in the field of medical books kept us on track; Laurie Orsek, whose fresh viewpoint enhanced the book greatly in its final stages; and Gail Kinn, whose meticulous attention to the details of copyediting and production made it all come together well and on time.

A group of hard-working assistants helped coordinate myriad details to keep the project moving. Special thanks to Amy Broderick, Letta Nealy, Arlyn Apollo, Ann Johnson, Nancy Palermo-Burgos, and Karen Gottlieb-White for everything from typing to chasing down references to keeping track of the whereabouts of the manuscript and all of us.

Finally, our gratitude goes to our spouses and children, who gave their moral support, offered practical suggestions, soothed frazzled nerves, and uncomplainingly went on without us many nights and weekends while this book was being completed.

—The Editors

Contents

How to Use This Book

As we look forward to major changes in health care for all Americans, we are already experiencing changes in the delivery of health care to women. One reason for the change is that more women are becoming doctors. In 1994, 20 percent of doctors and 40 percent of medical students are women, and an increasing number are specializing in women's health. The Johns Hopkins University School of Medicine has just accepted, for the first time in its 101-year history, a freshman class in which the majority of students are women. It did so without changing its criteria for admission.

The scope of services offered to women is changing, too. Heretofore, women usually turned to obstetricians and gynecologists for their medical needs, including treatment for diseases unrelated to reproductive health. Now, major medical centers across the country have opened or are planning special clinics devoted exclusively to women's health, offering everything from the traditional reproductive services to support groups for battered women.

It is clear that women must change, too. While our needs have sometimes been ignored by others, we have ignored them ourselves. We have always been the primary caregivers in our families, tending to husbands and children or sick or aging parents. We must begin to take more time for ourselves. Lifestyle factors contribute to, if not cause, the major chronic diseases that affect women and men alike, and we must take responsibility for changing any that are detrimental to our health.

One way to begin to take control of your health is to educate yourself, and that is why we wrote this book. It is designed to be informative, and practical and, because it comes from *Good Housekeeping*, always reliable.

Part One, "Color Atlas of the Female Body," is meant to provide a basic reference to female anatomy. While you will encounter many individual illustrations throughout the main chapters and in the Encyclopedia section, it is this first part that details each of the organ systems for a comprehensive look at how the body all fits together. It is a resource you should refer to frequently as you read the chapters that follow.

Part Two, "Understanding Your Body," begins with puberty and ends with the aging process. In between you will find basic information about all of the milestones that mark your life as a woman—menstruation, pregnancy, childbirth, and menopause, among others. While you may want to save some of these chapters for appropriate times in your life, or perhaps in your daughters' lives, we suggest that you read "The Female Body" as a foundation for the information contained in the rest of the book.

Part Three, "Taking Care of Your Body," is the heart of the book. Here our emphasis has been on prevention because we believe that there is so much you can do to have a positive impact on your health. This is where you will find answers to your nutrition questions, advice on losing weight once and for all, help in designing an exercise program you can stick to, tips for managing stress, resources for handling emotional problems, clues to why you feel tired all the time, and that one critical reason to quit smoking or abusing drugs—and sympathetic help in doing so. There is also practical advice on taking care of your body, and a provocative chapter on "Rethinking Body Image" that questions some of society's assumptions about women.

Part Four, "Women in the Workplace," delves into emerging issues in women's health. This part deals with issues that affect both physical and emotional health—occupational health and safety hazards and sexual harassment. "Women and the Health Care System" gives practical advice on navigating managed care, finding a doctor, and what to expect from your relationships with health care professionals. For young women who have not yet had a first gynecological exam, it takes you step-by-step through a typical exam, from making the appointment to what questions to ask when it's over. For older women, who may be facing responsibility for aging parents, it gives advice on arranging for care.

Domestic violence may not at first seem to fit into a book on health, yet more women are injured by men in their homes than by auto accidents, rapes, and muggings combined, and the aftermath of violence and rape can take a tremendous toll on a woman's emotional well-being. "Women and Violence" discusses the roots of domestic violence and how to protect yourself against rape.

Part Five begins with the Encyclopedia section— more than seventy entries in an alphabetical format giving concise descriptions of common ailments, tests, and treatments. We have concentrated on those disorders that exclusively affect women, that affect women more often than men, or that are manifested differently in women. A glossary of terms used in the book and a list of resources for further information, referrals, and self-help complete the volume.

Taken together, these five parts present a comprehensive guide to living a satisfying and more healthful life. We hope that you will refer to it again and again.

—The Editors

The Good Housekeeping Illustrated Guide to Women's Health

Color Atlas of the Female Body

The following pages are filled with color illustrations of female anatomy. They are intended as a companion to Chapter 1, "The Female Body," as well as an independent reference.

The major organs are grouped within systems in the Color Atlas. Through complex interrelationships, these independent organs act in concert to supply oxygen to each cell, process food into energy, remove waste, flex muscles, produce the menstrual flow, and accomplish the many conscious and unconscious functions that govern our daily lives. To add another layer to this intricate process, the signals that activate some of these functions may originate within other areas of the body entirely. Hormones produced by the endocrine system, for example, influence such diverse processes as the digestion of food, production of breast milk, timing of labor, and marshaling of the body's physical response to danger.

Most of the organs on these pages are identical to, if somewhat smaller than, those of men; others, primarily the urinary and reproductive organs, are very different. Some of the more subtle differences between men's and women's bodies are detailed on pages 14–15.

Developing a basic understanding of the organ system is fundamental to comprehending how the body functions in sickness and in health.

Color plate 1   The skeletal system
Color plate 2   The muscular system
Color plate 3   The heart and circulatory system
Color plate 4   The respiratory system
Color plate 5   The digestive system
Color plate 6   The urogenital system
Color plate 7   The endocrine system
Color plate 8   The reproductive system

THE SKELETAL SYSTEM

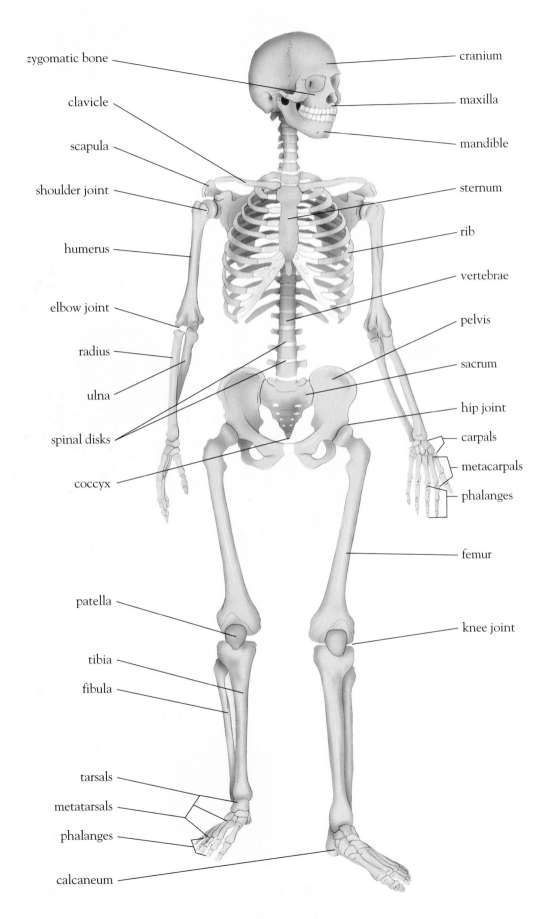

zygomatic bone

clavicle

scapula

shoulder joint

humerus

elbow joint

radius

ulna

spinal disks

coccyx

patella

tibia

fibula

tarsals

metatarsals

phalanges

calcaneum

cranium

maxilla

mandible

sternum

rib

vertebrae

pelvis

sacrum

hip joint

carpals

metacarpals

phalanges

femur

knee joint

Color Plate 1

THE MUSCULAR SYSTEM

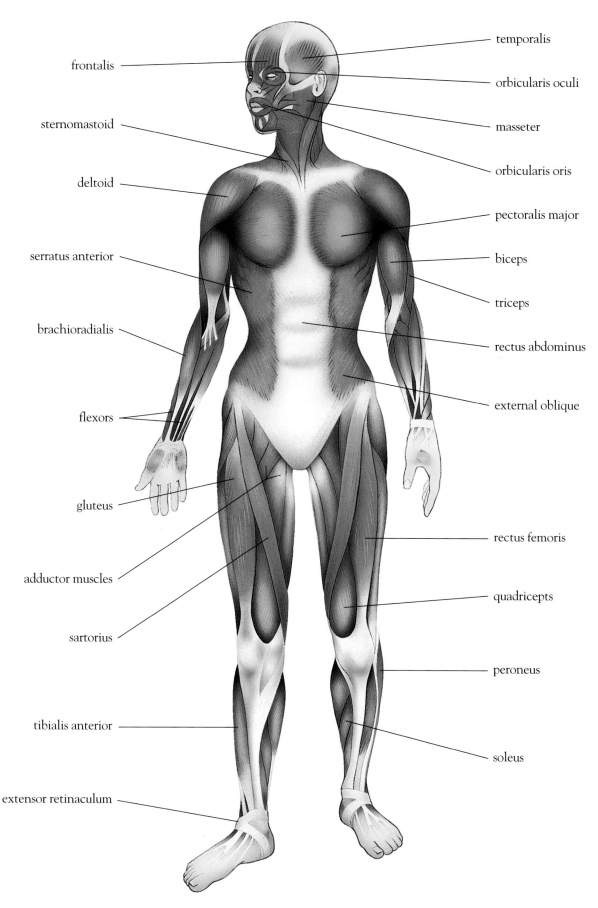

frontalis

temporalis

orbicularis oculi

sternomastoid

masseter

deltoid

orbicularis oris

pectoralis major

serratus anterior

biceps

triceps

brachioradialis

rectus abdominus

flexors

external oblique

gluteus

rectus femoris

adductor muscles

quadricepts

sartorius

peroneus

tibialis anterior

soleus

extensor retinaculum

Color Plate 2

THE HEART AND CIRCULATORY SYSTEM

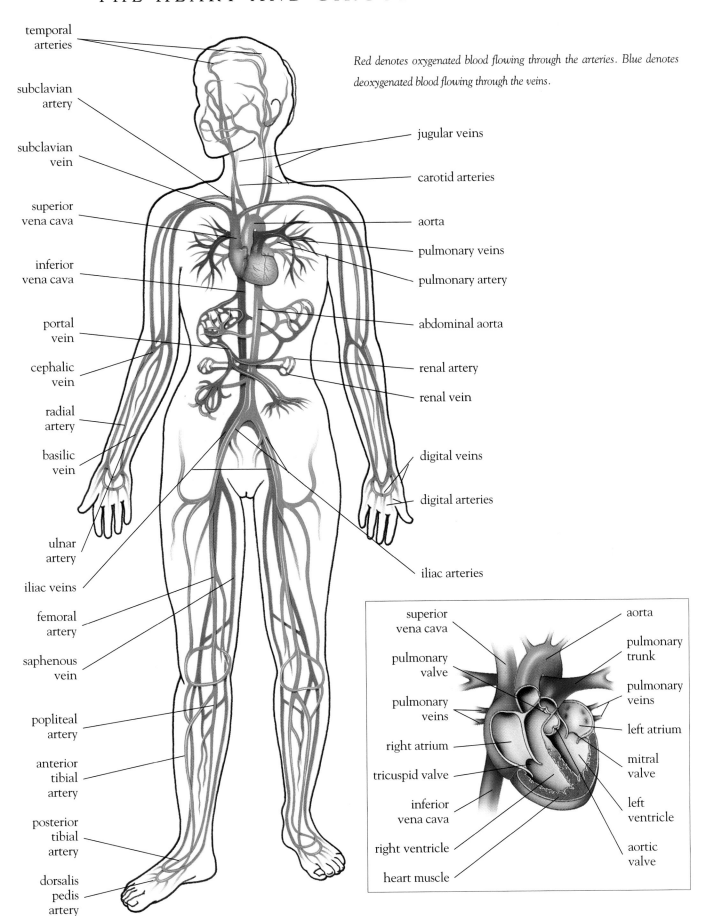

temporal arteries

subclavian artery

subclavian vein

superior vena cava

inferior vena cava

portal vein

cephalic vein

radial artery

basilic vein

ulnar artery

iliac veins

femoral artery

saphenous vein

popliteal artery

anterior tibial artery

posterior tibial artery

dorsalis pedis artery

Red denotes oxygenated blood flowing through the arteries. Blue denotes deoxygenated blood flowing through the veins.

jugular veins

carotid arteries

aorta

pulmonary veins

pulmonary artery

abdominal aorta

renal artery

renal vein

digital veins

digital arteries

iliac arteries

superior vena cava

pulmonary valve

pulmonary veins

right atrium

tricuspid valve

inferior vena cava

right ventricle

heart muscle

aorta

pulmonary trunk

pulmonary veins

left atrium

mitral valve

left ventricle

aortic valve

Color Plate 3

THE RESPIRATORY SYSTEM

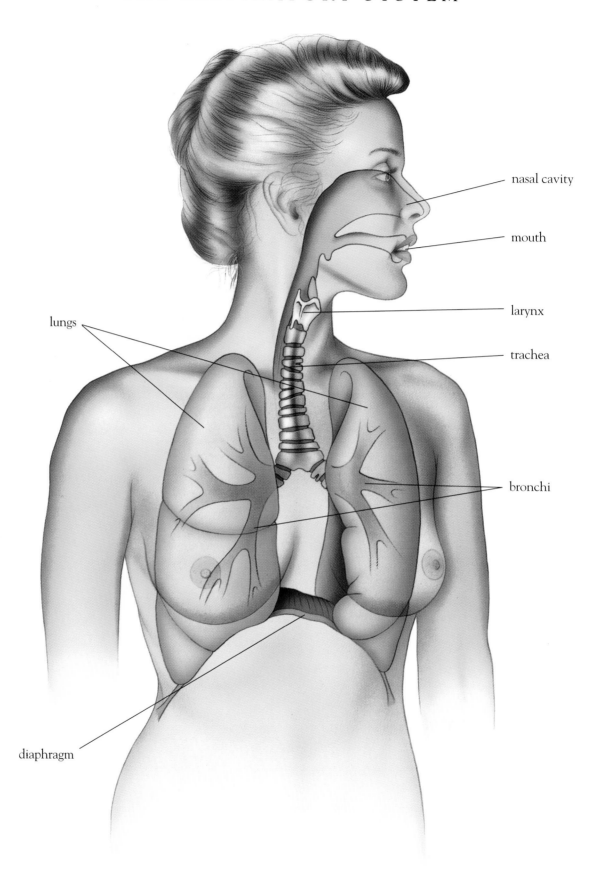

nasal cavity

mouth

larynx

trachea

lungs

bronchi

diaphragm

THE DIGESTIVE SYSTEM

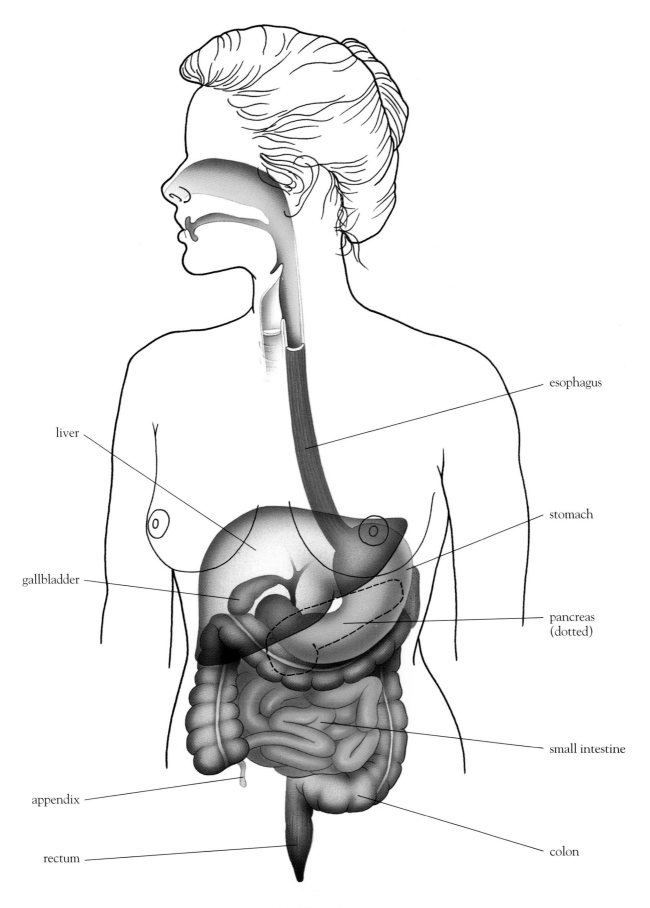

esophagus

liver

stomach

gallbladder

pancreas
(dotted)

small intestine

appendix

colon

rectum

Color Plate 5

THE UROGENITAL SYSTEM

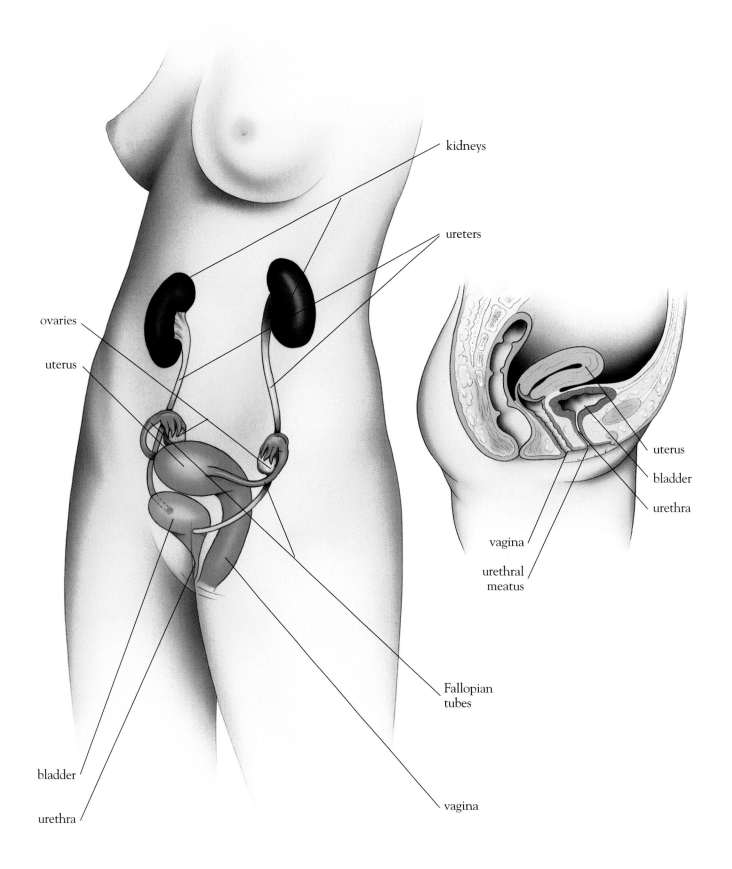

kidneys

ureters

ovaries

uterus

uterus

bladder

urethra

vagina

urethral
meatus

Fallopian
tubes

bladder

urethra

vagina

THE ENDOCRINE SYSTEM

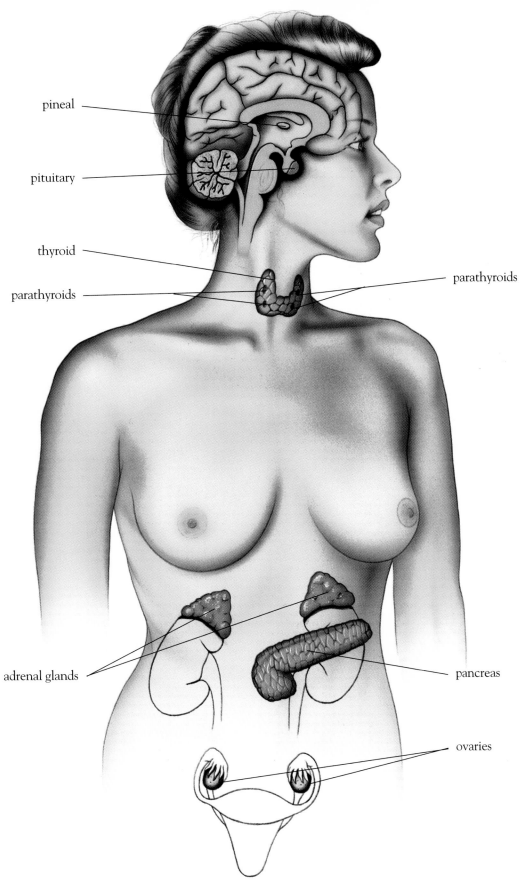

pineal

pituitary

thyroid

parathyroids

parathyroids

adrenal glands

pancreas

ovaries

Color Plate 7

THE REPRODUCTIVE SYSTEM

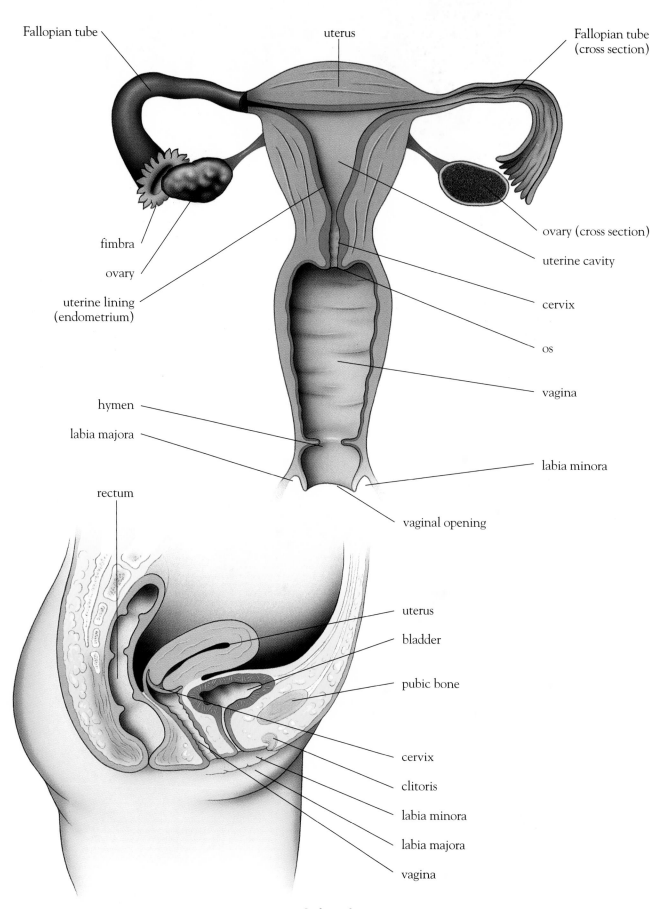

Fallopian tube

uterus

Fallopian tube
(cross section)

fimbra

ovary

uterine lining
(endometrium)

ovary (cross section)

uterine cavity

cervix

os

vagina

hymen

labia majora

labia minora

vaginal opening

rectum

uterus

bladder

pubic bone

cervix

clitoris

labia minora

labia majora

vagina

Color Plate 8

Understanding Your Body

CHAPTER

The Female Body

Throughout the centuries, women's concern about their bodies has centered on shape and appearance. It is only in the last 25 years or so, as women have grown more aware of the importance of protecting their own health and well-being, that they have become keenly interested in understanding how their bodies function. Men and women have virtually identical organ systems, although women's organs are usually smaller and there are some organs that are uniquely male or female. (See box, "Gender Differences.") This chapter describes those elements that are specific to women in their structure or function.

THE REPRODUCTIVE SYSTEM

The female reproductive system consists of the external organs, referred to as the genitals, or the vulva, and the internal organs, which include the vagina, uterus, Fallopian tubes, and ovaries.

THE VULVA In adult women, the upper part of the vulva is covered with pubic hair, which begins to grow at puberty and thins out after menopause. In some women, the hair is scant, while in others it is thick and spreads upward toward the navel and down to the inner thighs. Pubic hair grows on a soft, fatty cushion known as the mons pubis or mons veneris, Latin for "mount of Venus."

The bottom part of the mons has two folds of fatty tissue covered with skin, called the outer lips, or labia majora. Their size and color vary greatly among women. They may also change in size and shape during an individual woman's life, sometimes remaining somewhat open after childbirth, for example. Inside the outer lips are two folds of moist, hairless tissue known as the inner lips, or labia minora. The two sets of folds join in front and form part of the mons. Their purpose is to protect the opening of the urethra and the entrance to the vagina that lie inside them. The inner lips are particularly sensitive to touch. During sexual arousal, they swell and turn darker.

Above the opening of the urethra, the inner lips join to form a hood over the tip of the clitoris. Although it is this tip—about the size of a pencil eraser—that is commonly referred to as "the clitoris," the entire organ is in fact much larger and is mostly hidden under the skin. The tip is called the glans of the clitoris, and the firm, elongated part of the clitoris that extends upward under the skin of the hood is called the shaft. Running down from the shaft on each side are two bundles of erectile tissue called the bulbs of the vestibule.

The clitoris plays a major role in female sexual sensation and arousal and is involved in orgasms. It has a dense supply of nerve endings and some of its tissues are similar in structure to the erectile tissues of the penis. During sexual activity, the clitoris becomes firm and engorged with blood.

THE VAGINA An elastic, muscular tube 4 to 5 inches long, the vagina leads from the outside of the body to the uterus. It serves as a passageway for menstrual flow and as a birth canal. It is also the opening into which the penis is inserted during genital intercourse. Normally, the vagina is "closed," but because its walls are elastic, it accommodates a penis of any size and stretches greatly during childbirth. During intercourse, it may also lengthen.

The vagina is lined with mucous tissue that can range from almost dry to very wet. It tends to be dry in girls before puberty and in women after menopause. During the childbearing years, it can be drier during lactation and in the part of the cycle immediately following menstruation. Around the time of ovulation, during pregnancy, and when a woman is sexually aroused, the vagina is wet. Vaginal secretions keep the passageway clean, help prevent infection, and provide lubrication during intercourse.

In a young girl, the opening to the vagina is partially covered by a thin membrane called the hymen. As she matures, the opening in the center of the hymen gradually stretches from physical activity, insertion of tampons, or intercourse. In rare instances, the membrane may lack an opening or be very thick, and need to be opened by a physician. At both sides of the vaginal opening lie two mucus-secreting glands called Bartholin's glands. Some women may be able to feel them, but most become aware of their existence only if the glands become infected or swell because of a blockage of the drainage ducts.

The vagina has few nerve endings, and their pattern of distribution varies among women. In some women, most or all of the surface of the vagina is sensitive. In others, only the outer part of the vagina is sensitive, so they may not feel a tampon once it is in place, and they may experience sensations deep in the vagina only as pressure. Some women, particularly if they cannot feel a contraceptive sponge or a tampon in the vagina, may fear that these objects will somehow get "lost." This, however, is impossible,

since the vagina is relatively short and its opening into the uterus is so small that the vagina is virtually a dead end.

The walls of the vagina contain a layer of muscle that may contract spontaneously or at will. This action also involves a contraction of the pelvic floor muscles, which hold in place the organs of the pelvis. (To feel your pelvic floor muscles, try squeezing them to stop urination in midstream.) A woman whose muscles are weak may have difficulty controlling the flow of urine, but these muscles can be strengthened by exercise (see box, Chapter 2, "Sexual Health").

THE UTERUS The uterus, or womb, is a pear-shaped muscular sac that lies between the bladder and the rectum and is held in place by muscles and ligaments. The inner lining of the uterus, or endometrium, is shed each month during menstruation (see Chapter 4). In its nonpregnant state, the uterus is smaller than a fist and usually remains collapsed. Its main function is to hold and maintain a fetus during pregnancy, at which time it expands enormously.

The thick walls of the uterus, or myometrium, contain some of the strongest muscles in the body, which are constantly contracting and relaxing slightly. During intercourse, menstruation, and childbirth, they contract more forcefully to draw the sperm upward, allow menstrual blood to flow downward, and help push the baby through the birth canal. When they contract forcefully, a woman may experience cramps.

The upper part of the uterus is called the fundus, and the narrow neck at the bottom is called the cervix. The cervix has a smooth, firm, and rubbery surface. It projects into the vagina and has a tiny opening in the middle called the cervical os. This opening is lined with mucus-secreting cells, but the mucus is porous enough to allow sperm to travel upward to the uterus and menstrual blood to flow down. The os is normally about the diameter of a very thin straw, but during delivery it expands dramatically to allow the passage of the baby. Even in women who have had vaginal deliveries, the os measures only about ¼ inch long.

THE FALLOPIAN TUBES The Fallopian tubes are two delicate, narrow cylinders about 4 to 5 inches long. At one end, they are attached to the uterus; at the other, they extend toward the ovaries but are not attached to them. Instead, each tube ends in a funnel-shaped fringed opening with millions of minute feathery fingers called fimbriae that wrap around the outside of the ovary. The fimbriae move and create currents that trap the egg released each month through the ovary wall and channel it into the tube.

The walls of the Fallopian tubes contract slightly, pushing the egg toward the uterus. Fertilization occurs if the egg meets sperm somewhere along the way. The fertilized egg takes about 4 to 6 days to complete its journey to the womb and become implanted. If it implants itself in the wall of the Fallopian tube by mistake, the result is an ectopic pregnancy. In very rare cases, if the egg is not "trapped" as it leaves the ovary and is fertilized outside the tube, an ectopic pregnancy may occur elsewhere in the pelvic cavity. Any ectopic pregnancy is a serious condition usually requiring surgery.

THE OVARIES　The ovaries are a pair of organs usually about the size and shape of unshelled almonds. They lie on either side of the uterus, supported by ligaments near the open end of the Fallopian tubes, about 4 to 5 inches below the waist. A tough, white membrane covers the ovaries and protects some 350,000 to 400,000 follicles—tiny fluid-filled sacs containing immature eggs that are present in females at birth.

The ovaries perform two major functions: They produce mature eggs and manufacture female sex hormones. Estrogen, one of the major hormones released by the ovaries, is produced in the outer membrane of the follicles. In a fertile woman, one or more of the ovarian follicles begin to mature under the influence of pituitary hormones during each monthly cycle. Ovulation occurs in the middle of a 28-day cycle (or 14 days before the next period in a shorter or longer cycle) when the ripening follicle ruptures and the egg is released. Conception can occur if the mature egg meets with sperm within 12 to 24 hours. Although the time during which the egg can be fertilized is limited, sperm are usually viable for 1 to 2 days, and possibly as long as 5. In some cases sperm present in the genital tract from earlier intercourse can fertilize a just-released egg before a woman is aware that she has ovulated.

The empty follicle then turns into a small cyst called the *corpus luteum*, which produces the hormone progesterone for about 14 days. If no pregnancy occurs, the corpus luteum shrinks and stops producing progesterone, and the endometrial lining is shed. If the released egg is fertilized, the corpus luteum continues to secrete progesterone for 8 to 12 weeks until the placenta takes over this function.

THE BREASTS

Many women's breasts are very sensitive and play an important role in sexual response, but their main physiological function is to produce milk to feed a baby.

Milk is made in the part of the breast known as glandular tissue. This tissue consists of about twenty lobes arranged in a circular fashion around the nipple. The lobes are attached to a network of milk ducts—tubes that radiate from the nipple like spokes of a wheel and branch off into smaller tubes. Each lobe is made up of clusters of small lobules that contain tiny milk-producing units called acini. When the baby suckles, milk produced in the acini flows through the lobes into the system of ducts and to the nipple.

The breast also contains connective fibers and fat. The amount of fat, which is determined by heredity and body weight, significantly affects the size of the breasts, but size has no effect on the breasts' sexual responsiveness.

Nor is the ability to make milk affected by the size of the breasts: Even a very small breast has sufficient glandular tissue to perform this task. Moreover, glandular tissue expands during pregnancy, sprouting new offshoots. Women with very large breasts may in fact have some difficulty breast-feeding because their long milk ducts may become distorted as the breasts enlarge during pregnancy.

The breast sits on a layer of connective tissue called the fascia, which is firmly attached to the two underlying chest muscles, pectoralis major and pectoralis minor. Breast tissue is affixed to the overlying skin with fibrous straps called Cooper's ligaments.

The nipple is surrounded by a pigmented area called the areola, which may range in color from light pink to dark brown. During pregnancy the areola darkens, and may remain somewhat darker after childbirth. The surface of the areola contains Montgomery's glands, tiny pimplelike structures that secrete a fatty substance which lubricates the nipple to prevent cracking. These glands often enlarge during pregnancy, which is normal, as is the clear discharge (a forerunner of breast milk) that is often seen in the third trimester. A blood-tinged discharge at any time is not normal and should be reported to your doctor.

Nipples may be flat, protruding, or inverted. All shapes are normal, but a sudden change in a nipple—

particularly if a normally protruding nipple becomes inverted—may signal an abnormality and you should consult a physician promptly. The nipple contains erectile tissue, which may cause it to become erect in response to cold, sexual stimulation, or a baby's suckling.

CYCLICAL CHANGES During menstruation your breasts undergo cyclical changes. Glandular tissue expands in the premenstrual phase of the cycle in preparation for a possible pregnancy. The expansion occurs under the influence of increased estrogen and progesterone, which also leads to increased blood flow to the breasts and promotes retention of body fluids. Breasts often become tender and may develop cysts, sacs resulting from excess fluid accumulation. Some women need a larger bra during the premenstrual phase.

If no pregnancy occurs, hormone levels drop sharply, menstruation begins, and the breasts begin to shrink. They are usually at their smallest about 7 days after the onset of menstruation. Sometimes the glandular tissue does not shrink completely before expanding again the following month, leading to formation of small nodules or lumps. As a result, many women in their thirties and forties, who have gone through hundreds of cycles without becoming pregnant, notice their breasts becoming increasingly lumpy. This benign condition is known as fibrocystic breast disorder (see the Encyclopedia).

THE HORMONE SYSTEM

Hormones are chemical messengers that control numerous processes in the body—from growth to metabolism to sexual development and desire. The action of hormones is not fully understood, but biologists do know that they work by attaching to receptors, cells at special sites that are designed to respond to the hormone. The receptors then transmit a hormone's message to the appropriate area in the cell.

Hormones are secreted by several organs, including the kidneys, lungs, heart, and the lining of the intestines, but are mostly produced by the endocrine glands. In contrast to the exocrine glands, which produce sweat or saliva that is carried outside of the body, endocrine glands release their hormones directly into the bloodstream. The major endocrine glands include the following:

THE PITUITARY AND THE HYPOTHALAMUS The pituitary, a tiny gland located at the base of the brain, is often referred to as the master gland because it produces several hormones that control other parts of the endocrine system. These are known as trophic hormones, or tropins. The pituitary also releases other hormones, such as somatotropin, that affect body tissues directly. (See box, "Pituitary and Hypothalamus Hormones and Their Functions.")

Right above the pituitary, and connected to it by a short stalk, is the hypothalamus. This cherry-sized region of the brain regulates hormone production in the pituitary by sending nerve impulses and releasing its own hormonelike substances. Because the functions of the pituitary and the hypothalamus are closely interrelated, these glands are sometimes regarded as a single complex.

THE PINEAL The pineal, so called because it resembles a pine cone, is a tiny gland located deep within the brain. Long considered a mystery, the pineal is now known to secrete at least one hormone, melatonin. Melatonin is believed to suppress the electrical activity of the brain, producing a sedative effect and facilitating sleep.

THE THYROID This is a small, butterfly-shaped gland that lies over the windpipe just below the larynx. In response to the thyroid-stimulating hormone (TSH) released by the pituitary, it produces the thyroid hormones, triiodothyronine and thyroxine, or T_3 and T_4, which affect virtually all metabolic processes in the body and are necessary for normal growth. The gland also manufactures the hormone calcitonin, which promotes the storage of calcium in the bones.

The thyroid has a unique ability to absorb iodine from the bloodstream, which it needs for production of the thyroid hormones. Too much of these hormones speeds up the metabolism and can cause rapid heartbeat, weight loss, and other symptoms. Too little of the hormones slows down body processes and can cause lethargy and weight gain.

THE PARATHYROIDS The parathyroid glands, which are about the size of apple seeds, are located behind or inside the thyroid gland. Most people have two pairs of these glands, but this number can vary. Parathyroid hormone regulates the levels of calcium and phosphate in the body and the metabolism of the bones. While calcitonin lowers the concentration of calcium in the blood, the parathyroid hormone raises it. Excess amounts of the parathyroid hormone lead to hypercalcemia, an abnormally high concentration of calcium in the blood, which can cause kidney stones, brittle bones, and other symptoms. Low levels of the hormone can cause tetany, or severe muscle spasms.

THE THYMUS This gland lies at the base of the neck behind the breastbone. It grows during childhood, reaches its full size at puberty, and then shrinks gradually. Along with the lymph glands and spleen, the thymus produces white blood cells called lymphocytes. These cells play an important role in the body's immune system by producing antibodies and instructing other white blood cells to kill bacteria.

THE ADRENALS These glands are triangular structures about 2 inches long that rest atop the kidneys. Each gland has an inner part, the medulla, and an outer part, the cortex. The medulla produces catecholamines—adrenaline and noradrenaline—which help the body mobilize its resources in response to extreme conditions or perceived danger, in the so-called fight-or-flight response. Because these hormones are also produced elsewhere in the body, the medulla is not crucial for survival.

In contrast, hormones produced in the adrenal cortex are essential to a number of vital processes in the body. These hormones, called steroids, are divided into three classes according to their function. Aldosterone, the major hormone in the category of mineralocorticoids, helps maintain the body's balance of fluids. Among the category of glucocorticoids, the most abundant is cortisol, which transforms protein and fat into blood sugar and has an antiinsulin effect. Glucocorticoids maintain blood pressure and regulate the body's response to physical stress.

The third type of hormone produced by the adrenal cortex comprises the male and female sex hormones, androgens and estrogens, which supplement the ones released by the ovaries and testes. At puberty, the adrenal glands increase their secretion of androgens, particularly testosterone, in both males and females. In an average adult woman, about half of the androgens are released in the ovaries and half in the adrenal cortex. In normal amounts, androgens stimulate the growth of pubic hair at puberty and affect sex drive. Abnormally high levels may produce excessive hair growth on the body and face, acne, baldness, a deepened voice, increased muscular development, irregular menses, and fertility problems.

THE PANCREAS This long, narrow gland, which lies across the upper abdomen, is both an exocrine gland, producing digestive enzymes, and an endocrine gland, secreting insulin, somatostatin, and glucagon. These hormones are manufactured in the islets of Langerhans, which are specialized cells scattered throughout the pancreas. Insulin helps the body metabolize carbohydrates and use glucose (blood sugar). If insulin secretion is impaired, diabetes results. Glucagon stimulates the liver to break down glycogen, or stored blood sugar, and aids in the conversion of proteins to glucose.

THE OVARIES The ovaries begin releasing small amounts of the female hormone estrogen in the fetal stage of development and during childhood, but they substantially step up production at puberty. In menstruating women, the ovaries also manufacture the hormone progesterone. During pregnancy they produce relaxin, which loosens the pelvic ligaments to facilitate the birth of a baby. In addition, the ovaries release small amounts of the male sex hormone androgen.

Estrogen triggers the development of secondary sex characteristics, such as the "budding" of breasts. It is responsible for the maturing of the uterus and the Fallopian tubes, and affects numerous tissues and body processes. For example, it decreases oil secretion by the skin and gives a woman's bones and body their characteristic female shape. Estrogen is believed to protect menstruating women from certain disorders, such as heart disease and osteoporosis, which occur far more often after menopause when estrogen production sharply drops.

Progesterone prepares the lining of the uterus for pregnancy, increases protein formation, and affects liver and gallbladder function.

While men's sex hormones are produced at a fairly steady pace, those of women are released cyclically, at least during the childbearing years. This intricate cycle, lasting 28 days on average, involves varying levels of estrogen, progesterone, follicle-stimulating hormone and luteinizing hormone. (For more information, see Chapter 4, "Menstruation.")

The ebbs and flows of the female sex hormones have been credited with everything from energy spurts to temporary insanity. It is sometimes hard to separate fact from fiction when it comes to these hormones, but some women indeed find that certain moods are associated with specific parts of their menstrual cycles. In particular, mood swings, depression, and irritability are not uncommon during the premenstrual stage. Researchers have also suggested that some women experience a surge in sexual desire near the onset of ovulation.

PROSTAGLANDINS These are hormonelike substances originally thought to be produced by the prostate gland, hence the name. Researchers now know that prostaglandins are secreted by various tissues throughout the body, including the lining of the uterus. The substances are involved in a broad range of functions, including blood clotting, immune response, and metabolism. In the uterus, they stimulate muscle contractions and may be responsible for menstrual cramps. Antiprostaglandin drugs are used to alleviate the cramps, while prostaglandins (as injections, vaginal gels, or suppositories) are given to induce late abortions or to prepare the cervix for the induction of labor.

THE URINARY SYSTEM

In the urinary system, body fluids are filtered and stripped of waste products, which are then excreted in the urine. The system consists of the kidneys, ureters, bladder, and urethra. Except for the length of the urethra, the system is basically the same in men and women.

THE KIDNEYS The kidneys are two bean-shaped organs that lie on either side of the spine in the middle of the back. Each kidney is about 4 inches long and weighs about 5 ounces. The kidneys perform a host of vital functions: They control water balance, maintain the appropriate level of alkalinity of body fluids, keep bone marrow functioning, and remove the waste products of cell metabolism.

With every heartbeat, about one fourth of the blood expelled from the heart goes to the kidneys, where it is cleansed in over 2 million tiny filtering units called nephrons. Some 99 percent of the water, salt, and vital nutrients are reabsorbed into the circulation, while the rest is converted into urine.

THE URETERS These are two thin, muscular tubes about 10 inches long that transport urine from the kidneys to the bladder. While urine is stored in the bladder, valves at the entrance to the bladder prevent it from flowing back into the ureters.

THE BLADDER The bladder is a hollow sac that lies in front of the uterus in the pelvis. It is held in place by muscles and ligaments attached to adjacent organs and to the bones of the pelvis. When the bladder is empty, it collapses like a rubber balloon without air, but when it is full, it can expand to hold up to a liter of urine, or a bit more than a quart.

The walls of the bladder contain a layer of muscle that contracts to expel urine. The exit from the bladder into the urethra is surrounded by a muscular ring, the sphincter, which normally remains contracted to help prevent leakage of urine, but relaxes during urination.

THE URETHRA The urethra, about 1½ inches long in a woman, is a thin, slightly curved tube that connects the bladder with the meatus, the opening through which the urine leaves the body. The opening of the urethra is located between the clitoris and the vagina. Since it is usually closed and buried in the mucous tissues covering the clitoris, it may be hard to see, leading some women to believe that urine is expelled from the vagina. If you wish to see the opening, hold a mirror in front of your vulva and spread the folds surrounding the clitoris with your fingers.

URINE Urine consists of about 95 percent water and 5 percent dissolved solids—drugs, other chemicals foreign to the body, and the waste products of metabolism, including urea, uric acid, and creatinine. Normal urine is straw- or amber-colored. An adult generally passes 2 to 3 pints of urine in 24 hours. Alcohol, tea, and coffee increase the amount of urine, as does cold weather. In contrast, stress, sweating, and limited intake of fluids decrease the amount.

CONTROL OF URINATION Urination, referred to in medical literature as micturition, is regulated by an interplay of messages sent by the nervous system that coordinate the contraction and relaxation of various muscles in the urinary system.

When urine is formed in the kidneys, the ureters contract every 10 to 15 seconds and propel it in small amounts to the bladder. As the bladder fills up, nerve endings in its walls emit signals to a secondary micturition center in the lower part of the spine. Without external control, this center would send back a message to the bladder wall to contract and expel the urine. However, this action is suppressed by the main micturition center, located in the part of the brain stem known as the pons.

The pons micturition center makes temporary storage of urine possible, and it is responsible for voluntary control of urination: It prevents the bladder wall from contracting and increases the tone of the sphincter muscle, which keeps the bladder closed at the bottom. Eventually, the pressure in the bladder rises, it reaches its full capacity, and the pons receives powerful messages about the need to urinate. When you decide that you have to urinate, the pons removes its control, the bladder wall contracts, the sphincter is relaxed, and urine is expelled.

PITUITARY AND HYPOTHALAMUS HORMONES AND THEIR FUNCTIONS

VASOPRESSIN: regulates the body's fluid balance and constricts small blood vessels

OXYTOCIN: induces labor and promotes milk production and release

PROLACTIN: stimulates the breasts to produce milk

SOMATOTROPIN (growth-stimulating hormone): stimulates the growth of muscle and bone in children and adolescents

MSH (melanocyte-stimulating hormone): stimulates the skin cells to produce the pigment melanin

TROPINS: stimulate the production of other hormones

ACTH (adrenal-cortex-stimulating hormone): stimulates the adrenals to produce glucocorticoids and androgens

TSH (thyroid-stimulating hormone, or thyrotropin): stimulates the thyroid gland to secrete thyroxine

GONADOTROPINS: stimulate the ovaries and testes

FSH (follicle-stimulating hormone): in women, stimulates the ovarian follicles to produce eggs; in men, stimulates the testes to produce sperm

LH (luteinizing hormone): in women, stimulates the ovaries to secrete estrogens and progesterones; in men, stimulates the testes to release androgens

FEMALE SEXUAL DEVELOPMENT

Within about 8 weeks after conception, it is possible to recognize a fetus as distinctly male or female. Long before a baby girl is born, her reproductive organs are in place and her ovaries already contain their lifetime allotment of eggs.

From early childhood, a girl's body is shaped differently from a boy's. Her buttocks are generally more round, and her pelvis is relatively wider, which often causes the thigh bones to descend at an angle, turning inward toward the knees. This gives some girls and adult women a knock-kneed appearance. The characteristic female shape of the body becomes more apparent as girls approach puberty. (See Figures 1.1–1.5.)

PUBERTY

Puberty is a time of hormonal upheaval. The hypothalamus and the pituitary command the ovaries to step up their production of the female sex hormones, which cause the reproductive organs to mature in size and function and set off numerous other changes. These changes take place over 2 to 3 years and may begin anywhere between the ages of 8 and 14. (In boys, puberty usually starts approximately 2 years later and lasts about 4 years or longer. As a result, boys generally mature physically and sexually later than girls.)

The first physical sign of sexual development is the budding of breasts. In a young girl, the breasts usually consist of firm fibrous tissue and acquire their adult structure only when she begins to menstruate. The two breasts may grow at uneven rates, which some may find alarming, but it is completely normal. The second breast will usually catch up, although in many cases one breast remains slightly larger than the other. The discrepancy is rarely noticeable, but if it is significant enough to be disturbing, it can be corrected by plastic surgery.

Usually at about the same time breasts begin to develop, girls undergo a growth spurt. Their rate of growth during this period is comparable to that of early infancy. While at age 10 an average girl has achieved only 53 percent of her eventual weight, she has already reached 83 percent of her adult height.

Under the influence of the female hormones, the pelvis starts to expand in preparation for future childbearing, internal and external reproductive organs

Female sexual development

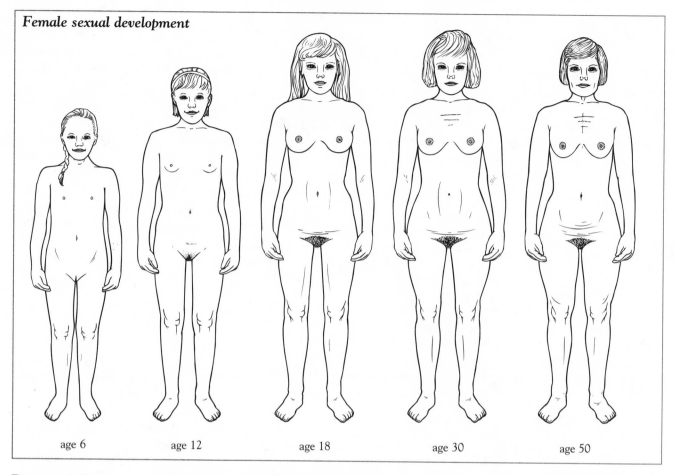

| age 6 | age 12 | age 18 | age 30 | age 50 |

Fig. 1.1–1.5 *Even at age 6 a girl's body is noticeably different in shape from a boy's: her buttocks are rounder, her shoulders narrower, her hips wider. By about age 12, the average onset of menstruation, she is already halfway through her growth spurt. Her breasts begin to bud, her pelvis widens, and pubic hair begins to appear. By age 18, most girls have attained their adult height, weight, and rounded shape. In middle age, fat deposits make the upper arms, hips, and thighs plumper and the breasts softer, giving a woman a mature shape. Weight gain later on tends to be around the middle. After menopause, calcium loss from the bones may result in loss of height.*

grow, vaginal walls thicken, and fat is deposited on the hips. Levels of male hormones also increase, causing the growth of pubic hair and, about a year later, hair in the armpits.

Even though other physical signs may appear first, the hallmark of puberty is menstruation. It generally occurs after the growth spurt is completed and girls have almost reached their adult height. In Western cultures, the average age for the onset of menstruation is 12½, but any time between the ages of 8 and 16 is normal. At the turn of the century, the average age was about 16, but better nutrition and other factors seem to have precipitated the earlier start. In one study, British researchers found that menstruation begins when a girl of average height reaches 105 pounds, although not all doctors agree with these findings. It also appears that the girl must experience a certain increase in body fat, which is why ballet

dancers, athletes, and others who have very lean bodies often have delayed menstruation.

For the first year or two, a girl may have irregular periods with either light or heavy flow, which may indicate that she is not ovulating regularly. Her body may be producing sufficient hormones to shed the inner uterine lining but not enough to bring eggs to maturity. Girls who engage in unprotected intercourse at this age and do not get pregnant may mistakenly assume they do not have to use birth control, but once they start ovulating regularly, pregnancy can occur very easily.

Other signs of puberty include a sharp rise in appetite and an increase in sleepiness. The increased appetite is designed to ensure that extra calories will be consumed to provide for the growth spurt, although this is unfortunately just about the time that many girls begin dieting. The changes in the sleep-wake cycle probably occur because the growth and other hormones that soar at puberty are released during sleep. Physical transformations are often accompanied by changes in temperament and unpredictable mood swings, these are also largely attributable to the influence of hormones.

Although the age at which puberty begins varies greatly, if a girl shows no sign of sexual development by age 13, she should be examined by a doctor. However, an extensive workup can be expensive and perhaps anxiety-provoking and should not be undertaken until after she is 15. She may be perfectly healthy and may eventually reach puberty without treatment, but she may also have a hormonal or other abnormality. Conversely, in very rare cases a girl may go through puberty prematurely—before age 8. This, too, may be normal and determined by heredity, but it may also signal an organic disorder.

ADULTHOOD

In young adult women, the physical and psychological turmoil of adolescence gives way to stability. Your heartbeat and breathing slow down, your body temperature falls, and in general you have better control of your emotions and sexual desire, although the monthly ebbs and flows of female hormones may affect your moods. The quality and duration of the menses may change. At the same time, the chances increase that you will experience what is called "premenstrual syndrome," uncomfortable physical and psychological symptoms that precede menstruation. Most often, the syndrome develops or worsens in women over 35. Menopause, which occurs on average at age 51, is precipitated by a dramatic drop in female hormones that results in a variety of physical changes and may require emotional adjustments.

THE LATER YEARS

Women experience many of the same age-related changes as men do, and some that are uniquely female. For example, both men and women begin losing bone mass at about age 35, but in women the loss of bone soars about a year after menopause. Since women have less bone mass to begin with, they are much more likely to have brittle bones in their later years.

Breasts grow softer and less dense with age because with the approach of menopause, they gradually lose their milk-producing glandular tissue. At the same time, the amount of fibrous connective tissue in the breasts increases. Breasts may lose some of their firmness and roundness, but the fat they contain often helps preserve their shape, even in older women.

On average, women put on weight with age, and the fat distribution changes. In your thirties and forties, you tend to gain weight on the hips and thighs; in your fifties and sixties, the fat is deposited more often at the waistline. (See Figures 1.4–1.5.)

As the level of female hormones declines, your uterus and ovaries decrease in size. Your vagina may grow smaller and less elastic, while its walls lose some of their protective layer. The clitoris may diminish in size, and the outer and inner lips may become thinner. Contrary to popular belief, you do not lose all your female hormones at menopause; rather, they continue to be produced by the adrenal glands, and the ovaries continue to release small amounts of estrogens for another 10 years or more. However, the relative proportion of male hormones in your body increases, which may cause hair to grow on the face and hair to thin on the head.

In both men and women, metabolism slows down with age, the digestive tract becomes less active, and lung capacity decreases. Your hair may turn gray, and individual hairs may grow thinner. Your skin loses thickness and elasticity, although much of the damage is due to the effects of the sun and can be avoided.

For reasons that are not fully understood, women outlive men by about 7 years. Thus, a baby boy born in 1986 could expect to live, on average, to age 71, while a baby girl born the same year could count on reaching the average age of 78.

GENDER DIFFERENCES

The obvious differences between men and women relate to their size and their reproductive functions. There are also some subtler variations between the sexes; some have implications for women's health, others remain a curiosity while scientists investigate their impact. Here is a rundown of some the lesser-known ways in which the average female differs from the average male:

THE SKELETAL SYSTEM. The most striking difference is the shape of the pelvis. In fact, the pelvic bone helps forensic specialists determine the sex of human remains with greatest certainty. In absolute terms, the male pelvis may be larger, but in relative terms, the female pelvis is usually wider with respect to her body. Most notably, its shape is different: In women, the bone is thinner and the space it forms in the center (the pelvic cavity) is relatively larger and rounder, rather than longer and more conical as in men—and thus easier for a baby to pass through.

Because her pelvis is wide, a woman's thigh bones descend from the hip joint at an angle. This may be why female athletes are more vulnerable to injuries in the knee joint.

Men also have broader shoulders and greater chest capacity than women, relative to the rest of their bodies.

In males, the cartilage of the larynx (the part of the windpipe that contains the voice apparatus) expands more at puberty and projects forward, forming a bulge called an Adam's apple. As a result, men have longer vocal cords that produce a deeper voice pitch than in women.

In terms of health, the structure and metabolism of the bones are the major distinguishing gender differences. Women's bones are lighter and thinner. Moreover, women begin losing bone mass as they approach menopause and their levels of estrogens, which help maintain bone density, begin to drop. Because men do not experience a correspondingly sharp drop in androgens, they are not at as great a risk for developing osteoporosis, or brittle bones.

THE MUSCULAR SYSTEM AND BODY COMPOSITION. Young men carry about 45 percent of their body mass in muscle; young women, 36 percent. Conversely, only about 15 percent of a young male's body weight is fat, while a trim, normal-weight young woman carries about 27 percent. In absolute terms, males have about twice as many muscle cells as women, and the muscle cells themselves are somewhat larger. Both sexes gain fat and lose muscle mass as they age.

Women generally collect fat on the thighs and buttocks, where it serves as a store of energy for pregnancy and breast-feeding, while men tend to have more abdominal fat, which can be quickly converted into energy in response to stress hormones.

The differences in body composition, as well as in the thickness of bones, explain why men on average have greater physical strength than women. The difference is particularly noticeable in the upper body, where women are about half as strong as men, while in the lower body they are about two thirds as strong. Women tend to lose strength faster than men as they age, possibly because they do not exercise as much. However, women have more flexible joints and exceed men in the range of all joint movements, with the exception of the knee.

THE CARDIORESPIRATORY SYSTEM. Women have smaller hearts than men, but their maximum heart rate is 10 percent greater. Their lung volume is about 10 percent smaller and their aerobic capacity (the maximum capability of an individual to use oxygen during physical exertion) is about 15 to 20 percent less.

Women also have a smaller blood volume and less body water than men. One effect of this disparity is a lesser tolerance for alcohol, which dissolves more readily in water than in fat. The same amount of alcohol is likely to result in greater concentrations and produce a stronger effect in a woman than it would in a man.

A woman's blood has about 5 percent less hemoglobin, the oxygen-carrying component, than a man's does, but this does not significantly affect performance in strenuous activities.

THE URINARY SYSTEM. Although both women and men have kidneys, ureters, bladders, and urethras, a woman's urinary system is completely separate from her genital and reproductive organs, and carries only urine. A woman's urethra is somewhat wider than a man's but only about 1.5 inches long, whereas a man's is 7 to 9 inches long. The shorter urethra makes women more prone to bladder infections because bacteria from outside the body have a shorter distance to travel to reach the bladder. Women are also at greater risk of urinary tract infections because their urethral opening lies relatively close to the anus, a source of bacteria.

Because of differences in anatomy and physiology, women are also more likely than men to develop incontinence. Part of the reason is their shorter urethra, which simply makes it easier for urine to escape. Certain types of incontinence are more common in women because the bladder and urethra are often displaced from their normal position during childbirth, disrupting effective storage of urine. Sometimes, older women become incontinent because the menopause-related drop in female hormones weakens the muscles that support various organs in the urinary system and nearby structures.

THE ENDOCRINE SYSTEM. In both sexes, the master gland of the hormone system, the pituitary, produces the same stimulating hormones, including the two gonadotropins FSH (follicle-stimulating hormone) and LH (luteinizing hormone), which affect glands of the reproductive system. In men, these hormones spur the production of sperm and the male hormones, androgens, while in women, they stimulate the production of eggs and the female hormones, estrogen and progesterone.

Both men and women have small amounts of hormones of the opposite sex. Thus men have a small amount of estrogens, but it is overshadowed by androgens, while women have a small amount of androgens, which are involved in the control of hair growth and sex drive, in addition to their estrogens. The genders differ markedly in the rhythm with which their sex hormones are released. In men, production of androgens is fairly steady, while in women, the levels of estrogen and progesterone, as well as those of gonadotropins, fluctuate in a closely synchronized manner in the course of the menstrual cycle.

THE SENSES. Men's visual acuity, especially their distance vision, is better than women's, perhaps a remnant of the need to spot distant prey. They are much more apt to have defective color perception, however. Women, in contrast, have better hearing and the difference becomes more apparent with age.

THE BRAIN. The similarities between the male and female brain are much greater than the differences, but subtle distinctions do exist. It is not known whether these differences are present at birth or a result of social conditioning, such as discouraging girls from taking math seriously.

In preliminary studies, scientists have found that parts of the corpus callosum, the bands of nerve tissue that connect the left and right hemispheres of the brain, are larger in women than in men. This suggests a stronger connection between the two halves of the brain, although scientists are unsure whether this translates into cognitive differences. According to one theory, better communication between the hemispheres may account for women's superior language skills, and perhaps for their fabled intuition.

On average, men's brains are about 10 percent larger than women's because men tend to be bigger. Scientists say, however, that when it comes to the brain, bigger is not necessarily better. In relative terms, women's brains are larger than men's in proportion to their body weight.

Sexual Health

Thirty years after the much-talked-about sexual revolution of the 1960s, the great majority of Americans are still largely uneducated about sex. According to a 1990 study by the Kinsey Institute and the Roper Organization, most Americans are seriously misinformed on topics ranging from sexuality, sexual problems, and birth control to AIDS and other sexually transmitted diseases. In fact, 55 percent of the survey respondents failed to answer at least ten out of eighteen questions correctly. (See box, "How Sexually Literate Are You?")

Achieving sexual "literacy" is crucial not only for enhancing your sexual pleasure but also to protect yourself against the growing array of sexual health hazards.

FEMALE SEXUALITY

Sexual feelings are something to be enjoyed and cherished—if not always acted upon—from puberty well into old age. In the two years prior to the onset of menstruation most young girls develop secondary sexual characteristics. The waist gradually narrows, the hips widen, and a padding of fat appears on the thighs and upper arms. Breasts start to develop and hair grows in the armpits and pubic region.

Adolescent girls begin to explore their sexuality, and many use masturbation as a way of learning about their bodies and their sexual responsiveness. Masturbation is a way of experimenting with and controlling the new urges and sensations they are feeling. This

is a normal part of sexual exploration and discovery and should not be discouraged. In fact, there is some evidence that young women who masturbate may experience fewer sexual problems later on than women who did not do so. Some girls have sexual fantasies when they masturbate, but not as often as boys of the same age.

Young adolescents are quite curious about the changes their bodies are undergoing, and girls tend to trade details of their menstrual periods or compare breast development. Just as some boys worry needlessly that their penises aren't big enough, girls may become obsessive about the perceived inadequacy of their breasts, convinced that they are too small, too large, peculiar in shape, or uneven in size. They may develop close, sometimes intimate relationships with another girl, or have a crush on an older female, often a teacher.

Later in adolescence young girls may develop crushes on and have fantasies about film and rock stars, as well as more accessible males. These are normal ways of exploring their feelings. Teenage girls are more emotionally mature than boys their own age, and it is not uncommon for them to be attracted to boys a few years older. They seek relationships that offer warmth, devotion, and nurturing as well as sexual attraction, an indication that they are beginning to separate from their parents.

Teenagers are having sex for the first time at increasingly younger ages—the average age is now 16 to 17—and almost one third of them forgo contraception. In general, even teenagers who use some contraceptive method are more likely than older women to become pregnant because they use it incorrectly. Four out of 10 adolescent girls who are sexually active will become pregnant before turning 20. Sex education is crucial to stemming the tide of teenage pregnancy and sexually transmitted diseases.

Men usually experience a sharp rise in sexual responsiveness in their teens, reaching the height of their sexual urges at age 17 or 18 and then starting a very gradual decline that by no means precludes sex well into old age. In contrast, women come to this point much later. By the time she reaches the peak of her sexual responsiveness in her late thirties and early forties, the average woman has been having sex for many years. She can be quickly aroused and her vagina lubricates easily. Many women experience multiple orgasms. This heightened period tends to last for many years, declining, if at all, only when she reaches her late sixties. If menopause dampens her interest in sex, it is usually only temporarily. In fact, many find that sex is more pleasurable now that they are freed of the necessity of contraception to avoid pregnancy. A 1984 study conducted by Consumers Union found that 65 percent of women and 79 percent of men were sexually active after the age of 70, and that half of those who were over 80 continued to engage in sex when it was available.

THE SEXUAL RESPONSE CYCLE Sexual expression differs for each woman, but the physiological process underlying it is consistent. The term "sexual response cycle" refers to the series of changes that most women experience, beginning with initial sexual contact, moving through orgasm, and returning to the original prearousal state. Researchers at the Masters and Johnson Institute divided the cycle into four stages—excitation, plateau, orgasm, and resolution. Of course, you need not pass through all stages to have a satisfying sexual encounter.

• **Sexual Arousal.** Stimulation plays a large part in sexual excitation, or arousal, but it is more than just physical. For women especially, anything that stimulates the senses and emotions can be sexually arousing: a certain song or an intimate look or innuendo from your partner. Another woman may feel like making love when she catches a whiff of a special scent. During this stage, stroking almost any part of the body can be sexually arousing if it is done by someone to whom you are attracted. However, certain areas, such as the internal and external genitals (see Figure 2.1), lips, buttocks, breasts, and nipples,

are inherently more sensitive than others. These areas, known as erogenous zones, have a rich supply of nerve endings and become engorged with blood when stimulated, further heightening sensitivity.

During this stage, also called foreplay, your pulse rate and breathing speed up and your blood pressure and sweating increase. Your vagina becomes lubricated as a mucuslike fluid, produced by the tissue lining the walls of the vagina, seeps into the vaginal canal. The Bartholin's glands, which lie alongside the vagina, also begin to secrete mucus. The clitoris and labia swell, and the uterus begins to elevate as its muscles start to tense.

You may experience a flush, or measleslike rash, on your abdomen that spreads upward to your chest and sometimes your face. Some women experience this flush at orgasm.

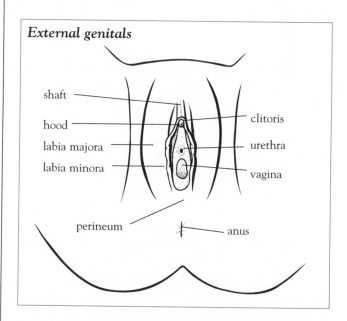

Fig. 2.1 *The external female sex organs, known collectively as the vulva, are all sensitive to physical stimulation. Chief among them is the clitoris, which contains a large concentration of nerve endings. During periods of intense sexual excitement, it becomes engorged.*

• **Plateau.** In the plateau stage, the labia and clitoris remain engorged at their peak as your body prepares for orgasm, with or without intercourse (see Figure 2.2). Generally speaking, the plateau stage lasts longer for women than it does for men, who tend to become aroused more easily but peak sooner and reach orgasm more quickly.

Physical stimulation is important during this stage, and different women require different kinds. In fact, the same woman may find a certain technique enjoyable one time and annoying the next. You should take time, alone and with your partner, to find out exactly what excites you. Stroking the breasts, clitoris, vagina, or skin are just a few of the techniques that work.

During the plateau stage, the clitoris slips under its hood. Direct clitoral stimulation can be uncomfortable now, but a generalized stroking or rubbing of the hood is often quite pleasurable. The nipples become erect and the breasts enlarge with increased blood flow. The upper part of the vagina increases in length and width by as much as 2 inches during the arousal and plateau stages. As blood flows into it, the outer third of the vagina swells so that later it will snugly surround the penis. The inner labia go from pink to red (or, in women who have had babies, from red to deep wine). Muscles all over the body tense up in anticipation of release. Some women reach this point within 10 minutes, while others may take up to an hour. Women who have not experienced orgasm may simply never have been stimulated long enough.

The controversial G Spot, named after Ernst Grafenberg who first reported it in 1944, has been hailed by believers as a new pathway to female orgasm and ridiculed by skeptics as nonsense. Grafenberg described the G Spot as a highly sensitive area on the upper wall of the vagina near the urethra. For some women, stimulation of this vaginal area seems to trigger orgasm or produce other pleasurable sensations. Grafenberg observed that upon sexual arousal, vaginal tissues become engorged and erect, much like in the male erection. Many experts feel that women should view the G Spot as another possible path to sexual pleasure and not feel pressured to respond one way or another.

• **Orgasm.** The sensations of orgasm, or sexual climax, are difficult to describe because they vary from woman to woman and even from experience to experience. While most people think of orgasm as an all-encompassing response, Masters and Johnson defined it as a series of contractions in the vaginal muscles, usually between three and twelve in number. The response can be localized in the vagina or clitoris, involving anything from modest to intense sensations, or it can extend to your entire body in an ecstatic wave. Engorgement and muscle tension peak; your body stiffens. Some women contort their faces or cry out involuntarily. Some moan or thrash around, while others lie perfectly still. With continued stimulation, some women experience more than one orgasm while others never reach it. (See section on "Sexual Dysfunction and Sexual Problems.")

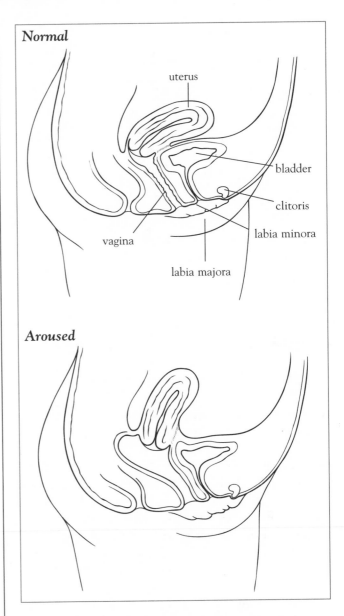

Fig. 2.2 *In the unaroused state the uterus lies horizontally above the bladder. During sexual arousal, the labia minora swell with blood and may protrude through the outer lips, the vagina increases in length and width, and the uterus ascends to a more upright position.*

Experienced couples are sometimes able to experience multiple orgasms together. The man must learn how to stimulate his partner almost to orgasm before entering, then start the thrusting that will bring her to her first orgasm. If he stops thrusting at this point and holds back until his excitement subsides, then begins thrusting again, he can not only bring his partner to orgasm again, but he will experience several peaks of intense pleasure before ejaculating. Many people believe that having both partners reach orgasm simultaneously is a desirable goal. It does foster the feeling of sharing a mutually fulfilling experience. However, achieving orgasm sep-

Pelvic floor muscles

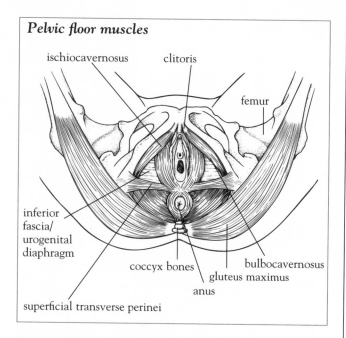

ischiocavernosus   clitoris

femur

inferior
fascia/
urogenital
diaphragm

coccyx bones

bulbocavernosus

gluteus maximus

anus

superficial transverse perinei

Fig. 2.3 *The pubococcygeal muscles encircle the pelvic floor in a figure 8, supporting the sexual organs and the bladder. Strengthening these muscles can enhance sexual pleasure and help prevent stress incontinence.*

arately is also satisfying, allowing you to experience your own orgasm fully and enjoy your partner's as well. The key consideration is whatever you both find pleasurable.

Sigmund Freud unduly burdened generations of women by declaring the vaginal orgasm to be superior to the clitoral orgasm. Then Masters and Johnson announced that the only way for a woman to reach orgasm is through clitoral stimulation. The debate continues as to whether there really are two distinct types of orgasm or whether vaginal orgasm results in part from stimulation of the clitoris. According to those who make the distinction, the clitoral orgasm, achieved through either direct or indirect stimulation, results in strong sensations in the clitoral area. Produced by stimulation by the penis, the vaginal orgasm causes heightened sensations in the vagina. Once again, what is important is not how you achieve orgasm, but that both you and your partner find pleasure in sex.

• **Resolution.** The resolution stage is a return to the prearousal condition. Engorgement subsides and the muscles relax. Many couples feel peaceful and connected as breathing and heart rate return to normal.

While this is the classic response cycle, there is no right or wrong way to engage in sex between mutually consenting adults. Whether you experience orgasm or receive pleasure simply from being close and intimate with your partner, your satisfaction should be the ultimate barometer of successful lovemaking.

The secret of having a satisfying sex life is to consider it a continuing learning experience. Sex manuals are helpful in understanding basic physiology and as a source of ideas, but in the end, you and your partner are responsible for finding different ways of pleasuring each other and for being receptive to new experiences. Talk openly with your partner about what pleases and displeases you, and be willing to keep on practicing. Consider doing the so-called Kegel exercises, which many women find adds to their own and their partner's pleasure. (See box, "PC Muscle Exercises for Sexual Enhancement.")

OTHER EXPRESSIONS OF SEXUALITY

• **Oral Sex.** Cunnilingus, the stimulation of a woman's genitals by her partner's mouth and tongue, and fellatio, stimulation of a man's penis by his partner's mouth and tongue, are common forms of sexual expression in both heterosexual and homosexual relationships. Some couples use it during foreplay, others instead of intercourse. It can be mutual or serial. Many women find both giving and receiving oral-genital sex pleasurable.

A man's tongue is softer than his fingers and can be used in a variety of gentle ways to stimulate the clitoris and vagina. If he doesn't have an erection or isn't physically up to intercourse, he can still give his partner pleasure without expending a lot of energy.

Some men who have trouble achieving an erection with manual stimulation are aroused with fellatio. You can run your tongue over the head and up and down the shaft of the penis or take the head into your mouth. It is not necessary, if you find it distasteful, to have your partner ejaculate in your mouth, although it is not harmful and some women enjoy it.

• **Anal Sex.** Although it is not nearly as popular as oral sex, 30 to 40 percent of American women have tried anal sex at least once. Some find it very pleasurable; others have responses ranging from distaste to extreme discomfort. If you want to try anal sex, remember that, unlike the vagina, the rectum has no natural secretions. Be sure to use a lubricant, such as K-Y jelly, liberally and ask your partner to go very slowly. Insertion should be gentle and his thrusts should not be as hard or as deep as vaginal thrusts. Also be sure that he washes his penis thoroughly before continuing with any oral or vaginal sex so that he doesn't spread the bacteria that normally live in the rectum.

PC MUSCLE EXERCISES FOR SEXUAL ENHANCEMENT

The pubococcygeal, or PC, muscle is a wide band of fibers shaped like a figure-8 that surrounds the openings of a woman's urethra, vagina, and rectum (see Figure 2.3). During orgasm the PC muscle convulses with rhythmic, involuntary contractions. It is also possible for a woman to contract this muscle voluntarily, enhancing both her own and her male partner's sensations.

In the late 1940s, Dr. Arnold Kegel reported that women could strengthen the PC muscle by contracting it for several seconds at a time, several times a day. These PC exercises not only helped stem urinary stress incontinence (leaking small amounts of urine during laughing, sneezing, or coughing), but they also enhanced sexual sensations. After several months of muscle toning, women who had never achieved orgasm before reported being able to reach climax. Those who were already orgasmic noted that by using voluntary contractions they could increase the strength of their orgasms or achieve multiple orgasms.

Here are some tips for doing Kegel exercises:

• Because your PC muscle also controls urine flow, you can locate it by partially emptying your bladder and then squeezing and releasing several times midstream. Always be sure to empty your bladder completely after you are done to avoid urine retention.

• Once you have located the PC muscle, begin tensing and relaxing it. To check if you are doing this correctly, insert a finger into your vagina and tighten the muscles to squeeze the finger.

• Start doing the Kegels by tensing and then immediately relaxing. Gradually increase the number of repetitions, and then progress to keeping the muscles tense for up to 10 seconds. Some experts recommend doing one hundred Kegels a day.

• You can perform Kegels anywhere—while cooking, watching TV, waiting for a light to change, standing in an elevator.

Since anal and rectal tissue is more vulnerable to small tears and bleeding than vaginal tissue, anal intercourse is more likely than vaginal intercourse to spread the HIV virus. If you are not in a mutually monogamous relationship, you should be taking precautions (see box, "Safer Sex Practices") anyway, but you must be especially careful with anal sex. This does not mean, however (as half of the respondents in the previously mentioned Kinsey survey believed), that AIDS can be transmitted through anal intercourse if neither partner is infected.

Couples who are not interested in anal penetration may nevertheless find anal stimulation pleasurable during foreplay. The anus is one of the erogenous zones and can be stimulated manually.

• **Masturbation.** Self-induced sexual stimulation is one of the most widely practiced and least discussed forms of sexual expression. Masturbation may begin as early as 4 months, when babies discover their genitals and the pleasurable feelings that come from touching them or rubbing them against something. By age 3 most children have masturbated; some will continue throughout childhood, while others will rediscover masturbation during adolescence.

Various surveys indicate that there is a greater acceptance of masturbation today than when Alfred Kinsey did his original studies in the 1940s and '50s. Masturbation is viewed as a pleasurable and safe alternative to casual sex and an important part of sexual therapy as well as a possible component of a sexually fulfilling relationship. Despite persistent myths, masturbation does not cause blindness, insanity, pimples, or other maladies. Although its practice is not essential to human sexual development, the only thing harmful about masturbation is the guilt that some people wrongfully feel when they practice it.

When women masturbate, they usually stimulate the clitoris either directly or indirectly through a circular or pressing motion. The strokes normally intensify and continue until orgasm is reached. Some women use the other hand to stroke their breasts, inner thighs, or stomach. Masters and Johnson found that, while masturbation is not preferred over sex with a partner, the orgasms are commonly more powerful.

Sometimes a vibrator or other sex aid (see box, "Sexual Enrichment") makes sexual stimulation easier or more pleasurable. In fact, some women who have never been able to reach orgasm during intercourse find that they can by masturbating with a vibrator. You may need to experience orgasm on your own, without feeling any pressure to perform, in order to get over any inhibitions. The vibrator need not be the type that is inserted into the vagina. A regular vibrator (the kind used for sore muscles) held lightly against your vulva is enough to produce a climax.

• **Sexual Fantasy.** It has been said that sex is mainly in the mind. Recent studies on the universality of sexual fantasy may prove the truth of that claim. These studies show that both women and men consciously use mental images to heighten sexual arousal. Fantasy can serve many purposes by creating an atmosphere and mood for sexual expression, alleviating sexual boredom, or focusing one's thoughts.

Women's fantasies tend to be more romantic than men's, but both can be very explicit and sometimes even violent. Women may feel guilty fantasizing about experiences that would embarrass them in real life. However, the Masters and Johnson researchers emphasize that sexual fantasies in women do not necessarily represent unrealized wishes; they may be a way for the subconscious mind to overcome inhibitions or indoctrinated beliefs such as the impropriety of enjoying sex. The most common fantasies include celebrity sex, sex with other partners, seduction, group sex, rape, sexual experimentation, sadomasochism, voyeurism, and romantic trysts.

• **Lesbianism.** Some women prefer to have sexual relationships with other women. As in the case of heterosexuals, lesbian relationships span a range of emotions and sexual involvements from casual to committed.

Lesbians have the same broad range of life-styles and relationships as do heterosexual women. Many lesbians are mothers divorced from heterosexual men who raise their children and eventually become mothers-in-law and grandmothers. Some lesbians co-parent with either homosexual or heterosexual men; others adopt or bear children through artificial insemination, either alone or in a committed domestic partnership. And, like many heterosexual women today, others choose not to have long-term relationships or children.

• **Bisexuality.** A bisexual person has relationships with partners of both sexes. Since gender is not an issue, many bisexual women choose their sexual partners on the basis of personal attraction. They simply feel that one can have different kinds of experiences with each sex and enjoy both types of interaction. As in the case of heterosexual and lesbian women, bisexual women engage in both casual and long-term committed relationships with members of either sex. For some women, bisexuality may be a period of experimentation or a stage or the way to celibacy.

• **Celibacy.** Another form of sexual expression is celibacy, or the voluntary decision not to engage in sexual interactions with others. The decision may be a religious one, or the individual may choose to take a temporary "time out" after a relationship ends or when a life situation makes it expedient. Or a married or committed couple may mutually decide to forgo sex as part of their relationship. Experts estimate that as many as one in ten American couples have sexless marriages, choosing to focus on friendship, affection, and common interests. When both partners subscribe to the celibacy, the relationship usually works and may even be stronger that those built on sexual ties.

SEXUAL ENRICHMENT

For many couples, greater intimacy begets better sex. As two people become more familiar and comfortable with each other, they often feel freer to experiment with other forms of sexual pleasuring and to try more playful ways to arouse each other, such as:

• Changes in atmosphere: candles, soft music, an intimate picnic dinner on the bedroom floor, a joint bubble bath with a bottle of wine

• Slowly taking each other's clothes off

• Massage (try scented oils)

• Changes in location; for example, renting a nearby hotel room, even for a few hours

• Playful teasers such as messengering a hotel key to your partner's office or arranging a date for a "pickup" in a local bar

• Positions or techniques you've never tried, such as oral sex

• Sexual aids and sexual toys such as vibrators, dildos, or ben-wa balls

• Sex workshops—these are not for everyone, but some couples report they give a real boost to their sex lives. To find out about workshops in your area, contact the American Association of Sex Educators, Counselors and Therapists. (See Resources.)

SEXUAL DYSFUNCTION AND SEXUAL PROBLEMS

Clinicians who work with women report that sexual dysfunction, or a problem with sex, is an extremely common concern that can have either physical or psychological causes. Some experts feel that the number of complaints would be even higher if women were less reluctant to discuss problems or if they knew how easily most difficulties could be resolved.

One thing to keep in mind, however, is that sexual dysfunction is a problem only if you are unhappy about it or feel that it is causing relationship difficulties. Unless you wish to change, you can live a full, rich life without sex or orgasm.

LACK OF DESIRE Inhibited sexual desire (ISD) is the most common complaint treated by sex therapists. People with ISD still engage in sexual activities. They can be sexually aroused and achieve orgasm. They simply lack the urge to engage in sex, rarely initiate it, and tend to have few sexual fantasies. Some people, for reasons not yet understood, simply do not have a high level of sexual desire; in other cases, external causes such as illness, medication, couple conflict, or emotional difficulties precipitate the loss of desire.

The first step in diagnosing ISD is a thorough examination to rule out physical causes. Diseases that can affect sexual desire include diabetes, endocrine and neurological disorders, heart problems, and any condition accompanied by chronic pain. Taking certain drugs, such as antidepressants, sleeping pills, tranquilizers, some heart disease medications, or excess alcohol, can lead to ISD. A hysterectomy with removal of both ovaries depletes the body's supply of testosterone, believed to affect the sex drive. An underactive thyroid gland can also reduce the sex drive. Treating these underlying conditions or changing or adjusting medication can often bring a return of sexual desire.

More often, ISD has a psychological cause: depression, anger, boredom, anxiety, fear of intimacy, or unresolved relationship problems. A woman may be subconsciously punishing herself or her partner by not allowing sexual feelings to arise, or she may fear disease or pregnancy, especially if her partner does not want to use contraception.

Some women who "have it all"—husband, children, home, and career—find themselves overwhelmed and unable to muster enough psychic energy for sex. Fatigue, worries, and preoccupation with responsibilities can blunt sexual responsiveness.

Factors such as childhood abuse or strong feelings of guilt because of family upbringing may also play a role in inhibiting desire. Many women have been taught that "good" girls dutifully pleasure their partners but do not enjoy sex themselves. Others find that their lack of knowledge or inexperience makes them hesitant about engaging in sex, or they are uncomfortable with a partner's desire for a sexual act they find wrong or perverse. If the underlying cause is emotional rather than physical, counseling, sex therapy, or a combination of both may prove helpful. (See section on "Sex Therapy.")

DYSPAREUNIA (PAINFUL SEX) Most women have experienced at least one instance when sex was uncomfortable or even painful; some find it painful every time. In more than half of cases, the cause of dyspareunia is physical and can be easily remedied. In other cases, there is a psychological reason for the physical pain. Or the two may be intertwined, as, for example, when an infection causes sufficient pain to make a woman dread intercourse and thus have trouble becoming aroused. Regardless of the cause, the problem most often manifests itself as a lack of sufficient vaginal lubrication.

• **Lubrication Problems.** The vaginal secretions that provide lubrication can be influenced by normal fluctuations in the hormonal cycle. Some women notice greater vaginal dryness after their periods, when hormone levels are at their lowest. Hormonal changes after childbirth cause a temporary decrease in lubrication and elasticity of the vagina. Estrogen levels also drop dramatically during breast-feeding.

The most long-lasting hormonal change occurs at menopause, when the female body stops producing estrogen altogether and vaginal dryness is a common complaint. Vaginal tissues may also become thinner and less elastic, making sex less pleasurable.

Decongestants that dry the mucous membranes lining the nose and mouth have the same effect on the vaginal membranes. Or the cause may simply be insufficient foreplay—not allowing a woman enough time to become fully aroused.

In any of these cases, sufficient stimulation and the use of a nonprescription, water-based lubricant, such as Koromex or K-Y jelly, may be all that is necessary. For postmenopausal women, prescription estrogen cream or estrogen replacement therapy may be advisable for more acute problems. (See Chapter 7, "Menopause.")

• **Vaginal Irritation.** The most common causes of irritation or burning sensations in the vagina are candidiasis (yeast infection), bacterial vaginosis (also called *Gardnerella vaginalis*), trichomonas, chlamydia, and cystitis (urinary tract infection). Vaginal warts may also cause irritation.

All of these conditions warrant prompt medical attention and can be treated easily with antibiotics or other medications. In some cases, a woman's partner must also be treated. (For specific infections, see the Encyclopedia.)

Other sources of irritation include an allergic reaction to bath or laundry soap or detergent, latex (in condoms or diaphragms), or douches or deodorants. Overuse of the latter products, which are generally unnecessary, may also cause vaginal irritation.

• **Vaginal and Pelvic Pain.** Some causes of pain are mechanical or anatomical. In younger women, a rigid, inflexible hymen may be responsible. A woman may experience pain when her partner thrusts his penis too deeply, hitting the cervix or bruising the urethral opening. A tipped or prolapsed uterus or bladder may also cause pain, as may an ill-fitting diaphragm. After childbirth, there may be gradually subsiding pain at the site of the episiotomy.

Deep dyspareunia, experienced as a pain in the lower abdomen during sexual intercourse, can be caused by a pelvic infection, endometriosis, a cyst (especially one that bursts), or a tumor. Once the physical problem is treated, dyspareunia usually disappears.

• **Vaginal Size Problems.** Although experts hold that all penises fit all vaginas, there are rare occasions when an incompatible fit causes dyspareunia. A thick penis that is too big for a vaginal opening can hurt upon penetration, while the thrusting of a too long penis can cause pain in the vaginal canal. Using extra lubrication can help relieve penetration pain. To alleviate thrusting pain, experiment with positions that don't use the entire shaft of the penis. For example, if a man lies on his back and the woman sits astride, she can control the amount of penetration.

If these measures aren't enough, dilation of the vagina may be recommended. Over a period of weeks, a set of plastic rods of increasing diameter is inserted into the vagina for 10 to 15 minutes at a time. This may be done by a gynecologist, or you can do it yourself or together with your partner.

• **Psychological and Emotional Causes.** The same emotional and psychological problems—anger, boredom, anxiety, fear of intimacy, depression, guilt, or unresolved relationship difficulties—that underlie inhibited sexual desire (ISD) can cause pain during intercourse. They are also often related to lack of arousal. In contrast to ISD, when sex is not painful but neither is it desired, a woman who experiences a lack of arousal desires to have sex but her vagina does not become lubricated.

In extreme cases, these problems can lead to vaginismus, a severe spasm of the perineal muscles and lower third of the vagina. While the roots of vaginismus are usually psychological, the manifestation is physical and completely involuntary. No amount of will or effort can cause these muscles to relax. Vaginismus is typically treated with a combination of psychotherapy, muscle relaxants, and dilators (see section on "Other Expressions of Sexuality").

PREORGASMIA Preorgasmia is the inability to reach orgasm. Women with this complaint usually experience arousal and even reach the plateau stage, but they do not continue on to sexual climax. They are called *pre*orgasmic because more than 90 percent do learn to achieve orgasm. Causes for failure to reach orgasm are similar to those for many other sexual problems—anxiety, lack of knowledge, improper technique by a partner, guilt, or low self-esteem.

Between 10 and 50 percent of women, depending on the source of the estimate, achieve orgasm but not through intercourse. They may have orgasms only with masturbation or manual stimulation by their partners, or some may experience orgasms with one partner but not with another.

If you are satisfied with your sex life as it is, no problem exists. However, if you desire an orgasm, you may want to consider sex therapy, either with or without your partner.

SEX THERAPY To change certain aspects of your sexual behavior or functioning you have several options. Some women find the solutions in one of the many self-help books in bookstores or libraries. Others are more comfortable consulting sex therapists, who are trained to assist people in achieving sexual fulfillment.

Sex therapy involves changing learned beliefs and behaviors, but it does not mean you have to abandon morals or become sexually promiscuous. In the therapeutic sessions, you outline your goals and the therapist works within those guidelines. Most sex therapists understand how difficult it is to discuss sexual problems, and they offer slow, gentle guidance in exploring new techniques, discussing possible underlying causes, and breaking old, unsuccessful patterns of behavior. In addition to individual treatment, couple therapy and group therapy have achieved excellent results. Most sex therapists encourage anyone who is in a long-term relationship to explore the problem with her partner because the education process is enhanced when both partners participate.

As a first step, the sex therapist typically rules out physical causes by requesting that you first consult a doctor, either your own or one recommended by the therapist who is familiar with sexual problems. If no physical problem exists, the counselor tries to help pinpoint such emotions as resentment, inhibition, guilt, or anger that may be blocking your response at some point in the sexual cycle. He or she will also provide exercises tailored to a couple's particular problem. You and your partner may be instructed to explore each other's responsiveness through touch, while avoiding sexual consummation, or to abstain from physical interaction while you attempt to resolve problems within your relationship. Most techniques involve a series of sensate exercises that gradually progress to orgasm during sexual activity.

Unfortunately, some people who call themselves sex therapists have not received formal training. It is often difficult to check their credentials because not all states have licensing requirements. Sex therapists may have such disparate academic credentials as an M.D. in psychiatry, a Ph.D. in psychology, an M.S.W. in social work, or an M.S. in marital and family therapy.

One reliable group that certifies sex therapists is the American Association of Sex Educators, Counselors and Therapists (AASECT), although certification does not necessarily indicate competence. You can also consult the American Association of Marriage and Family Counselors and the Association of Humanistic Psychology. (See Resources.) A local university, medical school, or social services organization, such as a family service agency, Planned Parenthood, or a community mental health center, may suggest sex therapists with appropriate credentials.

Another key consideration in choosing a therapist is personality. Schedule a preliminary consultation to see if you feel you can trust and respond to the coun-selor. You should also ask the therapist about the course of treatment as well as his or her qualifications and training in sex therapy techniques. Qualified practitioners usually do not mind such questions. Actual sexual activity should be reserved for at-home assignments. Under no circumstances should sex with the counselor be part of the therapy.

SAFER SEX IN THE AGE OF AIDS AND OTHER STDS

The term "sexually transmitted diseases" (STDs), which has replaced the term "venereal diseases," covers more than thirty conditions caused by bacteria or viruses that range from the annoying to the fertility-threatening or life-threatening. Diseases that can be transmitted sexually include AIDS, chlamydia, genital warts, gonorrhea, herpes, pelvic inflammatory

WARNING SIGNS OF SEXUALLY TRANSMITTED DISEASES

The following symptoms may indicate you have a sexually transmitted disease (STD) that should be reported to your doctor:

• Blisters, sores, bumps, or warts around the vulva or rectum

• Pain or burning on urination or moving your bowels

• Copious or foul-smelling vaginal discharge

• Itching around your vagina, vulva, pubic hair, or rectum

• Painful intercourse or bleeding after intercourse

• Pelvic or lower back pain

• Tenderness in the pelvic area when you cough or jar your pelvis

• Unusually severe menstrual cramps or abnormal bleeding

These symptoms may be accompanied by chills, fever, or a feeling of general malaise. Or you may be infected and have no symptoms. If you think you may have been exposed to an STD, tell your doctor so that you can be tested.

HOW SEXUALLY LITERATE
ARE YOU?

The following test was developed by the Kinsey Institute and administered by the Roper Organization to a representative sample of almost 2,000 American adults, most of whom failed. How would you have done?

1. Nowadays, what do you think is the age at which the *average* or *typical* American *first* has sexual intercourse?

   a. 11 or younger   e. 15   i. 19
   b. 12   f. 16   j. 20
   c. 13   g. 17   k. 21 or older
   d. 14   h. 18   l. Don't know

2. Out of every ten married American men, how many would you estimate have had an extramarital affair—that is, have been sexually unfaithful to their wives?

   a. Less than one out   g. Six out of ten
       of ten   (60%)
   b. One out of ten   h. Seven out of ten
       (10%)   (70%)
   c. Two out of ten   i. Eight out of ten
       (20%)   (80%)
   d. Three out of ten   j. Nine out of ten
       (30%)   (90%)
   e. Four out of ten   k. More than nine
       (40%)   out of ten
   f. Five out of ten   l. Don't know
       (50%)

3. Out of every ten American women, how many would you estimate have had anal (rectal) intercourse?

   a. Less than one out   g. Six out of ten
       of ten   (60%)
   b. One out of ten   h. Seven out of ten
       (10%)   (70%)
   c. Two out of ten   i. Eight out of ten
       (20%)   (80%)
   d. Three out of ten   j. Nine out of ten
       (30%)   (90%)
   e. Four out of ten   k. More than nine
       (40%)   out of ten
   f. Five out of ten   l. Don't know
       (50%)

4. A person can get AIDS by having anal (rectal) intercourse even if neither partner is infected with the AIDS virus.

   True   False   Don't Know

5. There are over-the-counter spermicides people can buy at the drugstore that will kill the AIDS virus.

   True   False   Don't Know

6. Petroleum jelly, Vaseline Intensive Care, baby oil, and Nivea are *not* good lubricants to use with a condom or diaphragm.

   True   False   Don't Know

7. More than one out of four (25 percent) of American men have had a sexual experience with another male during either their teens or adult years.

   True   False   Don't Know

8. It is usually difficult to tell whether people *are* or are *not* homosexual just by their appearance or gestures.

   True   False   Don't Know

9. A woman or teenage girl can get pregnant during her menstrual flow (her "period").

   True   False   Don't Know

10. A woman or teenage girl can get pregnant even if the man withdraws his penis before he ejaculates (before he "comes").

    True   False   Don't Know

11. Unless they are having sex, women do not need to have regular gynecological examinations.

    True   False   Don't Know

12. Teenage boys should examine their testicles ("balls") regularly just as women self-examine their breasts for lumps.

    True   False   Don't Know

13. Problems with erection are most often started by a physical problem.

    True   False   Don't Know

14. Almost all erection problems can be successfully treated.

    True   False   Don't Know

15. Menopause, or change of life as it is often called, does *not* cause most women to lose interest in having sex.

True   False   Don't Know

16. Out of every ten American women, how many would you estimate have masturbated either as children or after they were grown up?

a. Less than one out of ten
b. One out of ten (10%)
c. Two out of ten (20%)
d. Three out of ten (30%)
e. Four out of ten (40%)
f. Five out of ten (50%)
g. Six out of ten (60%)
h. Seven out of ten (70%)
i. Eight out of ten (80%)
j. Nine out of ten (90%)
k. More than nine out of ten
l. Don't know

17. What do you think is the length of the average man's *erect* penis?

a. 2 inches   e. 6 inches   i. 10 inches
b. 3 inches   f. 7 inches   j. 11 inches
c. 4 inches   g. 8 inches   k. 12 inches
d. 5 inches   h. 9 inches   l. Don't know

18. Most women prefer a sexual partner with a larger-than-average penis.

True   False   Don't Know

Answers

(In some cases, more than one answer is correct or the answers represent a range, e.g., 30 to 40 percent.)

1. f, g   7. True   13. True
2. d, e   8. True   14. True
3. d, e   9. True   15. True
4. False   10. True   16. g, h, i
5. True   11. False 17. d, e, f
6. True   12. True   18. False

Source: Copyright © 1990 by the Kinsey Institute for Research in Sex, Gender, and Reproduction. From the book, *The Kinsey Institute New Report on Sex*, June M. Reinisch, Ph.D., with Ruth Beasley, St. Martin's Press, New York. Used with permission.

disease (PID), syphilis, and trichomonas. (For specific diseases, see the Encyclopedia.)

Some STDs are extremely uncomfortable; others exhibit relatively few symptoms until they cause their damage or are transmitted to others. Many STDs can be successfully treated with antibiotics or other medications, but drugs are not as effective against those caused by viruses. Clearly, the best course is to avoid all these diseases in the first place by practicing "safer sex." Although the common term was originally "safe sex," no method, barring celibacy or long-term monogamy, is entirely safe. (For specific recommendations, see box, "Safer Sex Practices.")

Chlamydia is the most common sexually transmitted disease in the United States today. Left untreated, it can lead to pelvic inflammatory disease, or PID, a serious infection of the upper reproductive tract. PID can also be caused by gonorrhea and other bacterial STDs that have spread into the pelvic area. Diseases such as diabetes and medications such as cortisone can lower the body's defenses against infection. If a woman using an intrauterine device (IUD) gets gonorrhea or chlamydia, the presence of the IUD may allow the infection to develop more quickly into PID. (See box, "Warning Signs of Sexually Transmitted Diseases.")

The most dangerous and deadly viral STD is acquired immune deficiency syndrome (AIDS), a disease in which the body's immune system breaks down. AIDS is caused by the human immunodeficiency virus (HIV), which is transmitted through sexual intercourse—anal, vaginal, or oral—with an infected person or by sharing drug needles with an infected person. Pregnant women with HIV can pass the virus to their babies, although this risk can be reduced dramatically, from 30 percent to 8 percent, if HIV-positive women take the AIDS drug AZT (Retrovir) during pregnancy and immediately after childbirth. There is also some evidence that HIV-positive babies may fare much better if they are identified shortly after birth and started on AZT immediately. These new findings make HIV testing all the more important for any woman considering pregnancy who suspects she has been exposed to the virus.

People receiving infected blood in transfusions can also acquire AIDS, although donating blood poses no risk. The risk from transfusions has been reduced considerably now that the blood supply is more carefully screened.

Normal household contact with an AIDS patient does not seem to transmit the virus, although such practices as sharing toothbrushes or razors, which might contain blood, should be avoided.

Women seem to be less effective than men at transmitting the HIV virus, which means that lesbians are at much lower risk for getting it than are heterosexual women, although they are by no means risk-free. In the United States, more men than women are infected at the present time, so heterosexual women are more likely to encounter an infected male than vice versa.

Women are the fastest-growing group of AIDS patients. According to the Centers for Disease Control and Prevention, women made up 2 percent of the AIDS population in 1990 and 16 percent in 1993. Two thirds of the heterosexually transmitted AIDS cases reported in 1993 were women.

Other viral STDs include genital warts (human papilloma virus, or HPV), herpes II, and hepatitis B. Some viral STDs are linked to a greater risk of cervical cancer. Where AIDS is concerned, monogamous relationships of at least 10 years' standing are considered virtually risk-free unless one or both of the partners is a drug user with a history of sharing needles.

SAFER SEX PRACTICES

- Do not have sex with someone whose sexual and drug history is unknown. Do not be afraid to ask questions, but remember that people are not always honest, or are simply unaware they may have an STD. When in doubt, abstain.

- Do not think that just because a partner is nice, he or she does not have an STD. Nice people get STDs, too.

- Avoid sex with a large number of partners. If each of your partners also engages in intercourse with others, this multiplies your potential exposure to an STD.

- Avoid sex if you or your partner have any symptoms of an STD, even mild ones. Visit your doctor or clinic immediately.

- Condoms are effective for reducing the risk of both pregnancy and disease. Other contraceptive methods are not. Even if you use an IUD, diaphragm, cervical cap, or the pill, you still need to use a condom to reduce the risk of getting STDs.

- For maximum risk reduction, be sure the condom covers the entire penis. If it does not, as in the case of some novelty condoms, it will not provide the protection you want. (See Chapter 3, Contraception, Sterilization, and Abortion for instruction on putting on a condom.)

- If your partner says no to condoms, you should say no to sex.

- Always use a latex (rubber) condom, since natural or lambskin condoms have been shown to allow viruses through. Make sure the package indicates that the condoms were designed to prevent disease and always check the expiration dates.

- Along with a condom, use spermicides containing nonoxynol-9, which help reduce the risk of both pregnancy and STDs.

- If the condom isn't already lubricated, apply a water-based lubricant, such as K-Y jelly or Koromex, to reduce the risk of breakage. Never use baby lotion, hand or body lotion, or cold cream as a lubricant. Avoid products that contain fats, oils, or petroleum jelly. These substances can weaken latex and cause it to break. If you are unsure, check with your pharmacist.

- If you are not in a mutually monogamous relationship, do not participate in anal sex, which can cause tissue in the rectum to tear and bleed, facilitating disease transmission. Because of greater friction, a condom is more likely to break during anal intercourse.

- While the risk of contracting AIDS and other STDs from saliva is low, you should still use a condom for oral sex. If your partner is a woman, use a latex barrier for the vagina.

- If a condom is sticky or gummy, discard it. Never reuse a condom.

- Do not use mood-altering drugs such as alcohol or cocaine that can impair your judgment and cause you to forget to practice safer sex.

Contraception, Sterilization, and Abortion

Birth control is now an issue of such widespread concern in our country that we sometimes forget the relative newness of its development and use. In fact, this chapter would not have existed 50 years ago. The reasons for its importance are clear: Unplanned pregnancies account for about half of all pregnancies in the United States. More than half of these are aborted. In the United States, women under age 25 become pregnant far more often than do their European contemporaries, and American women age 20 to 34 have a higher percentage of aborted pregnancies than those in any other country in the world. Couples no longer expect coitus and conception to go hand in hand, and contraception, sterilization, and abortion enable them to delay parenthood.

Contraception itself is an ancient phenomenon, probably predating our writing about it. The earliest written records contain references to intravaginal sponges, plugs, and spermicidal substances, such as different spices and oils, seaweed, honey, and lemon juice. Legend has it that a Dr. Condom, who supposedly practiced in England in the 1600s, invented the barrier method that carries his name to accommodate Charles II, who wished to limit the number of his illegitimate children. By the late 1800s, intrauterine devices, diaphragms, and cervical caps had been invented, and the era of modern contraception began with the marketing of oral contraceptives in the 1960s. Today, women have a variety of choices (see Figure 3.1).

METHODS OF CONTRACEPTION

NATURAL FAMILY PLANNING Also referred to as fertility observation or periodic abstinence, natural family planning involves using hormonal changes in the body to predict periods of fertility, then abstaining from sex during those times. The abstinence period usually starts several days before and continues

Methods of contraception

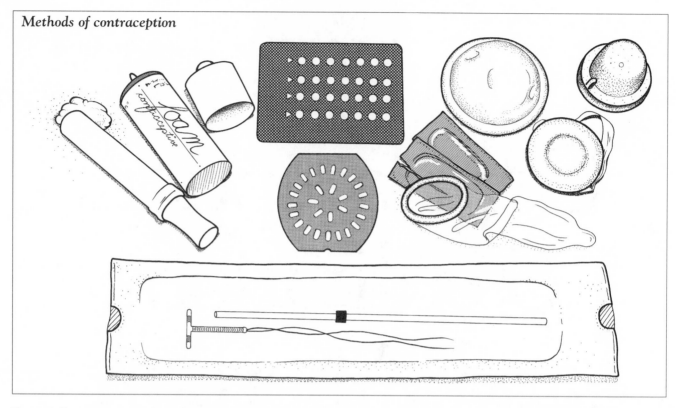

Fig. 3.1 *Shown are some of the methods of birth control currently available in the United States.*

for several days after ovulation—the time when an ovary releases an egg and you may become pregnant.

Natural family planning is not a new name for the rhythm method, which used information from past cycles to determine fertility. This newer method uses careful observation of the body to detect physical changes that are more accurate predictors of fertility.

Three recognized methods of natural family planning are the *ovulation method*, the *temperature method*, and the *symptothermal method*, which is a combination of the first two methods. In the ovulation method, changes in the cervical mucus indicate the period of fertility. You ovulate once during each cycle, at which time the amount of mucus increases, it becomes clear and slippery, and it stretches. You can observe this by taking a sample of vaginal mucus, pressing it between your thumb and forefinger and then spreading them apart. (See Figure 3.2.) These mucus changes help sperm glide in the right direction. Under optimal conditions, sperm that would otherwise die or swim in circles may survive as long as 5 days within your body. At other times, the mucus is more cloudy, has a thicker consistency, and clumps instead of stretching.

Cervical mucus test

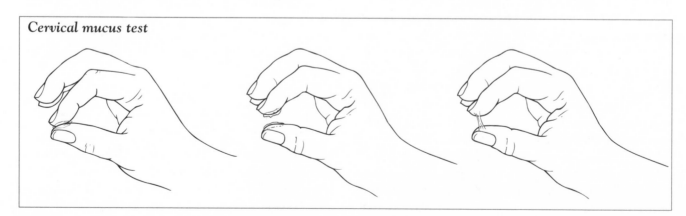

Fig. 3.2 *Normally, the cervical mucus is small in quantity and tends to clump together. During ovulation, the mucus increases in quantity and becomes clear, slippery, and stretchy.*

The temperature method requires monitoring body temperature with a special finely calibrated oral thermometer called a basal thermometer. You take your basal, or resting, temperature each morning, generally before getting out of bed, then record it on a graph. When ovulation has occurred, the temperature increases by about 0.4°F to 0.8°F. (For more information, see Chapter 5, "Infertility.")

The problem with this method is that it cannot predict when ovulation will occur, only that it has already happened, so you must chart your pattern over several months, then begin abstaining from intercourse a few days before you believe you will ovulate.

The symptothermal method involves monitoring at least two signs of ovulation, usually the changes in cervical mucus and the basal body temperature. Although more complicated, this combination of techniques is more effective than either method alone.

Many clinicians are not well trained in these procedures, so it is best to receive instruction from someone at Planned Parenthood, a women's center, or an organization such as the Ovulation Method Teachers Association (OMTA). (See Resources.)

• **Pros.** The natural method is a form of birth control without chemicals, mechanical devices, pills, or prescriptions. Hence, some consider it the most simple method, and it is acceptable to people whose religious beliefs forbid using other forms of birth control. It is also the safest method available, causing no medical difficulties (except, it can result in pregnancy if done improperly). If sharing birth control responsibility with your partner is important, this process is an easy way to do so. Note: Some women may be tempted to use natural family planning to pinpoint their fertile periods, in order to limit the days on which they must use a contraceptive method, such as condoms, that they may find intrusive. But using these other methods instead of abstaining can interfere with the body's physiology, thus making changes such as mucus secretion harder to detect and possibly lessening the accuracy of the natural method.

• **Cons.** The major disadvantage of the natural method is that it requires a period of abstinence, meaning *no* genital-to-genital contact. Although it may allow for more spontaneity than any of the barrier methods of contraception, natural family planning does require more work than just taking a pill or inserting a diaphragm. Also, it may be nearly impossible for women with irregular cycles to use natural family planning effectively.

• **Effectiveness.** The efficacy of natural family planning depends on the care and skill with which it is practiced. If you know your body well, keep accurate daily records, and understand the fertility detection process, it can be a very effective birth control option, equally as successful as the combined use of a diaphragm and spermicide. (See chart, "Birth Control Methods Compared.") In some studies, it has been shown that more than nine out of ten couples used the method successfully. To achieve such success, however, you must be committed to sticking to the regimen without fail. The average couple is generally much less successful, with the typical success rates anywhere from 53 to 86 percent.

• **Ease of Use, Availability, and Contraindications.** There is nothing particularly difficult about using natural family planning, and the cost is practically nothing—the price of a thermometer and calendar, readily available at most drugstores. Information about natural family planning methods can be obtained from Planned Parenthood, OMTA, most Catholic hospitals and churches, and other family planning clinics. There are no medical contraindications for these methods, but if you have irregular cycles, you should consider other birth control options.

SPERMICIDAL AGENTS Until the advent of the pill and the intrauterine device, creams, jellies, foams, and sponges containing spermicides (chemicals that kill or impede sperm) were widely used in combination with condoms and diaphragms. Because of their protective properties, barrier methods have again increased in popularity, causing a rise in the use of associated spermicides.

This type of contraception involves vaginal insertion of spermicides that form a mechanical barrier at the cervix and kill sperm as well. These preparations consist of a spermicidal agent, such as nonoxynol-9 or octoxynol, and a base that holds the agent in the vagina.

• **Types.** Creams or jellies are inserted into the vagina with an applicator before intercourse. Although they can be inserted up to an hour beforehand, they are most effective used immediately before having sex. These preparations must be reinserted for protection if sex is repeated. Aerosol foams are inserted with an applicator immediately before sex and must be reinserted before intercourse is repeated.

Foaming tablets are moistened and then inserted with an applicator deep into the vagina 5 minutes

BIRTH CONTROL METHODS COMPARED

Efficacy rates given in this chart are estimates based on a number of different studies. They should be understood as yearly estimates, with those dependent on conscientious use subject to a greater chance of human error and reduced effectiveness. For comparison, 60 to 85 percent of sexually active women using no contraception would be expected to become pregnant in a year.

TYPE	MALE CONDOM	FEMALE CONDOM	SPERMICIDES USED ALONE	SPONGE	DIAPHRAGM WITH SPERMICIDE	CERVICAL CAP WITH SPERMICIDE
Estimated Effectiveness	About 85%	An estimated 74–79%	70–80%	72–82%	82–94%	At least 82%
Risks	Rarely, irritation and allergic reactions	Rarely, irritation and allergic reactions	Rarely, irritation and allergic reactions	Rarely, irritation and allergic reactions; difficulty in removal; very rarely, toxic shock syndrome	Rarely, irritation and allergic reactions; bladder infection; very rarely, toxic shock syndrome	Abnormal Pap test; vaginal or cervical infections; very rarely, toxic shock syndrome
STD Protection	Latex condoms help protect against sexually transmitted diseases, including herpes and AIDS	May give some protection against sexually transmitted diseases, including herpes and AIDS; not as effective as male latex condom	Unknown	None	None	None
Convenience	Applied immediately before intercourse	Applied immediately before intercourse; used only once and discarded	Applied no more than 1 hour before intercourse	Can be inserted hours before intercourse and left in place up to 24 hours; used only once and discarded	Inserted before intercourse; can be left in place 24 hours, but additional spermicide must be inserted if intercourse is repeated	Can remain in place for 48 hours, not necessary to reapply spermicide upon repeated intercourse; may be difficult to insert
Availability	Nonprescription	Nonprescription	Nonprescription	Nonprescription	Rx	Rx

Source: *FDA Consumer*, September 1993.

PILLS	IMPLANT (NORPLANT)	INJECTION (DEPO-PROVERA)	IUD	PERIODIC ABSTINENCE (NFP)	SURGICAL STERILIZATION
97–99%	99%	99%	95–96%	Very variable, perhaps 53–86%	Over 99%
Blood clots, heart attacks and strokes, gallbladder disease, liver tumors, water retention, hypertension, mood changes, dizziness, and nausea; not for smokers	Menstrual cycle irregularity; headaches, nervousness, depression, nausea, dizziness, change of appetite, breast tenderness, weight gain, enlargement of ovaries and/or Fallopian tubes, excessive growth of body and facial hair; may subside after first year	Amenorrhea, weight gain, and other side effects similar to those with Norplant	Cramps, bleeding, pelvic inflammatory disease, infertility; rarely, perforation of the uterus	None	Pain, infection, and, for female tubal ligation, possible surgical complications
None	None	None	None	None	None
Pill must be taken on daily schedule, regardless of the frequency of intercourse	Effective 24 hours after implantation for approximately 5 years; can be removed by physician at any time	One injection every 3 months	After insertion, stays in place until physician removes it	Requires frequent monitoring of body functions and periods of abstinence	Vasectomy is a one-time procedure usually performed in a doctor's office; tubal ligation is a one-time procedure performed in an operating room
Rx	Rx; minor outpatient surgical procedure	Rx	Rx	Instructions from physician or clinic	Surgery

before having sex. They must dissolve completely, similar to antacid tablets dissolving in water. Another tablet must be inserted before having sex again.

The waxy, cone-shaped vaginal suppositories are inserted with an applicator 10 to 15 minutes before having sex to allow them time to melt. As with other spermicides, a fresh suppository must be used for each act of intercourse.

None of these methods works particularly well when used alone. Each can, however, boost the effectiveness of diaphragms and condoms. Creams and jellies are especially recommended.

The contraceptive sponge is soft, round, and filled with spermicide. It is inserted into the vagina to fit over the cervix (see Figure 3.3). Once the sponge is moistened and thus activated, it acts as a sustained release system for the sperm that can be used for a 30-hour period. The sponge must stay in place for 6 hours after the last act of intercourse, but can be inserted up to 24 hours ahead of time and is safe for repeated intercourse during the first 24 hours, which gives you a certain flexibility. For example, if you insert it 2 hours before the initial act of intercourse, sex can safely be repeated any time in the next 22 hours and the sponge can be left in place for 6 hours after that.

• **Pros.** All of these products are easily obtainable at most drugstores. They are relatively inexpensive and require no prescription. When used alone, they do not interfere with sensation during sex and may actually increase lubrication. They are easy to use, and, with the exception of the sponge, there is nothing to remove later.

No major health risks occur with spermicides. In fact, their use may be beneficial. Studies have concluded that they provide some protection against sexually transmitted diseases (STDs), such as gonorrhea and pelvic inflammatory disease (PID).

• **Cons.** Creams and jellies are messy, and tablets or suppositories that do not fully dissolve can cause friction. In addition, all of these products must be applied before sex and must be left in the vaginal tract for at least 6 hours afterward, during which you cannot bathe, although you may shower. About 1 to 5 percent of all users have some minor allergic reaction or irritation to the products. Switching brands may help. Four percent of sponge users suffer an allergic reaction, and 8 percent complain of vaginal dryness, soreness, or itching.

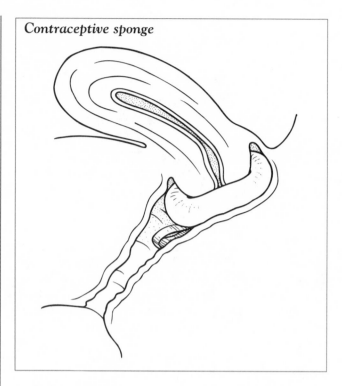

Contraceptive sponge

Fig. 3.3 *The contraceptive sponge contains a spermicide that is effective for 24 hours, even with repeated intercourse.*

• **Effectiveness.** Failure rates for spermicidal preparations vary widely according to the population studied. When inserted alone, regularly, and correctly, they are usually effective in preventing pregnancy in seven to eight out of ten women. When used with a condom, they are even more effective.

The sponge is more effective than spermicide preparations alone, but less so than diaphragms and condoms. Some studies indicate that its failure rate doubles in women who have had children, which may indicate that one size does not fit all.

• **Cautions.** A 1981 study linked spermicides with increased risk of miscarriage and congenital disorders, but since then a number of follow-up studies showed there is no such correlation.

Aerosol, foams, and foaming tablets should not be used with diaphragms. They do not form the required seal between the cervix and the diaphragm membrane because they do not adhere to the latex in the same way a jelly or cream does. For repeated intercourse, however, within 8 hours after the insertion of a diaphragm and cream or jelly, an applicator full of foam may be used for renewed spermicidal protection.

Shake aerosol foam cans vigorously before use to ensure an even distribution of the spermicidal chemical. All spermicidal products should be inserted as close to the cervix as possible for maximum protection.

CONDOMS The condom (rubber or prophylactic) has become part of everyday small talk now that acquired immune deficiency syndrome (AIDS) and other STDs are causes of such widespread concern. "Safer sex" is seemingly synonymous with using a condom. Even though its protective aspect is the one most touted these days, the condom is still a viable means of birth control when used properly.

Condoms come in all shapes, sizes, and colors. (In fact, there are enough products on the market that stores in several large cities sell almost nothing else.) Some things have not changed, however. Usually, condoms are made of a thin, strong latex rubber. (Those made of sheepskin do not offer protection against STDs.) They come rolled up and unroll to about 7½ inches, although there are larger and smaller sizes available. A rubber ring at the open end keeps the condom from slipping off the penis. The closed end often has a nipplelike tip, called a reservoir, that holds the ejaculated semen.

Some condoms are prelubricated with jellies or spermicides, making them less likely to tear. They may be more comfortable. They may also slip off more easily, but this is unlikely once a couple becomes experienced in their use. (For more information, see Chapter 2, "Sexual Health.")

You or your partner can put the condom on at any time after he has an erection. Place it, rolled up, over the head of the penis and gently but firmly unroll it down the shaft. If the condom has a sperm reservoir, squeeze it to remove the air before unrolling. If it doesn't, make your own by pinching the tip together as you put the condom on so that when it is completely unfurled you have about ½ inch at the end to catch the semen and keep the condom from bursting.

After intercourse the loss of erection will quickly loosen the fit, so be sure that your partner withdraws before his penis is completely flaccid. Grasp the base of the condom to keep the semen from spilling out as you take it off. Always check it for tears before disposing of it. If you discover that the condom has leaked, insert some spermicidal foam, cream, or jelly into your vagina immediately. If none of these is available, you may want to call your physician within 24 hours to discuss taking morning-after hormones or having an IUD inserted (this may keep the fertilized egg from implanting in your uterus if conception has taken place).

• **Pros.** Condoms are an effective, readily available, and relatively inexpensive form of birth control. Both men and women can buy them; no prescription is necessary. They require little practice to be used correctly, and they can be carried discreetly.

There are few if any health concerns in using condoms. The effects are completely reversible in case you want to become pregnant. Perhaps the most positive aspect of using condoms, however, is the fact that they serve a dual purpose: preventing pregnancy and STDs.

• **Cons.** The disadvantages of condoms is that using them takes away some spontaneity, and there is a slight loss of sensation for the man. The break in action that occurs can be minimized and made more pleasurable if both partners make putting on the condom a part of their foreplay. It is unfortunate that little emphasis has been placed on producing a condom that interferes less with the man's physical pleasure, but this may not always be a disadvantage: Men who ejaculate too early may find that diminished sensation gives them more staying power.

Because condoms are so compact, they fit in a purse or wallet. Even so, many people find it embarrassing or difficult to pull one out at the opportune moment, especially if it is the woman asking the man to use the condom. A woman who feels uncomfortable doing this should try to look beyond that moment. It will pass quickly, and the sexual experience will be much more satisfying if both partners feel protected from unwanted risks.

There are no contraindications to using condoms, but if their disadvantages interfere with your commitment to use them, it is better to choose another form of birth control rather than take the risk of going without.

• **Effectiveness.** When used properly, good-quality condoms fail only about 2 percent of the time. For the general population, however, the failure rate is about 15 percent. The best protection is provided by a condom that is lubricated with spermicide or used along with a separate spermicidal foam, cream, or jelly.

•**Cautions.** To prevent tearing and for maximum comfort, use a lubricated condom, or a nonlubricated condom in conjunction with a water-based lubricant such as K-Y jelly. Never use petroleum jelly or other oil-based mixtures because they can damage the rubber. Never reuse a condom.

Condoms should not be kept around for too long. They have a shelf life of about 5 years, but only if they are kept away from heat. Carried around in a wallet, a condom may be good for only a year.

THE DIAPHRAGM A diaphragm is a round, soft rubber dome with a flexible metal-spring rim (see Figure 3.4). It covers the cervix, where it acts as a barrier against invading sperm. Diaphragms are used with a spermicidal jelly or cream that would kill any sperm that might get around the rim of the diaphragm before they reached the cervix.

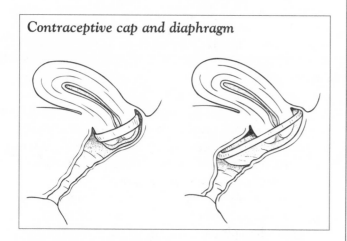

Fig. 3.4 *The cervical cap may be left in place longer than the diaphragm and does not require the use of a spermicide, but it is not available in as many sizes.*

Diaphragms come in sizes ranging from about 50 to 105 millimeters (mm) in diameter, the one most often prescribed being 65 to 80 mm (or about 2½ to 3¼ inches). There are three basic types: flat spring, coil spring, and arcing. Both the flat-spring (the earliest type made) and the coil-spring designs fold flat for insertion. (See Figures 3.5–3.6.) The flat-spring diaphragm has a metal band in the rim, and the coil-spring type has a wire spiral. The arcing diaphragm, the most popular in the United States, has a rim that folds into an arc, allowing easier insertion. The best type for you depends on your size, vaginal muscle tone, and other factors, but this determination must be made by a health professional.

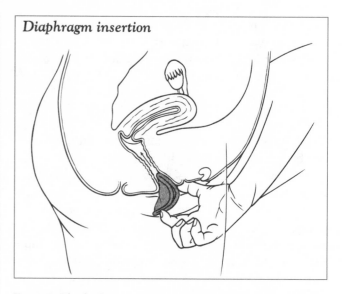

Fig. 3.5 *The diaphragm is folded in half for insertion, which can be done while squatting, lying down with knees raised, or standing up with one foot propped on a chair.*

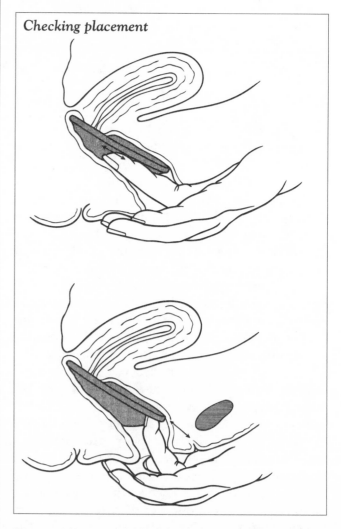

Fig. 3.6 *After inserting a diaphragm, always check its position by pulling lightly on its forward rim to be sure that it is snug and does not slide. Then run your finger back and forth to find the rim and the bulge in the center that indicates it is covering the cervix.*

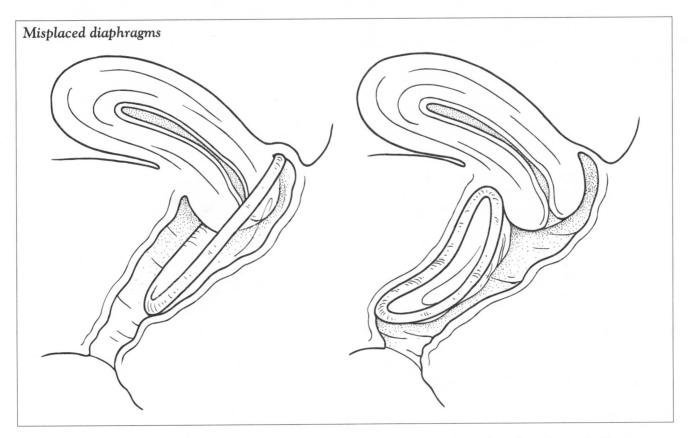

Misplaced diaphragms

Fig.3.7-3.8 *A diaphragm that is too small may be displaced by the penis, while one that is too large will not fit snugly enough to keep sperm out. Even a well-fitted diagphragm may be improperly inserted so that the cervix is not completely covered (left) or, in the most common error, not covered at all.*

• **Pros.** Used correctly, the diaphragm is a safe, reasonably effective method of birth control, although it is not as effective as birth control pills or an IUD. (See Figures 3.7–3.8.) It offers some protection against gonorrhea, PID, and tubal infertility, possibly because it acts as a mechanical barrier to infections that may be transmitted by the male, and because the spermicide has some antibacterial properties. It does not require taking hormones. The initial cost is relatively low (about $20 to $25) and, with proper care, a diaphragm can last for many years.

• **Cons.** The main disadvantage to a diaphragm is that it must be inserted every time before you have sex, along with the spermicidal cream or jelly, which is placed inside it and along the rim. (It can, however, be inserted up to 6 hours in advance.) This can cause a messy discharge and make oral sex less enjoyable. A spermicide must be reapplied to the outside of the diaphragm if intercourse is repeated. Some women may not be suited physically for the diaphragm, causing room for error in its use.

A diaphragm usually presents few if any health risks for most women. It may shift around, especially if it is improperly fitted, causing cramps in the uterus or discomfort in the urethral or rectal area. The diaphragm cannot get "lost" in the vaginal canal, as the vagina ends about an inch beyond the cervix.

The spermicidal cream or jelly may cause irritation in some women, but it may be possible to alleviate this by switching brands. (For more information, see section on "Spermicidal Agents.")

Urinary tract infections are about twice as likely to occur in women who use diaphragms than in those who use oral contraceptives. This can be attributed to several factors: the diaphragm rim pressing against the urethra; the interference of the spermicide with the vaginal chemistry, causing bacteria growth; or incomplete emptying of the bladder. The best preventive action is to urinate completely before and after having sex. For some women, switching to a different type of diaphragm or a smaller size will reduce infections.

• **Effectiveness.** Because the efficacy of the diaphragm depends on the skill and knowledge of the user, the failure rate ranges from 6 to 18 percent, with older, more experienced users having the most success. No adequate studies have determined how use or nonuse of the spermicide affects this rate. To be effective, the diaphragm must be left in place for 8 hours after intercourse.

• **Ease of Use and Availability.** The diaphragm must be prescribed and fitted by a doctor, nurse-practitioner, or other health care professional. The person fitting the diaphragm will choose the type of diaphragm that is most suitable, depending on the size and shape of your vagina and the muscle tone in the vaginal wall. He or she will use a fitting ring or the actual diaphragms, which are disinfected, trying different diameters until a match is made. You should practice inserting and removing the chosen diaphragm in the practitioner's office. (See Figure 3.9.) This will help you determine if there are any potential problems and allow you to raise questions that can be discussed and resolved before you actually use the diaphragm as a birth control device.

If a diaphragm is uncomfortable during use, talk to your health care provider about other options, such as using a different type of diaphragm or one that is larger or smaller.

• **Contraindications.** Women with uterine displacement, such as severe prolapse, cannot use a diaphragm. It is also contraindicated for any woman whose bladder protrudes through the vaginal wall or who has other openings, called fistulas, in the vagina.

THE CERVICAL CAP The cervical cap is shaped like a thimble and works something like the diaphragm. (See Figure 3.4.) It attaches to the cervix like a suction cup and keeps sperm from passing through. The cap is used with a spermicidal cream or jelly, which both increases the suction and kills any sperm that might break through the seal.

Although the cervical cap has been in use in Europe for many years and was actually used in the United States in the early 1900s, it was approved by the FDA less than a decade ago. While there are several types of cervical caps, the only type approved in the United States is the Prentif cavity rim, which is made of flexible rubber and comes in four sizes, from 22 mm to 31 mm in diameter. It is about 1½ inches long.

• **Pros.** The cervical cap is about as effective as the diaphragm and may be left in place for up to 36 hours. A spermicide is not absolutely necessary, but a teaspoonful placed in the cap before insertion helps combat the unpleasant discharge that may occur with such long-term wear. This small amount of spermi-

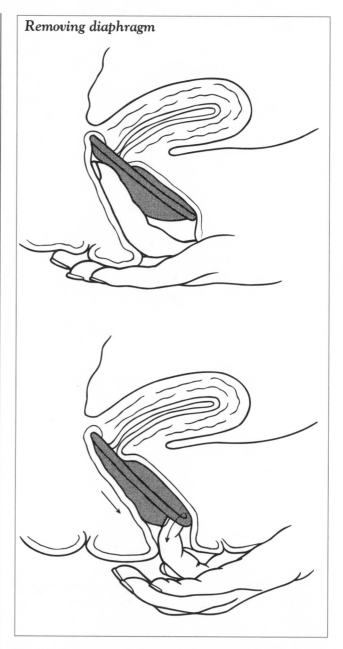

Removing diaphragm

Fig. 3.9 *To remove a diaphragm, hook your index finger under the forward rim and pull down and out.*

cide makes the cervical cap less messy to use than the diaphragm.

There are not enough data to determine conclusively that the cervical cap causes no risk to health, but most experts agree that it is as safe as the diaphragm. It also has the advantages of low cost and long wear.

• **Cons.** Although it has advantages over the diaphragm, the cervical cap is harder to fit because it comes in only four sizes. Only about 50 percent of women are able to find a proper fit. Insertion of the cervical cap is also more difficult because it must fit firmly over the cervix. It must stay in place for at least 6 hours after having sex.

• **Effectiveness.** Data from U.S. trials of the cervical cap show that it is as effective as the diaphragm. The failure rate during the first year of use ranges from 6 to 18 percent. The most common reason the cervical cap fails is that it sometimes becomes dislodged during intercourse.

• **Ease of Use and Availability.** The cervical cap is readily available in most areas, although some practitioners may not have all four sizes. Once the cervical cap has been fitted, you must learn how to insert it. You must locate your cervix, slide the cap into your vagina and up its posterior wall, and push it onto the cervix. Its position must be checked after insertion and after sexual intercourse.

To remove a cap, you must exert pressure with a fingertip to break the seal, then hook your finger over the rim of the cap and pull it down out of the vagina.

• **Contraindications.** If you have a long or irregularly shaped cervix or a deep vaginal canal, you may have a problem getting a good fit, which makes the cap ineffective. If there is cervical erosion or laceration, you should choose another method of birth control.

ORAL CONTRACEPTIVES In the early 1900s, it was discovered that hormones extracted from ovaries and given orally could prevent fertility in mice. The problem with mass-producing an oral contraceptive for humans was linked to the difficulty of making large quantities of the hormone itself. In the 1940s, the production of progesterone from plants became possible, but it was not directed toward the development of a contraceptive preparation until 1951, when Margaret Sanger, then president of the International Planned Parenthood Federation, provided research grants for that purpose. Three pharmaceutical companies began producing the birth control pill, which became readily available by prescription by the early 1960s.

Combination pills, which contain synthetic forms of both estrogen and progestin, are prescribed most often. (Natural estrogen and progesterone would not be effective if taken as a pill.) These pills work by inhibiting the maturation and release of eggs from the ovaries. Normally, during your menstrual period, your low estrogen level causes the pituitary gland to secrete a hormone called follicle-stimulating hormone (FSH), which in turn causes eggs to begin ripening in the ovaries. The estrogen component in the pill raises the body's estrogen level enough to inhibit the release of FSH and thus the release of an egg. This is similar to what happens during pregnancy to prevent fertilization of a second egg; thus, the action of the birth control pill simulates pregnancy.

A progestin component, such as norethindrone or norgestrel, is added to the pill to produce a second fertility-reducing effect. It increases the thickness of the cervical mucus and ensures that the uterine lining that normally develops during each menstrual cycle never develops fully. Thus, if by chance an egg is released to be fertilized, the cervical mucus will help prevent sperm from reaching it, and the uterine wall will not be a suitable place for the fertilized egg to attach. Some preparations, called minipills, contain only progestin and rely on this hormone's effects alone to prevent pregnancy.

Birth control pills usually come in 21- or 28-day packs. The pills containing hormones are taken in the first 21 days of the cycle. The other 7 days, either you take no pill or one that does not contain hormones.

The latest development in oral contraception is the multiphasic pill. The hormone dosage is altered periodically throughout the pill cycle. These preparations and low-dose monophasic pills (containing less than 50 micrograms of estrogen) were produced to reduce the pill's ill effects by lowering the dose (a lower dose of estrogen does not decrease the effectiveness of the pill).

• **Pros.** As a method of birth control, oral contraceptives are almost completely fail-safe. Their other advantages include the regulating effects they have on the menstrual cycle: The menstrual period occurs during the week that you are off the pill or taking pills that contain no hormones. The menstrual flow is usually lighter, and cramps rarely occur. Women who were previously plagued by cramps and premenstrual tension often report an improvement once they are on oral contraceptives.

Sexual intercourse may be more enjoyable for some couples who choose oral contraceptives, since there is no interruption of the sexual act and a diminished fear of pregnancy. As explained later in this chapter, the birth control pill also reduces the risk of certain cancers and some other gynecological problems.

• **Cons.** Aside from the safety concerns mentioned in the next section, you must remember to take the pill at approximately the same time every day. This can be more difficult than it sounds for women who are forgetful or lead very busy lives.

The pill may also have some uncomfortable side effects, such as weight gain, bloating, nausea, fluid retention, and mood changes. However, these and other side effects, such as having no period at all (amenorrhea) or breakthrough bleeding, can often be alleviated by changing to a different type or brand of pill.

Depending on when in the cycle you start the pill, it may take up to a month for it to become completely effective, so during that time, you must use another form of birth control. If you do not want to become pregnant and decide to discontinue the pill, another form of birth control should be used right away, even though your menstrual cycle may not return to normal for a few months. Even if you want to become pregnant, it's a good idea to wait a couple of months before trying to conceive so that you can accurately identify when you had your last menstrual period, thus allowing for a more precise dating of the pregnancy.

Oral contraceptives are more expensive than most other birth control methods, running about $20 a month (unless your physician prescribes a generic oral contraceptive) plus medical checkups every 6 to 12 months to be sure there are no detrimental side effects.

• Safety, Contraindications, and Health Benefits. The safety of birth control pills has been debated from the time they were first marketed. They continue to be a controversial form of contraception. The results of three studies, two British and one American, that began in 1968 and continued for approximately 10 years, have had a large impact on users and the clinicians who prescribe the pills. Later studies may be more accurate because they provide data on the effects of lower-dose preparations used by women who have been more carefully screened than those who participated in the original research.

The studies have shown the following:

• The occurrence of deep-vein blood clots in the leg is four times greater in users of higher-dose oral contraceptives than in nonusers, and the risk of superficial blood clots for these pill users is two times greater. There is no connection between varicose veins and these other, more serious problems in women who take birth control pills. For women on low-dose pills, blood clots are rare and usually occur only when an underlying circulation problem is exacerbated by pill use.

• Women with insulin-dependent diabetes should be encouraged to use other forms of birth control because they may be at risk for developing blood clots, but this effect in low-dose users who are under 35 and have no other health risks is probably minimal. Changes in insulin and glucose levels in the blood for women who take low-dose pills and do not have a history of diabetes are not considered clinically significant.

• Women with liver or gallbladder disease should use another method of birth control.

• High blood pressure (hypertension) as a result of taking oral contraceptives occurred in approximately 5 percent of higher-dose pill users. Lower-dose pills may cause a slight increase in blood pressure, but a higher incidence of hypertension has not been reported. Women who already are hypertensive should not use the high-dose pill because they may be at increased risk for heart attack. Results are inconclusive with the low-dose pill.

• The first British studies found that the risk of heart attack increases in women who are over 35 and does so significantly when obesity, hypertension, and, most dramatically, smoking are present. In a 1983 British report, however, only women who were over 35 and smoked had significantly increased odds of developing heart disease. Two U.S. studies did not find an increased risk of heart disease in users of oral contraceptives who did not smoke. In fact, during a study in the Seattle area, there were no cardiovascular deaths among users, but there were eleven mortalities in the nonusers. The ongoing Nurses' Health Study, known for its accuracy and long-term follow-up of a large number of subjects, found no increase in risk of cardiovascular disease linked with the duration of oral contraceptive use. Some physicians advise patients to take a children's aspirin each day with their pill to further reduce the possibility of hypertension and heart disease.

• The risk of stroke, according to the 1983 and 1984 British studies, approximately doubled in women who used the high-dose pills, although the 1984 report also noted that not a single patient on the low-dose pills had suffered a stroke. Two U.S. studies involving healthy patients on low-dose pills found there was no significant link between developing stroke and taking birth control pills.

• Women who experience migraine headaches may find that using oral contraceptives affects this condition, either negatively or positively.

• To prevent any potentially dangerous side effects or drug interactions, a woman who wishes to take birth control pills should inform her doctor about any health conditions she has or medication she is taking.

Early studies showed that women who take the high-dose pills and smoke are up to thirty-nine times more likely to have a heart attack and at least twenty-two times more likely to have a stroke than women who neither smoke nor use birth control pills. More recent studies on women taking low-dose pills seem to indicate that the increased risk from smoking is not as high. However, since the risk of developing heart disease triples for women who smoke five to fourteen cigarettes a day, this finding should not be considered a green light for smokers.

• **Cancer Risk and Prevention.** The risk of certain cancers in oral contraceptive users is frequently debated, and current findings conflict. Taking oral contraceptives—either low dose or high dose—for at least 12 months reduces the risk of developing endometrial cancer by 50 percent, and the protective effect is most pronounced in women who use the pills for 3 years or more. The protection lasts for at least 15 years after a woman stops taking the pills.

Oral contraceptives also protect against ovarian cancer, reducing the risk by 40 percent of that of nonusers. The protective effect increases with duration of pill use, and it continues for at least 10 to 15 years after the birth control pills are discontinued. An 80 percent reduction in risk can occur in women who take the pills for more than 10 years.

There are conflicting reports concerning the incidence of cervical cancer in women who use oral contraceptives. Some studies indicate there is an increase of invasive cervical cancer in women who use the pills for more than 5 years, and a twofold increase in women who take them for more than 10 years. Another study, completed by the Centers for Disease Control and Prevention (CDC), found no such evidence. There are some other factors that might be responsible for the increased risk, but they are hard to assess: number of sexual partners, age of first sexual intercourse, exposure to the human papillomavirus (which can cause genital warts, some types of which are thought to be related to cervical cancer), use of protective-barrier contraception, and smoking. A Pap smear every 6 months can detect early cervical disease, which is why many physicians require that this test be done before they renew prescriptions for birth control pills.

The possible connection between breast cancer and oral contraceptive use is a leading concern among women and their physicians. While early studies showed no significant differences in breast cancer rates in users of oral contraceptives compared with nonusers, the original participants in those studies were mostly married women who were using the pills to space out the births of their children. Many of them had already had a child, which itself is a protective factor against breast cancer.

Oral contraceptives have since become the primary birth control method of younger women, who use them to delay an initial pregnancy and take them for a longer period of time. Studies of these women, who have just reached or have yet to reach menopause, have only been able to assess the risk of premenopausal breast cancer (diagnosed before the age of 45), which accounts for 13 percent of all breast cancers. These later studies have differed in their results: Some indicate there is a higher risk of developing the cancer; some indicate no such danger exists. All of the research has been hampered by the problems of studying a difficult subject that has many risk factors and few long-term participants.

The largest of these case-control studies was performed by the CDC. Its results indicate a slightly increased risk of breast cancer diagnosed before the age of 35, no increased risk between the ages of 35 and 44, and a reduced risk for ages 45 to 54. There is no evidence of any latent effect, that is, breast cancer developing many years later.

In juxtaposition to these studies of breast cancer risk, other data show that taking high-dose pills for more than 2 years helps protect against benign breast disease. Current and recent users are one fourth as likely to develop it as nonusers. There are no data that say the same is true of low-dose preparations.

It is difficult to sift through all the study data and come to any steadfast conclusion. The fact of the matter is that many more studies of accurate design and long duration will be necessary to fully determine the breast cancer risks associated with oral contraceptive use. In the meantime, the medical community is fairly united in its belief that the benefits of the birth control pills overshadow their possible risks for healthy women.

• **Effectiveness.** All the combination preparations—high dose, low dose, multiphasic—are highly effective in preventing pregnancy. The annual failure rate for women who take the pill every day is less than 1 percent. The failure rate for the general population during the first year of use is about 3 percent, most often because women fail to take the pills as directed. This rate increases significantly with progestin-only minipills because they do not inhibit ovulation.

• **Ease of Use and Availability.** The pills are small and easy to swallow. The only tricky part may be remembering to take them. They are available only by prescription, but most drugstores carry several brands. Most physicians require that you have a Pap smear and a physical exam every 6 months to a year before renewing a prescription, which means that you should plan ahead and make an appointment with your doctor before your prescription runs out.

LONG-ACTING STEROID METHODS These methods rely solely on low doses of progestins for contraception and thus provide an advantage for women who should not use estrogen. They are virtually as effective as sterilization in preventing pregnancy and have no serious health effects. They can, however, have some minor but bothersome side effects.

The most popular method is the hormone implant. The first, and so far only, such implant on the market is Norplant, in which six small capsules of progestin are inserted surgically into the upper arm. Another method that is less popular in the United States, but has been used for more than 20 years in many other parts of the world, is medroxyprogesterone acetate, known as Depo-Provera. This form of progestin is administered by injection with protection that lasts 4 to 6 months but, for safety's sake, the injections are usually repeated every 3 months. Norethindrone enanthate is similar to Depo-Provera and is injected every 2 months.

Implants and injectables share the same method of action and pros and cons. Although the following information relates only to Norplant, the only difference, from the user's standpoint, is that the implants are good for up to 5 years, while the injections must be repeated four to six times a year.

In Norplant a low-dose progestin called levonorgestrel is encased in six matchstick-size capsules made of flexible tubing. A clinician inserts the capsules through an incision just under the skin of the upper arm. The hormone is released into the bloodstream within hours of the procedure.

The progestin prevents the release of an egg from the ovaries in about two thirds of a woman's menstrual cycles, increases the thickness of the cervical mucus, thus impeding the sperm trying to fertilize the egg, and causes the uterine wall to be a less inviting place for the egg to embed itself and mature if fertilization does occur.

• **Pros.** The implant method is the most effective reversible form of birth control available. Its period of effectiveness lasts up to 5 years, but it may be removed at any time fertility is desired. The implants require no daily routine or interruption of intercourse and can be used by women who cannot take birth control pills containing estrogen.

• **Cons.** Norplant requires a minor surgical procedure under local anesthesia that takes approximately 15 minutes for insertion and 15 to 30 minutes for removal. About 13 percent of women experience problems with removal that may be painful, require longer surgery, and result in scarring. Side effects of progestin can include irregular menstrual bleeding, depression, and weight gain. The data on safety are not conclusive because Norplant is a recent product, but there may be fewer risks than with the pill. As with the pill, Norplant does not protect against STDs, so a barrier method must still be used for those at risk.

• **Effectiveness, Cost, and Availability.** Studies by the Population Council, the nonprofit research group that developed Norplant, show that in the first year of use, fewer than 1 percent of women became pregnant.

The cost of Norplant and its insertion and removal is comparable to the price of birth control pills over 5 years. However, that amount must be paid in a lump sum, which is difficult for some women. For short-term use, it is much more expensive than other methods.

While Norplant is available in most areas, if you are considering it, you should find out if your health care provider has experience in the surgical procedure and knowledge of the implant's action and side effects.

• **Contraindications.** If you have a blood clotting disorder, vaginal bleeding for which no cause can be found, acute liver disease, a liver tumor, or breast cancer, you must use another form of birth control.

THE INTRAUTERINE DEVICE (IUD) The IUD prevents pregnancy in a number of ways, some of which are not completely understood. First of all, it acts as a foreign body within the uterus, causing an inflammatory response that kills sperm or inhibits their migration to the Fallopian tubes. The inflammation also

Inserting an IUD

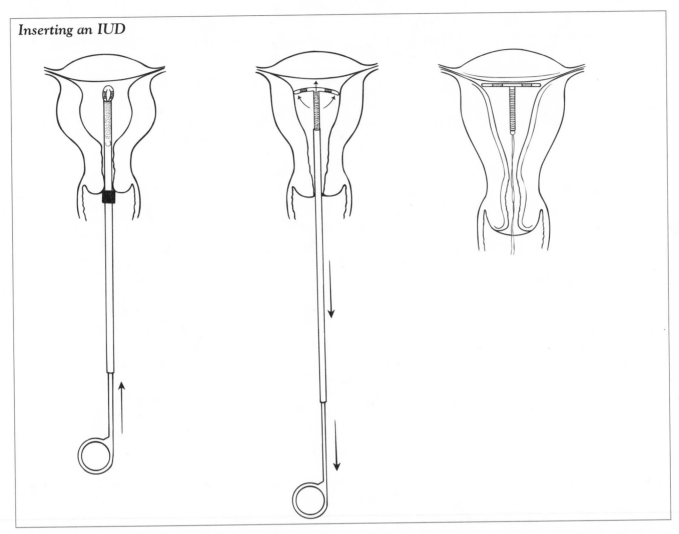

Fig. 3.10–3.12 *An IUD is put into place by pinching together the two wings of the T-shaped device and placing it in a hollow tube that is inserted through the vagina into the uterus (left). A plunger releases the IUD (center), which then sits in place against the fundus of the uterus. A string attached to the bottom (right) allows periodic checking for position and is ultimately used for removal.*

creates a second line of defense, should an egg become fertilized: It interferes with the normal buildup of the uterine wall necessary for egg implantation.

Only two IUD models are available in the United States. The Copper T380A, marketed by ParaGard, produces an additional contraceptive effect: By releasing free copper and copper salts, it causes an increase in the production of prostaglandin and a decrease in the action of some endometrial enzymes.

The Progestasert, available since 1976, is an IUD that contains a hormone delivery system: A reservoir slowly releases progesterone, creating sperm-impeding thick cervical mucus as well as other contraceptive effects. It must be replaced annually.

The IUD is one of the oldest forms of birth control (legend has it that camel drivers used intrauterine stones to prevent pregnancy in their animals) and is a leading method in countries other than the United States. For instance, in 1988, 59 million Chinese women used it compared with 0.7 million American women.

The decline in its use in the United States is a result of several factors, but primarily because of consumer fears engendered by an IUD called the Dalkon Shield. Introduced in 1970, the Dalkon Shield had a locator string that acted as a wick, providing a pathway for bacteria to enter the uterus. In some cases, sexually transmitted bacteria spread into the uterus and Fallopian tubes, which resulted in PID. Within 5 years, sales of the shield were discontinued, but the existing devices were not recalled until the early 1980s. By then, many Dalkon Shield users had been rendered infertile from pelvic infections, and the large number of lawsuits caused the bankruptcy of the pharmaceutical company producing them.

Subsequently, two other pharmaceutical companies, Ortho, maker of the Lippes Loop, and Searle, maker of the Tatum T and the Copper 7, voluntarily removed their products from the market. These IUDs were shaped differently from the Dalkon Shield, their strings did not seem to enable bacteria to enter the uterus, and they were never judged unsafe by the FDA. Their removal represented a marketing decision based on reduced financial return and the growing expense of product liability insurance and lawsuits. Nevertheless, American women were left with lingering doubts about the safety of the devices in general and, until 1988, with Progestasert as their only choice if they wanted an IUD.

• **Pros.** The IUD is an extremely effective and safe device that is best suited to women who are over 30, have already had a child, have no history of PID, and are at low risk of contracting an STD. The perfect candidate is someone who does not wish to have any more children, but would like a reversible form of birth control in case she changes her mind. Others who may benefit from IUDs are women over 40, or those who breast-feed, smoke, or have preexisting conditions such as hypertension.

Like the long-term hormone implant, the IUD does not require any daily regimen, nor does it interrupt the sexual experience. Once in place, it can pretty much be forgotten. According to the FDA, for example, the Copper T380A is effective for 10 years. Hence, over the long haul, the cost of the copper IUD is less than oral contraceptives, for example. The progesterone-releasing IUD, however, must be replaced each year because its reservoir is emptied in 12 to 18 months.

The IUD is available in all parts of the United States, and many physicians believe the time has come for a revival in its use in appropriate candidates.

• **Cons.** The IUD must be inserted and removed by a clinician (see Figures 3.10–3.12), making its initial cost high. The average cost is about $300, which, for the Copper T380A over 10 years, is less than many other forms of birth control. Some women experience heavy bleeding or increased pain from cramps. In fact, these are the most frequent reasons for the removal of the device. Others who worry about implanting a foreign object in their bodies should avoid the IUD.

• **Effectiveness.** The failure rate in the first year of use of all IUDs is approximately 4 percent, with a 10 percent expulsion rate and a 15 percent removal rate. The failure rate decreases with age and duration of use, making it as effective as oral contraceptives in some segments of the population.

• **Safety and Contraindications.** There is no evidence that use of the currently available IUDs increases a monogamous woman's risk of PID or infertility. Most IUD-related infections are now believed to be the result of the spread of bacteria at the time of insertion or of having contracted an STD. Using condoms with new partners decreases the latter risk. The use of IUDs only by women who are completely monogamous decreases the risk further.

IUDs do not increase the risk of ectopic (tubal) pregnancies. In fact, a World Health Organization study concluded that women who had used IUDs were 50 percent less likely to have an ectopic pregnancy than women who had used no contraceptive methods. The copper IUDs offer even more protection—users are 90 percent less likely to experience this problem. However, women who become pregnant with an IUD in place have an unusually high risk of having an ectopic pregnancy.

The IUD should not be used by anyone who has had a previous history of PID, or bacterial endocarditis (inflammation of the lining of the heart or heart valves), or is at increased risk of endocarditis because she has rheumatic heart disease or artificial heart valves.

Because the IUD does not stop ovulation, it is possible to become pregnant, although the failure rate is quite low—one to five pregnancies per one hundred users per year. If a woman becomes pregnant with an IUD in place and wants to continue the pregnancy, she should have the IUD removed immediately. Spontaneous abortion occurs 50 percent more often when the IUD remains in place. Even after removal, spontaneous abortion occurs approximately 30 percent of the time.

STERILIZATION

More than one third of married couples in the United States have opted for sterilization of one partner or the other, making this the most common form of birth control in this group. Whether performed on man or woman, sterilization is virtually 100 percent effective. (See box, "Factors in Choosing Sterilization.")

Sterilization methods

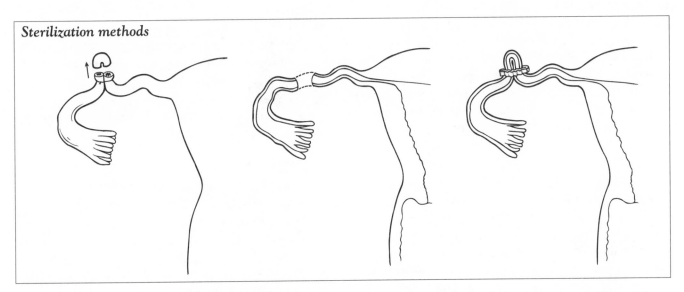

Fig. 3.13-3.15 *In one popular method of female sterilization, a small loop of each Fallopian tube is tied off and then severed. Alternatively, the Fallopian tubes may be coagulated using an electric current or clamped off using a clip or band.*

Laparoscopy for sterilization

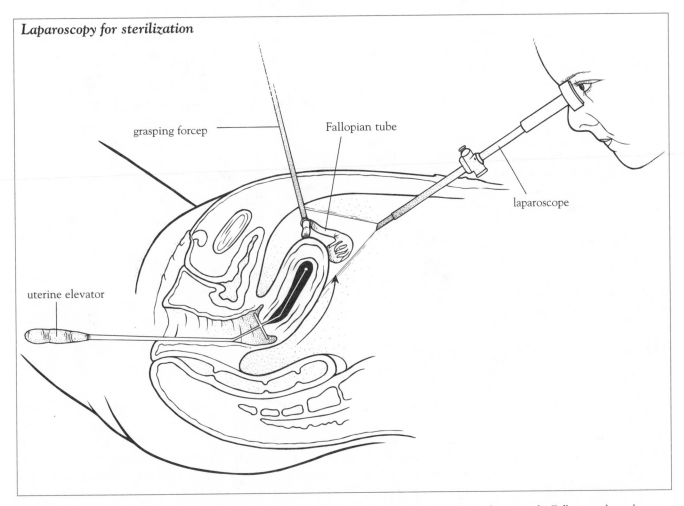

grasping forcep

Fallopian tube

laparoscope

uterine elevator

Fig. 3.16 *During laparoscopy for sterilization, one instrument elevates the uterus while a second is used to grasp the Fallopian tube and perform the sterilization. The doctor is guided by a laparoscope, a lighted tube that is inserted through a small incision just under the naval, which gives the procedure its common name, "belly-button surgery."*

FEMALE STERILIZATION PROCEDURES In all cases, the Fallopian tubes are cut or blocked, thus preventing the egg from traveling from the ovary to the uterus. Instead, the egg dissolves and is absorbed by the body. Several types of surgical procedures are used to achieve this result either by cutting the tubes and tying them off (ligating), coagulating the tubes by use of an electric current (electrocautery), or sealing the tubes using clips or bands(see Figures 3.13–3.14).

• **Laparoscopy.** This procedure (also called "belly-button surgery") is the most common form of female sterilization in the United States. A tiny incision is made just below the navel through which a long, lighted tube called a laparoscope is inserted to view the Fallopian tubes (see Figure 3.16). Tools inserted through the laparoscope or through a second tiny incision lower in the abdomen grasp the Fallopian tubes and perform the sterilization.

Laparoscopy is usually performed on an outpatient basis under either local or general anesthesia. The entire procedure takes less than an hour, although the patient may be recovering in the hospital for several hours. Recuperation is generally quick; most women experience little discomfort and return to work within a few days.

• **Laparotomy.** This requires a standard surgical incision in the abdomen, usually at the pubic hairline, and general anesthesia. Through the incision, the Fallopian tubes are cut and tied. A hospital stay of several days is usually necessary afterward. Some pain is experienced during the first 24 to 48 hours, and a longer recuperation period is required. Because laparotomy is more complicated, it is usually reserved for cases where other methods have failed, or when there is scarring from previous surgery, or where surgery is already necessary for another condition.

• **Minilaparotomy.** This is the most popular type of female sterilization in many countries and is gaining in popularity in the United States. A small incision is made above the pubic hairline. The Fallopian tubes are threaded up through the incision and then cut and cauterized, clipped, or banded. The operation can be done under local anesthesia on an outpatient basis. It is as safe as laparoscopy, but may produce more postoperative pain. Unlike laparoscopy, a minilaparotomy can be performed shortly after childbirth or an abortion. It is not recommended for women who are obese, or have adhesions or scarring from previous surgery, or have pelvic infections.

FACTORS IN CHOOSING STERILIZATION

You are a good candidate if you are absolutely certain you want to terminate your fertility and you have been well informed about the procedure and its effects.

You may want to think about having tubal sterilization if:

• You have all the children you want.

• You and your partner cannot use or do not want to use other methods of family planning.

• You have health problems that may make pregnancy unsafe.

• You know you do not want any more children and you do not want to face the need for an abortion if your temporary methods fail.

• You want to enjoy sex without fear of unwanted pregnancy.

• You do not want to pass on a hereditary disease or disability.

Tubal sterilization may not be right for you if:

• You are very young.

• You are unsure about having children in the future.

• Your current relationship is not stable.

• You are considering the operation because you are having a difficult pregnancy.

• You are undergoing stress in your life.

• You are considering the operation just to please your partner.

• You are counting on having the operation reversed if you change your mind later on.

Source: "Female Sterilization: Answers to Your Questions About Permanent Birth Control," the Association for Voluntary Surgical Contraception, New York, 1990. Used with permission.

• **Culpotomy and Culdoscopy.** These methods use the vagina as an entryway. In culpotomy the tubes are cut and tied as in a laparotomy, but the incision is made inside the vagina. Culdoscopy, similar to laparoscopy, involves inserting the magnifying instrument through the vagina, then clipping and cauterizing the Fallopian tubes. Both procedures may be performed under local or general anesthesia during an average 1-day hospital stay. Both have the advantage of not leaving a scar (although the laparoscopy and pubic-hairline scars are nearly invisible). They carry a higher risk of failure (subsequent pregnancy) than the methods described earlier and because there are always bacteria in the vagina, they can cause infection. Although it is rare, sometimes sexual intercourse is painful after this procedure, which is thought to result from sensitivity or scarring in the area of incision.

• **Pros and Cons.** Sterilization is the most cost-effective contraceptive method because it is a one-time procedure that is effective for the duration of the fertility cycle. Although it is almost ten times safer than childbirth, it does carry a mortality rate of 1.5 deaths per 100,000 procedures, while other methods of contraception have none.

With the exception of those who have undergone laparotomy, most women are able to resume normal activities within a week. Other contraception must be used until the next menstrual period to make sure an egg has not passed the point where the tubes were blocked. In some cases, menstrual changes occur, but generally they do not.

The average risk of becoming pregnant after sterilization is less than 1 percent (slightly higher if the operation is performed in conjunction with childbirth, when changes in blood vessels associated with pregnancy may make the severed tubes more viable and likely to reattach).

Terminating fertility is a drastic measure, and no woman should undertake it believing that it can be easily reversed. About 2 percent of sterilized women in the United States express regret 1 year after having been sterilized, and almost 3 percent after 2 years.

Most of those who regret their decision are under age 30 or were sterilized at the time of a cesarean section because the timing was convenient. Change in marital status is a common reason for discontent.

• **Sterilization Reversal.** About 2 in 1,000 sterilized women have their Fallopian tubes reconnected. The best results (70 to 80 percent pregnancy rates) occur when the tubes are closed off with clips or rings or when surgical methods are used that involve cutting and tying. The worst results occur when the tubes have been sealed with electrocautery because a longer section of tube has been damaged.

Reversal is a major operation for which many women are rejected. Candidates are usually in their late thirties or younger, in good health, have a fertile partner, ovulate regularly, have only a small section of their tubes damaged, and have been sterilized within the previous 10 years. Even when all these signs are positive, only about 60 percent of women who undergo sterilization reversal are able to become pregnant. (See box, "Questions to Ask Yourself About Sterilization.")

MALE STERILIZATION Male sterilization, called a vasectomy, is safer, easier, more effective, and less expensive than female sterilization, yet few men undergo the procedure. Vasectomy involves cutting and tying or cauterizing the vas deferens, the tubes that transport sperm from the testes to be mixed with seminal fluid. Postoperative complications such as infections occur rarely and are easily treated. There is no decrease in the volume or velocity of the ejaculation. Once all the sperm that can be stored in the vas deferens at the time of sterilization are eliminated (which takes about 6 weeks or 15 ejaculations), virtually all men who have vasectomies are sterile. Although there seem to be slightly higher rates of prostate cancer in men who have had a vasectomy, no study has shown any cause-and-effect relationship.

About 50 percent of men who undergo vasectomy reversal are able to father a child. This rate decreases with the time elapsed between the procedure and the reversal.

ABORTION

Fifty percent of all pregnancies in the United States are unplanned, and half are terminated by abortion. In fact, since 1980, abortion has been the most frequently performed surgical procedure in this country, and it certainly has caused the most controversy.

QUESTIONS TO ASK YOURSELF ABOUT STERILIZATION

Would you regret your decision to become sterilized if:

• Your current relationship ended in divorce and your spouse received custody of your children?

• Your current relationship ended and you had a new partner who wanted children?

• One or more of your children died?

• Your financial situation improved significantly?

• You felt lonely after your adult children left home?

METHODS OF ABORTION The first step in any abortion is confirmation of the pregnancy and determination of the gestational age. Failure to date the pregnancy accurately is the most common reason for later complications.

If the pregnancy is in the first trimester, the most usual method of termination is *vacuum curettage*, or vacuum aspiration, performed under local anesthesia (often accompanied by a tranquilizer). The cervix is dilated, either before the procedure by inserting *Laminaria japonicum*, a sterile seaweed preparation that swells as it absorbs fluid, or during the procedure by using small rods of progressively increasing diameter. Once the cervix is dilated, a hollow plastic tube attached to a suction pump is inserted and the uterine cavity is suctioned for a few minutes. After the procedure, you stay in recovery for observation for 1 to 2 hours before being sent home.

Complications may possibly occur within the first week, so it is wise to schedule a postoperative visit if any of the following symptoms occur. These include increased bleeding, pain, fever, and continued symptoms associated with pregnancy, and may indicate a perforated uterus, infection, or a pregnancy that has not been completely terminated.

Heavy bleeding due to incomplete aspiration and retained tissue occurs in up to about half of 1 percent of cases. Moderate to severe bleeding and severe pelvic pain are signs of infection, which occurs in an equal number of cases. Treatment is a combination of prompt uterine reaspiration and antibiotics. Antibiotics are sometimes prescribed as a preventive measure after the abortion.

Two methods are used in second-trimester abortions, which can be performed up to 24 weeks: *dilation and evacuation* (D&E) and *instillation*. For a D&E, the cervix is dilated using sterile seaweed or metal rods (see previous section). Because greater dilation is required than with a vacuum curettage, the procedure can take several hours and may be performed on the evening before the procedure. The doctor then uses surgical instruments to remove the fetal tissue and placenta and may follow up with curettage—scraping of the uterus. Although a sedative and local anesthesia are preferred because they carry less risk, at some facilities you may have the option of general anesthesia.

In the instillation, or induction, procedure, prostaglandin (a hormonelike fatty acid found normally in the body) or a saline solution is injected through the abdomen into the amniotic sac. Alternatively, prostaglandin may be given as a vaginal suppository.

The prostaglandin induces premature labor, and the resulting uterine contractions help expel the fetal tissue and placenta. The synthetic hormone pitocin may be given to continue the contractions until all the tissue has been expelled.

The most important factors determining the success of second-trimester abortions are the surgeon's skill and the accurate evaluation of the age of the fetus. The gestational limit at which a doctor will perform a second-trimester abortion may depend on the practice at the local medical facility and the availability of emergency medical support should there be complications. After 20 weeks' gestation, instillation abortions are more common than D&Es.

• **Safety.** Surprisingly, the death rate from legal abortion is less than that from childbirth. Death rates in 1985, for example, were 1 in 200,000 legal abortions compared with 20 per 200,000 births. Abortions performed after the first trimester under general anesthesia involve higher risks, but nearly 89 percent of the procedures are performed before that cutoff. Even in difficult cases, an experienced surgeon, aided by ultrasonography, will probably be able to perform the procedure without any complications arising. There is no evidence of problems with later childbearing among women who have had uncomplicated first-trimester vacuum-aspiration abortions.

• **Cautions and Contraindications.** Although many women feel secure about their decision to have an abortion, recognizing it is the best option for their personal circumstances, others have reservations and, sometimes, regrets afterward. Because the decision can be an emotional one, you should discuss it thoroughly with your doctor and, if appropriate, with your partner.

Women who have some uterine malformations, severe cardiorespiratory disease, severe anemia, or clotting disorders, or who have already experienced difficulties with a first-trimester abortion should carefully assess the need for an abortion and the risks of continuing the pregnancy.

RU 486 RU 486 is a French-developed drug that blocks the action of progesterone, a hormone that is a necessary component of an ongoing pregnancy. Without progesterone, the fertilized egg is unable to implant in the uterus, the uterine lining breaks down, and a miscarriage occurs. The drug, also referred to as mifepristone or mifegyne, is combined with a prostaglandin agent that causes uterine contractions. The success rate of this dual process is more than 85 percent. As an alternative to surgical abortion, mifepristone shows promise, but it is not yet approved for use in the United States. The patent for the drug has now been transferred to the Population Council, which will test it in clinical trials.

The drug has been approved for use in France, after a long battle that climaxed in October 1988, when the French company responsible for the development of RU 486 chose to take it off the market, citing pressure from antiabortion groups in the United States and Europe. The French health minister, Claude Evin, responded by ordering the company to return RU 486 to the market. He declared it "a product that represents medical progress" and should therefore be available to women.

• **Ease of Use.** A common misconception of RU 486 is that it is simply a pill that can be taken to avoid getting a surgical abortion. The current regimen in France is far more involved: First, a pregnancy test and physical examination are performed. Then, after a required waiting period of 1 week, the woman is administered an oral dose of three RU 486 tablets (totaling 600 milligrams) in a clinic or hospital that is licensed to perform abortions. (The drug is not available in pharmacies or through private physicians.) The woman returns to the medical facility 2 days later to receive an injection or vaginal suppository of prostaglandin. Usually, the uterine lining has already begun shedding, and within a few hours, the mild contractions triggered by the prostaglandin cause the expulsion of the embryo. A follow-up exam, performed at the medical facility 8 to 12 days later, assures that the procedure is complete. In the event that the pregnancy has continued, a vacuum-aspiration abortion is usually performed within the following week, to which the woman has already consented before taking RU 486. The cost is about the same for both methods.

• **Effectiveness.** RU 486 is most effective when taken during the first 7 weeks of the pregnancy. It is the method used in approximately one in four abortions performed in France. By early 1991, the RU 486 regimen had been used in 65,000 cases, with an effectiveness rate of 96 percent, about the same as for a surgical abortion.

• **Side Effects.** The primary side effect is bleeding, which has been severe in about 1 percent of all cases. Usually, the bleeding is less than during menstruation or with a spontaneous abortion, but it lasts for about 8 to 15 days (similar to that following a vacuum-aspiration abortion).

If pregnancy continues following the RU 486-prostaglandin method, fetal deformities may occur. Of the two continued pregnancies so far, one resulted in the birth of a normal healthy baby and the other was terminated in the second trimester after a sonogram showed deformities that may or may not have been due to the termination regimen.

Cardiovascular problems may occur in women who are at risk of heart disease. In France one woman had a heart attack and another had ventricular fibrillation. Both cases involved heavy smokers over 35, and the events occurred within 2 hours of receiving the prostaglandin.

• **Contraindications.** Women who have blood clotting disorders, chronic adrenal-gland failure, and those who are on long-term corticosteroid therapy must not use RU 486. In addition, the use of prostaglandin is discouraged for women who are over 35, smoke, or have cardiovascular problems, and it is contraindicated for those who have asthma, have become pregnant with an IUD in place, have had a cesarean section within the previous year, or have fibroid tumors.

THE FUTURE

Although the current political climate, lack of research funding, and concern about product liability have curtailed contraception development, some new options, such as the female condom, have become available. This condom, a polyurethane pouch inserted into the vagina, is held in place by an inner ring while an external ring covers the outer lips. Although it is not as effective against STDs as a male condom, it offers some protection to a woman if her partner will not use his condom. Early reports show that the female condom is not as effective a birth control measure as many other contraceptive options. As women become more adept at using it, this may improve. The response so far, however, has been lukewarm.

Farther in the future are such emerging contraceptive methods as biodegradable progestin implants, injectable contraceptive preparations, vaginal rings that release hormones, and other ovarian suppressors.

Menstruation

Part of being a woman means living a life of cycles. Moods, physical well-being, and even body temperatures can waver in a predictable manner during the cycle of the months. Of course, the most noticeable sign of the cyclical nature of the female is the menstrual period. The "menstru" in menstruation, in fact, means monthly. Whether it is something you dread, merely tolerate, or celebrate, the monthly ebb and flow of hormones is a reaffirmation of your womanliness and reproductive health.

Your menstrual period first becomes part of your life sometime between the ages of 10 and 16, takes time off when you are pregnant or nursing a baby, then tapers off into menopause between the ages of 45 and 55. The cycles are considered to be over when you have not had a period for a year.

Although it might seem like more from the number of tampons or sanitary napkins you use, the chief physical manifestation of your monthly period amounts to merely about one quarter of a cup of discharge. The menstrual flow looks like blood, but it also contains mucus and tissue (containing tiny blood vessels) that has built up in the uterus. This substance is a lining that developed to nestle a tiny ball of cells that would have become an embryo if pregnancy had occurred.

"The curse," "on the rag," and other vernacular terms for menstruation indicate that this is not a favorite time for many women. Antimenstrual feelings, however, go far beyond schoolgirls' snickering. Many cultures have banished women during their menstrual periods. For example, the Old Testament states that a woman cannot touch her husband at all during her period and for 7 days thereafter, and then must undergo a ritual cleansing bath, a practice still followed by married Jewish Orthodox women.

Fortunately, a mere menstrual period rarely stops an active woman today. She can do virtually anything during her period—work out, make love, even have a pelvic exam should that be necessary. Many women report heightened sex drives during this time.

HORMONES AND THE MENSTRUAL CYCLE

Your monthly cycle is activated by communication among the brain, ovaries (where the eggs are formed), and uterus (the pear-shaped organ that stretches to accommodate a fetus). This communication is carried out by hormones—chemical messengers that are produced in one part of your body and travel in the bloodstream to other parts, where they exert various effects.

The menstrual cycle is complex because several hormones are involved. It is easiest to follow by labeling the days of a typical cycle, which lasts about 28 days. (See Figure 4.1.)

Day 1 is when bleeding starts. The levels of the hormones estrogen and progesterone in your bloodstream are not very high at this time. Deep in your brain, a tiny, pea-shaped gland called the pituitary receives signals from another part of the brain, the hypothalamus, telling it to secrete follicle-

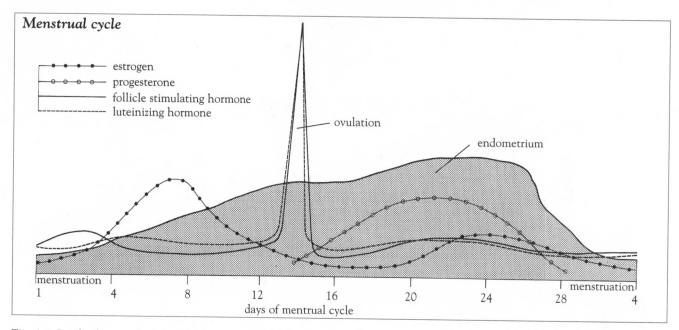

Menstrual cycle

estrogen
progesterone
follicle stimulating hormone
luteinizing hormone

ovulation

endometrium

menstruation

menstruation

1   4   8   12   16   20   24   28   4

days of mentrual cycle

Fig. 4.1 *Levels of various hormones fluctuate throughout the 28 days of the average menstrual cycle, building up to trigger the ripening of an egg, preparing for pregnancy, and then declining if no pregnancy occurs, which triggers the shedding of the uterine lining and starts the cycle all over again.*

stimulating hormone (FSH). This hormone causes a few of the hundreds of minuscule, undeveloped eggs in one ovary to mature. One egg, or maybe two if twins are in the offing, leads the pack. As the egg "ripens," the cells surrounding it form a structure called a follicle and another hormone, estrogen, is released. (See Figure 4.2.) Estrogen is a messenger that heads for the uterus, where it stimulates the growth of tissue in the lining. Here, cells divide, arteries extend, and a home for an eventual embryo is readied—just in case.

The estrogen level mounts until it peaks at day 14. The FSH level is also high. This hormonal milieu prompts the secretion of a very important pituitary hormone called luteinizing hormone (LH). A great surge of LH on day 14 causes the ripened egg to burst from the ovary. This event, called ovulation, occurs 14 days, plus or minus 2 days, before your next period begins, no matter how long your cycle is.

Between the 15th and 28th days, the egg, having left the ovary, is captured by waving fingerlike projections (fimbriae) leading into one of the paired Fallopian tubes that connect to the uterus (see Figures 4.3–4.4). If conception takes place—that is, if the egg meets and merges with a sperm in the tube—it continues its journey to the uterus, dividing a few times to form a ball of cells. This preembryo then nestles into the uterine lining 5 to 7 days after conception (see Figures 4.3–4.4). However, if the egg is not fertilized, it is absorbed painlessly by your body.

Meanwhile, the follicle left in the egg's wake is busy. It matures into a structure called a corpus luteum that secretes large amounts of progesterone, which further readies the uterus for occupancy. Progesterone is the pregnancy hormone. It sees to it that the uterine lining has plenty of mucus and a starch-like substance called glycogen, which are necessary for the embryo-to-be to be implanted. If you become pregnant, progesterone will continue to be secreted, maintaining the uterine lining and suppressing menstruation.

By about day 26, the corpus luteum stops secreting progesterone, shrivels up, and is absorbed by your body. Progesterone levels plummet, as do estrogen levels, which have already fallen quite a bit. These declining hormone levels trigger the shedding of the uterine lining, a sure sign that pregnancy is not to be. As you reach for a pad or tampon, your brain is already sending out the hormonal signal to start the process all over again.

The first half of the menstrual cycle is called the preovulatory, or follicular, phase because this is when the follicle matures. The second half of the cycle is called the postovulatory, or luteal, phase because this is when the corpus luteum functions.

Before the 1930s, it was thought that women were at their most fertile during and right after their periods, since some other mammals have a period of bleeding called estrus. Estrus, however, is not the same phenomenon as menstruation. Women are

Egg maturation and release

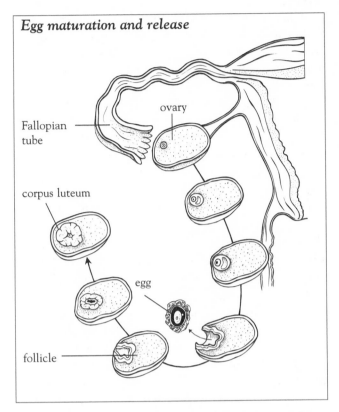

Fig. 4.2 *On day 1 of each cycle, an egg begins to mature within a cell structure called a follicle. The follicle enlarges and moves toward the ovary wall until day 14, when the egg bursts through the wall of the ovary, ready to be picked up by the Fallopian tube. The ruptured follicle then transforms into the corpus luteum and secretes progesterone in preparation for pregnancy, only to degenerate on day 26 if none occurs.*

Route of egg

Fertilization and implantation

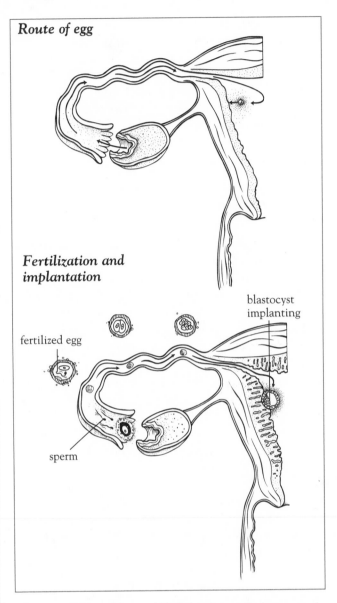

Fig. 4.3–4.4 *After bursting through the ovary wall, the egg travels through the Fallopian tube to the uterus. If it is penetrated by a sperm on the way, it begins the process of cell division and implants itself on the wall of the uterus.*

most fertile right in the middle of a 28-day cycle, when LH surges and a ripe egg pops out of the ovary. Female apes and certain female monkeys have menstrual cycles similar to human females.

OTHER PHYSICAL CHANGES

Besides bleeding, there are many other predictable physical manifestations of the monthly hormone cycle. Basal body temperature drops slightly just before ovulation and rises slightly just after it. The mucus glands that line the birth canal are exquisitely sensitive to hormonal changes. They increase their activity just before ovulation, and on the day of ovulation, produce a wet, clear, slippery secretion that probably eases the way for sperm on their journey toward the egg. This secretion can be distinguished from mucus present at other times by its stretchability, a quality described medically as *spinn-*

barkeit. At other times, the vaginal discharge is more likely to be absent or thick and cloudy but scant.

Some women feel a sharp pain in the lower abdomen at ovulation. This may last from a few minutes to a day, and is called *mittelschmerz*, which is German for midcycle pain. About 10 percent of women bleed very slightly ("spot") at ovulation.

The cervix, which is the mouth of the uterus, shifts position during the monthly cycle. Some women can detect the change by placing a finger in the vagina. When you are at midcycle, your cervix is high and difficult to reach, and softer than at other times.

If you wish to practice natural family planning (see previous chapter), are trying to become pregnant, or just want to know what stage of the menstrual cycle you are in, you can keep a record of cycle changes. This record is called charting, which can include changes in body temperature, position of the cervix, consistency of the cervical mucus, weight, appetite, sex drive, and frequency of certain symptoms, such as headaches.

CRAMPS

It is a rare woman who has never experienced menstrual cramps. This discomfort is called dysmenorrhea (see box, "Menstrual Cycle Problems"). Along with it you may also experience diarrhea, frequent urination, sweating, abdominal bloating, backache, nausea and vomiting, and pain radiating down your upper thighs and back. These unpleasant feelings are caused by body chemicals called prostaglandins, which are similar to hormones but act where they are produced rather than traveling in the bloodstream. Prostaglandins are also responsible for labor pains, which are often described as very intense menstrual cramps.

Fortunately, a number of nonprescription drugs, such as aspirin, ibuprofen, and naproxen sodium (Advil, Midol 200, Motrin, Nuprin, and Aleve), contain antiprostaglandin agents and are usually quite effective in treating cramps. (See section on "Premenstrual Syndrome.") Many women find that mild exercise also helps relieve menstrual cramps.

When cramps are especially intense, as they can be between the ages of 15 and 25, getting bed rest and placing a heating pad or a hot water bottle wrapped in a towel over the abdomen may provide some relief.

Constipation can make cramps worse. Avoiding constipation by getting regular exercise and including good sources of fiber (fruits, vegetables, and grains) in the diet is important at any time but especially so during premenstrual days.

If cramps are so severe that they disrupt your daily routine, you should see your doctor, who may prescribe a stronger analgesic, such as mefenamic acid (Ponstel) or naproxen sodium (Anaprox). A woman past her teens may be helped by taking birth control pills or other hormone treatments that suppress menstruation.

Intense menstrual cramps that begin within the first 3 years of the onset of menstruation are called primary dysmenorrhea, and in most cases they do not signify that anything is wrong. In fact, the cramps confirm that ovulation is taking place. If severe cramps and accompanying symptoms begin later in life, an underlying condition could be the cause. Common causes are benign tumors called fibroids that grow in the uterus, and endometriosis, a condition in which endometrial tissue, normally found lining the uterus, builds up in and on other sites, such as the ovaries, Fallopian tubes, bowel, and bladder.

BLEEDING BETWEEN PERIODS

Bleeding from the vagina that occurs other than during a period is called metrorrhagia. There are several possible causes of abnormal bleeding: an early miscarriage, a polyp growing on the cervix (see Figure 4.5), or an infection or inflammation of the uterus or cervix. A dislodged intrauterine device (IUD) may also cause bleeding. Any unusual bleeding should be reported to your physician, because it may be a sign of cancer in the cervix or uterus, although in the majority of cases cancer is *not* the cause.

HEAVY OR FREQUENT BLEEDING

A sign that menstrual periods are dangerously heavy is when you need to wear more than one sanitary napkin or tampon at a time. An excessive flow of blood at the time of the period or a period that lasts more than a week are both forms of a condition called menorrhagia.

MENSTRUAL CYCLE PROBLEMS

NAME	SYMPTOMS
Dysmenorrhea	Severe cramps and other pains
Menorrhagia	Heavy or frequent menstrual periods
Metrorrhagia	Breakthrough bleeding
Oligomenorrhea	Irregular or unusually light menstrual periods
Primary Mmenorrhea	Failure to begin menstruating
Secondary Amenorrhea	Cessation of menstrual periods

Vaginal cysts and polyps

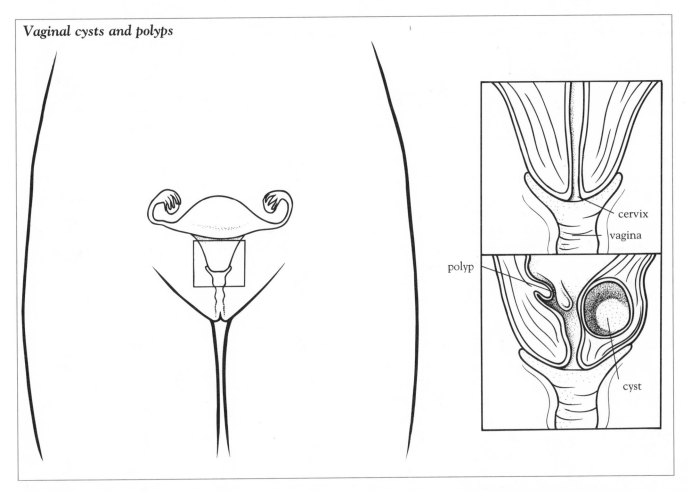

Fig. 4.5 *Endometrial polyps are growths that are usually benign but may be premalignant or malignant. Ranging from a fraction of an inch to almost an inch in size, they may arise from the uterine lining or be attached to it by a slender stalk. They may be a cause of abnormal vaginal bleeding, in which case they can easily be removed by hysteroscopy or a D&C. Cervical cysts are benign growths that may arise if the mucus-secreting glands in the cervix becomes obstructed, causing mucus to collect in the glands.*

Heavy or prolonged periods may have any of several causes. You may just have a thicker uterine lining than other women, so you bleed more. In an older woman, it may mean that menopause is imminent. Recently inserted IUDs often cause heavy periods for a few months. Fibroid tumors growing in the uterus may also cause excessive bleeding, simply because they increase the surface area, providing more sites for bleeding. Too heavy periods may also result from pelvic inflammatory disease, a hormonal imbalance, or a blood clotting problem. An early miscarriage can produce a single episode of heavy bleeding, often with painful cramps. Abnormal bleeding may be a sign of uterine or cervical cancer.

Consult your doctor if your periods are too heavy or frequent. He or she may prescribe birth control pills or other hormonal therapy, most commonly a synthetic form of progesterone. If fibroids are the culprit, they may have to be removed. Often dilation and curettage (D&C) is performed to scrape the uterine lining clean. A D&C not only helps pinpoint the cause of heavy bleeding, but frequently alleviates the problem.

A heavy loss of blood from anywhere is dangerous because over a period of time it can cause anemia, an inadequate number of red blood cells. Because these cells ferry oxygen throughout the body, anemia can cause profound fatigue. Menorrhagia can cause anemia if it continues for more than a few months.

All women lose blood during menstruation, so anemia is always a possibility (a simple blood test will confirm it). Being certain to obtain enough iron in the diet can make anemia less likely. Meats, dark green leafy vegetables, and egg yolks are high in iron. Drinking a glass of orange juice with these foods increases the amount of iron that the intestines absorb from them. If your menstrual blood flow is heavy, talk with your physician about taking iron supplements.

MENSTRUAL IRREGULARITY

Your menstrual cycle may be irregular and infrequent in its first few and last few years. A preteen may have three or four cycles a year, as might her mother, if she is old enough to be approaching menopause. This type of menstrual irregularity is called oligomenorrhea, and it is defined as having fewer than eleven menstrual periods a year.

Irregular periods may have a physical cause, such as pregnancy, thyroid disease, an acute illness, or the use of birth control pills. However, the menstrual cycle is known for being exquisitely sensitive to emotional stress. This is not surprising because both the emotional state and the menstrual cycle are controlled by chemical messengers in the brain. Stress probably activates parts of the brain that send signals to the hypothalamus and pituitary, which secrete the hormones that control the menstrual cycle.

Many events can throw the menstrual cycle temporarily out of kilter: leaving home, taking final exams, travel to a different time zone, a job change, a relationship problem, or a family crisis. To determine whether the cause of menstrual irregularity is physical or emotional, it may be helpful to note the dates of your periods on a calendar along with important events. If they coincide, chances are that emotionally provoked brain chemistry is at fault. It is important to consult a physician if pregnancy is desired because an unpredictable menstrual cycle can interfere with conception.

Irregular menstrual periods can, in rare cases, indicate a serious medical problem. If continuing irregularity cannot be explained by the fact that a woman has just begun to menstruate or is nearing menopause, a doctor should be consulted.

A fascinating menstrual-regularity phenomenon is synchronization, which tends to occur in all-female environments. Typically, twenty young women, each with a distinct menstrual cycle, begin to share a college dormitory floor in September. By May chances are that many of them will have their periods at the same time! Synchronization has also been documented in convents and prisons. It is disrupted if men come to live with the women. Menstrual synchronization may be caused by pheromones, which are hormonelike substances secreted by one organism and perceived by another. Pheromones have not yet been definitively identified in humans, but are known to send sexual signals in some other animals.

FAILURE TO MENSTRUATE

Menstruation that never begins is termed primary amenorrhea. Usually, this is due to late puberty, a tendency that may be inherited, and is not a cause for alarm. To be sure, if you have reached the age of 16 and have not yet menstruated, you should see a physician. Where heredity is not involved, a number of hormonal problems may be behind the lack of menstruation. The pituitary, thyroid, or adrenal glands or the ovaries may be the source of the problem, and hormonal treatment may be necessary. Rarely, the problem can be a missing part of the reproductive tract, such as the ovaries or uterus, or a chromosomal abnormality.

The cessation of menstrual periods for 4 months or more after a regular cycle has been established is called secondary amenorrhea. This occurs much more often than primary amenorrhea, and it is more easily prevented and treated. Other causes of secondary amenorrhea are pregnancy and breast-feeding. A woman who discontinues birth control pills may find that her period does not return for up to a year. Chronic diseases, such as thyroid disorders, and long-term use of certain drugs, such as tranquilizers and antidepressants, can also cause secondary amenorrhea.

Too little body fat may also be responsible for secondary amenorrhea. This may be the result of drastic dieting, as in cases of anorexia nervosa, or extremely rigorous exercise, in which case the condition is called exercise or athletic amenorrhea. Many female Olympic athletes with very trim physiques experience menstrual abnormalities. Running is the sport most often associated with cessation of menstrual periods, but the extent of running sufficient to stop periods varies from woman to woman. If exercise is the cause of amenorrhea, cutting back restores the menstrual cycle. Likewise, menstruation usually resumes with more normal eating habits.

A combination of low body fat and hard physical work can lead to delayed onset of menstruation, lowered fertility, and early menopause. Your body-fat level must be equal to or greater than 17 percent for menstruation to begin, and greater than 22 percent for it to continue. This may be your body's way of ensuring that you do not become pregnant unless you have enough stored energy to support a developing baby.

Menstrual periods also may stop in times of extreme stress. This is called environmental amenorrhea, and tends to occur with severe to catastrophic changes in a life situation. War, famine, emotional stress such as a divorce, rape or job loss, or psychological disturbances may all lead to temporary cessation of periods. Severe stress is thought to disrupt interactions between the pituitary gland and the hypothalamus region of the brain that produce and regulate the luteinizing hormone necessary for ovulation.

Menstruation often resumes spontaneously after secondary amenorrhea. It is not necessarily a problem unless you want to become pregnant. However, if your periods do not return after 4 months and pregnancy is not the cause, you should see your doctor. Life-style changes or adjustments in medication may be necessary. If not, your doctor may want to check the hormone levels in your blood. A low level of estrogen may place even a young woman at risk for osteoporosis. In this case, he or she may recommend birth control pills or estrogen replacement therapy. If you want to get pregnant, it may be necessary to take fertility drugs.

TOXIC SHOCK SYNDROME

Toxic shock syndrome (TSS) has been around for many years, but came into prominence in the early 1980s, when it peaked sharply among menstruating women using new, superabsorbent tampons. The menstrual connection helped researchers close in on the nature of TSS fairly quickly. Today we know that tampons containing polyacrylate rayon or polyester foam with carboxymethylcellulose—no longer on the market—prompt bacteria of a strain of *Staphylococcus aureus* that may be already present in the reproductive tract to produce the toxin that causes TSS (see Figure 4.6). The superabsorbent fibers take magnesium away from the bacteria, which produce the toxin in response.

TSS begins with a sudden high fever greater than 102°F, accompanied by diarrhea, vomiting, muscle aches, and inflamed eyes. A day or two later, a rash resembling a sunburn appears all over the body. Although these symptoms may seem like those of the flu, you should see a physician immediately if you are menstruating because TSS can quickly develop complications. These include a severe drop in blood pressure (the "shock" part of TSS); kidney, heart, or liver failure; and blood clotting problems. Toxic shock syndrome is treated in a hospital with antibiotics, intravenous fluids, and possibly corticosteroid drugs.

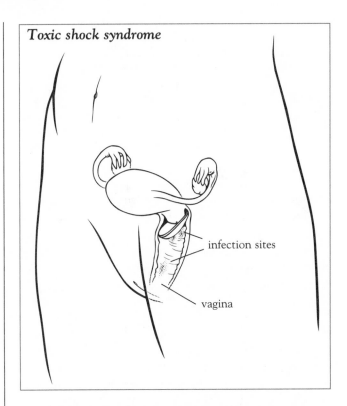

Fig. 4.6 *Toxic shock syndrome is much less common now that high-absorbency fibers are no longer used in tampons. But it does occur in a small number of women who use tampons or contraceptive sponges.*

Prompt medical attention is called for because TSS is fatal 2 to 3 percent of the time.

Nowadays TSS is very rare. Annually it strikes 5 in every 100,000 women while they are menstruating, and 1 in 100,000 who are not actively menstruating. It tends to recur, usually within 6 months, in an estimated 5 to 33 percent of women. The decline in TSS is largely attributable to the fact that high-absorbency fibers are no longer used in tampons, and because women are aware of its symptoms, they stop using tampons if any occur.

Several risk factors must be present for TSS to develop. You must already be infected with the strain of *Staphylococcus aureus* that causes toxic shock. This is not unusual because many people harbor these bacteria without any symptoms at all. Conditions must be just right for the bacteria to manufacture the toxin and for you to react to it. (See box, "Lowering the Risk of TSS.")

High-absorbency tampons are not the only objects that can create cozy conditions for the bacteria that produce the TSS toxin. Used properly, contraceptive sponges can spend several hours in the reproductive tract. Eight in 100,000 sponge users develop TSS, a

LOWERING THE RISK OF TSS

To significantly lower your risk of contracting toxic shock syndrome (TSS):

• Do not use tampons.

• Remove a diaphragm or contraceptive sponge promptly, but no sooner than 8 hours after intercourse.

• Do not use a diaphragm or vaginal sponge during your period or in the first 3 months after giving birth.

• Do not use a tampon, diaphragm, or vaginal sponge if you have ever had TSS.

• Inform your doctor if you think you may have had a mild case of TSS.

If you must use tampons:

• Do not use superabsorbent brands that may have been left over from before these products were banned, or that are imported from abroad.

• Do not keep one tampon in for more than 8 hours.

• Wash your hands before inserting a tampon, and do not touch your vagina as you insert it.

• Do not use tampons continuously. Change off by wearing a sanitary pad at night.

figure higher than for tampon users. A few cases of TSS have been linked to a diaphragm that was left in place for more than the suggested time. Taking birth control pills lowers the risk of contracting TSS by one half, perhaps because the menstrual flow lessens.

PREMENSTRUAL SYNDROME

The fluctuations of hormones can drastically affect how you feel. Distinct physical, mental, and behavioral changes that take place during the last 3 to 14 days of the menstrual cycle—anytime in the 2 weeks preceding your period—constitute premenstrual syndrome (PMS). From 25 to 100 percent of women have PMS at one time or another, according to various studies, but only about 3 to 15 percent of menstruating women experience it as debilitating.

PMS is difficult to study because women interpret discomfort in different ways, and perceptions of

symptoms are influenced by portrayals of the premenstrual woman as raging, irrational, or an emotional wreck. Some women may be conditioned to expect certain feelings at this time of the month, making PMS for them more of a self-fulfilling prophecy than a bona fide illness. Nevertheless, there is a large enough body of evidence to suggest that it is a very real if complex condition.

PMS is diagnosed more by its cyclical nature than by the symptoms themselves, which number more than one hundred. (See box, "A Sampling of PMS Symptoms.") Physical symptoms include headache, vertigo (dizziness), backache, nausea, vomiting, and constipation. Some women develop acne in the latter half of their cycles (2 days to 2 weeks before the start of the menstrual flow), and many crave sweets, particularly chocolate. Fluid retention occurs, so you may put on a few pounds and your breasts and belly may feel bloated. A fierce headache may signal an impending period.

The emotional hallmarks of PMS are not only more well known but are more common than physical complaints. Studies have documented dramatic manifestations of PMS: increased rates of suicide attempts, psychiatric hospital admissions, and violent crimes by women during menstruation. These are unusual, however. More frequently, the premenstrual

A SAMPLING OF PMS SYMPTOMS

Some of these symptoms are more common than others, and they represent only a fraction of a wide-ranging list that have been recorded.

Acne	Headache
Anxiety	Intolerance of alcohol
Backache	Irritability
Bloating	Mood swings
Breast tenderness	Sensitivity to light
Cramps	Sleeplessness
Depression	Tearfulness
Difficulty in Concentrating	Throbbing varicose Veins
Fatigue	Vaginal itching
Food cravings (especially chocolate and salty foods)	Weight gain

time of the month brings irritability, extreme sensitivity, or sudden and inexplicable tears or depression. You may feel lethargic and anxious. Changes in sleep patterns are also associated with PMS.

Some women experience a related disorder known as premenstrual exacerbation. They have an underlying, sometimes undiagnosed, chronic condition that may be troublesome all month long but that intensifies premenstrually. Conditions that can be affected by the menstrual cycle include anorexia, anxiety, bulimia, depression, epilepsy, panic disorders, substance abuse, and thyroid dysfunction. Many women are able to handle the physical or emotional symptoms the rest of the month, but find that the mood changes they undergo as their periods approach become unbearable. Identifying and treating the primary condition can have a positive effect on the premenstrual symptoms.

There is some debate over the cause of PMS. Prostaglandins, the body chemicals behind menstrual cramps, probably play some role. The syndrome was once thought to be the result of a hormone imbalance, but it now seems that women with symptoms have the same hormone levels as those without—they may simply have abnormal reactions to those levels. The hormone progesterone, which helps maintain the uterine lining, is known to calm the central nervous system and help the kidneys secrete salt, which lowers fluid retention. A study in England seemed to indicate that progesterone vaginal suppositories were helpful in alleviating PMS symptoms. However, a large study in the United States found that they were of no use in alleviating either physical or psychological symptoms.

Another possible cause of PMS is a deficiency of vitamin B_6, also known as pyridoxine. Vitamin B_6 is involved in the synthesis of the nerve-cell messenger dopamine, and somehow the regulation of dopamine may trigger some of the behavioral symptoms of PMS. Being careful to get sufficient B_6 in the diet may help alleviate PMS in some women. This vitamin is found in meat, poultry, fish, shellfish, green and leafy vegetables, whole grains, and legumes. Or check with your doctor about taking a B_6 supplement: A dose of 50 to 100 milligrams (mg) a day is sufficient; doses above 500 mg can be toxic.

Finally, PMS symptoms may reflect a sudden drop in endorphin levels. Endorphins are small brain molecules that mediate perceptions of pain and pleasure, among other activities. Fluctuating ovarian hormones may cause a decrease in endorphin levels, leading to feelings of tension, irritability, and anxiety.

What can you do about PMS? First, you must determine whether your symptoms are actually due to PMS. To do this, you should chart these symptoms for at least 3 consecutive months. Record the dates of your menstrual flow as well as a daily assessment of moods, physical symptoms and their intensity, eating habits and food cravings, and any stressful events and your reactions to them. It is likely that you have PMS if symptoms are absent for at least 7 days in the first half of the cycle but recur predictably in the second half. Premenstrual exacerbation is probable if your symptoms don't disappear the rest of the month but do increase in intensity before your menstrual flow begins. In both cases, the symptoms should lessen or disappear when your flow begins or reaches its height.

The very act of keeping a diary can be helpful. What may have been a vague set of symptoms begins to take on predictable regularity, and this in itself offers some small comfort. Recognizing patterns and triggers makes it easier to cope by planning and adjusting schedules and avoiding additional stress where possible.

There is no miracle cure for PMS, but some symptomatic relief is possible. Getting more exercise may help alleviate symptoms by increasing endorphin levels. Very careful attention to diet, including reducing sugar, caffeine, alcohol, and processed foods, may also be helpful. Limiting your salt intake sometimes helps avoid fluid retention. Taking vitamin E supplements can reduce breast tenderness in some cases. Physical pain, such as headache or backache, can be relieved with aspirin, ibuprofen, or acetaminophen. Over-the-counter preparations to counter fluid retention and bloating include ammonium chloride, pamabrom, and pyrilamine maleate. Midol PMS and Premesyn PMS combine a mild diuretic with an antihistamine and acetaminophen, to work on cramps, swelling, and aches and pains.

If these measures do not help, there are stronger prescription medications to alleviate pain and hormone therapy to alter the menstrual period itself. Ponstel and Anaprox are prescription analgesics. Propranolol (Inderal), a beta-blocking cardiac drug, is sometimes prescribed for premenstrual migraine. Antidepressants and antianxiety drugs may also be used. Low-dose oral contraceptive pills may alleviate PMS in some women. In women close to menopause, low-dose estrogen replacement therapy may be helpful.

CHAPTER 5

Infertility

Infertility appears to be an increasingly common problem, as a growing number of couples are seeking medical help in conceiving a child. Every year Americans spend at least $1 billion to achieve pregnancy and pay about 2 million visits to doctors for infertility. Between 15 and 20 percent of couples in the United States are infertile.

Several explanations have been proposed for these statistics. Many women are postponing having children until they are in their thirties, when their fertility begins to decline. (See box, "Fertility and Age.") Age may increase the likelihood of having had multiple sexual partners, thus increasing the risk of exposure to sexually transmitted diseases (STDs) that can result in pelvic inflammatory disease (PID) and infertility. Advancing age increases the likelihood of exposure to environmental and industrial toxins, which may affect fertility. Finally, with the recent development of new treatments for infertility, people are more aware that the condition can be treated and are seeking help.

Definitions of infertility vary. When all age categories are considered together, approximately 60 to 70 percent of the couples trying to conceive will succeed within 6 months, and an additional 20 percent will conceive within 1 year. Some doctors believe that a couple who fail to conceive after having unprotected intercourse for a year should be considered infertile. Others think the cutoff point should be 2 years.

If the couple have never been able to conceive a child, infertility is referred to as primary, but if they already have one or more children but are unable to conceive again, the condition is known as secondary. People who are completely unable to have children are considered to be sterile, but except for obvious cases—as for example, when a woman has had a hysterectomy—it is impossible to know with absolute certainty that a person is infertile.

Both infertility and the treatment for it can be emotionally devastating. People unsuccessfully trying to conceive a child may experience envy toward friends who have children or get depressed during child-centered holidays. They may feel like failures or develop exaggerated feelings of guilt over past behaviors that may have impaired their fertility. Adding to the stress, the most intimate details of their lives are scrutinized as their doctors try to establish the cause of infertility, and lovemaking often turns into a chore. Moreover, treatment for infertility is expensive and not always covered by medical insurance. However, for a couple who are eager to have a baby—or to find out whether they can—the effort is worthwhile because most causes of infertility can at least be diagnosed.

About one fourth of all couples who believe they are infertile conceive while undergoing tests for infertility. Many others can be helped once the cause is established. When there seems to be no possibility of a couple having children, many have turned to adoption as a solution. Although the number of children available for adoption has decreased, numerous public and private agencies throughout the country provide information and assistance in this area.

A more recent and highly controversial alternative to adoption has been surrogate motherhood. When the husband is fertile but the wife is not, another woman is impregnated with the husband's sperm and surrenders the baby to the couple after giving birth. Surrogate mothers are generally paid by the infertile couple, but some also agree to participate because they enjoy the experience of pregnancy. There have been cases, however, when a surrogate mother has decided to keep the baby, resulting in a court case. When surrogate parenthood is planned, therefore, the feelings of all three participants must be carefully discussed and considered. The surrogate mother in a small number of cases has actually been the baby's grandmother—a youthful mother willing to undergo pregnancy again to help a daughter or daughter-in-law unable to conceive.

CAUSES OF INFERTILITY

In order for pregnancy to take place, the man must produce sperm of sufficient quality and quantity and the woman must produce a healthy egg, or ovum. The sperm must travel through the vagina and uterus to meet the ovum while it is in one of the Fallopian tubes. (The timing of intercourse is important because although sperm usually live for a few days, an ovum can be fertilized only during a 12- to 24-hour period. If the sperm reach the tubes too long before or after ovulation, they will not enounter any eggs to fertilize.) Once the egg is fertilized, it must travel to the uterus and become successfully implanted in its lining. A disruption in any stage of this delicate process can lead to infertility.

In the past, when a couple could not have a child it was automatically assumed that the woman was "barren," but doctors now believe that it is just as often the man who is infertile. In about 40 percent of cases, the cause of infertility lies with the female partner and in another 40 percent with the male. In the rest, both partners have a fertility problem or no cause can be found, although this number is decreasing as better diagnostic methods are being developed.

Not long ago, unexplained infertility was often attributed to psychological factors, but it is now known that many cases were due to organic causes that were not understood at the time. The psychological condition of the partners probably affects reproductive

FERTILITY AND AGE

Women are most fertile in their midtwenties. Their fertility begins to decline after that and drops more rapidly after age 30. While you can become pregnant as long as you are menstruating, the chances of pregnancy diminish greatly as you near menopause.

The following table demonstrates the relationship between age and female fertility:

AGE	CHANCES OF CONCEPTION WITHIN 6 MONTHS
25 years	74.6%
35 to 39 years	25.5%
After 40 years	22.7%

A man's fertility also decreases gradually with time, but the more rapid drop generally occurs after age 40. However, men have no cutoff point equivalent to menopause to mark the end of their reproductive phase, and some remain fertile throughout their lives.

Adapted from *Gynecologic Endocrinology and Infertility for the House Officer*, Williams & Wilkins, Baltimore, 1988, p. 142.

activity, but scientists are not sure to what extent. For example, stress can temporarily suppress ovulation and sperm production. Unfortunately, the infertility itself may be a cause of significant emotional stress to the couple. In particular, the man may feel that being infertile somehow makes him less virile, although there is no connection between fertility and sexual drive and performance. To help the couple deal with these and other difficulties, an infertility workup often includes consultations with a psychologist.

CAUSES OF INFERTILITY IN MEN Male causes of infertility fall into the following major categories:

•Low Sperm Count. This is the most common cause of male infertility. Generally, the count is considered low when a milliliter of semen contains less than 20 million sperm, although some physicians believe that a man will have difficulty impregnating a woman if his semen contains less than 80 million sperm per milliliter. In fewer than 2 percent of infertile men, the semen contains no sperm at all—a condition known as azoospermia.

Sperm production is most often disrupted by infection of the prostate gland or the ducts of the man's reproductive system. Once the infection is treated, sperm count usually returns to normal. Another common cause of low sperm count is a varicocele, a varicose vein in the testicle. The dilated vein is believed to affect sperm production by raising the temperature in the testicle. About 10 to 15 percent of all men have a varicocele, but not all of them are infertile. When the vein is tied off in a surgical procedure, sperm counts improve in about 70 percent of cases.

Among other factors, the production of sperm may also be suppressed by temporary illness such as the flu, chronic disorders such as colitis and rheumatoid arthritis, hormonal and genetic diseases, and severe stress. Contracting mumps after puberty permanently disrupts sperm production in about one fourth of

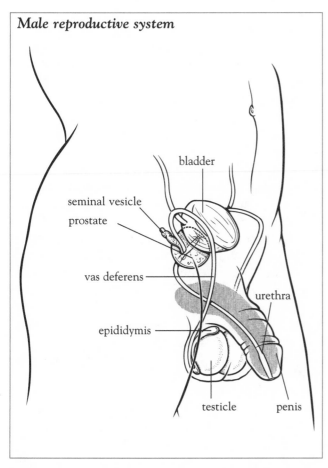

Male reproductive system

bladder

seminal vesicle

prostate

vas deferens

urethra

epididymis

testicle   penis

Fig. 5.1 *Sperm is manufactured in the testes, stored in the epididymis, and then passes through the vas deferens to the seminal vesicle, where it mixes with semen and secretions from the prostate. From there the sperm travels via the urethra to the penis, where it is ejaculated during orgasm. Shown are some of the problems that can interfere with this process.*

cases. Severe injury to the testicles, STDs, and tumors may also reduce or eliminate sperm in a man's semen.

• **Poor Sperm Quality.** The quality of sperm is no less important than its quantity. All men produce some sperm that are abnormal in shape or structure. When *most* sperm are defective, however, a man is unlikely to be fertile. Doctors believe that more than half of the sperm must be normal in order to achieve pregnancy. The sperm must also be able to move rapidly and easily in order to travel along the female reproductive tract and reach an egg.

The quality of sperm, as well as its ability to move (motility), may be reduced as a result of chronic illness, infection (particularly in the prostate gland), or when a man takes certain medications, such as those used to treat emotional disorders. Motility may also be affected if the semen is too viscous or thick.

• **Sperm Delivery Problems.** Sperm may not be reaching the penis (see Figure 5.1) if the vas deferens, the tubes through which they travel, are blocked. The obstruction can be caused by injury, accident, or scar tissue resulting from previous infections or STDs. If the penis has a structural abnormality—for example, if the opening is on the top or bottom rather than the tip—the semen may have difficulty reaching the cervix. A small number of men have a condition called retrograde ejaculation, in which sperm are released into the bladder instead of traveling down the urethra.

If a man has a sexual dysfunction, such as impotence, premature ejaculation, or inability to ejaculate, he may be unable to deposit sperm in the vagina. These conditions often have a psychological cause that may be resolved by sex therapy.

CAUSES OF INFERTILITY IN WOMEN A woman may be infertile because she is not producing eggs, or because she has a structural abnormality or disease that prevents normal fertilization and pregnancy (see Figure 5.2). The following are the major causes of female infertility:

• **Lack of Ovulation and Hormone Problems.** Ovulation—the release of a mature egg by the ovary—is a necessary step for pregnancy. Women in their twenties generally ovulate twelve or thirteen times a year, but with age the number of ovulatory cycles decreases. A woman who has irregular menstrual periods or no menses (regardless of age) may not be ovulating at all.

Ovulation can be hindered, at least temporarily, by numerous illnesses and behaviors, which is per-

Female fertility problems

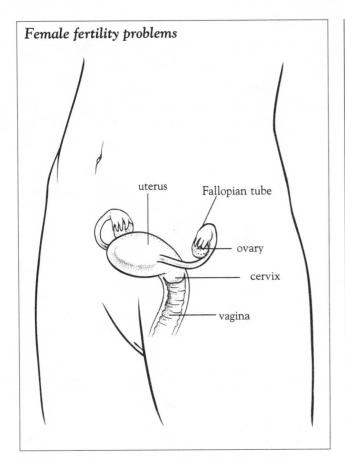

uterus

Fallopian tube

ovary

cervix

vagina

Fig. 5.2 *A variety of illnesses, behavioral factors, and hormonal problems can suppress ovulation; in women who do ovulate, structural abnormalities may prevent fertilization or implantation.*

haps the body's way of ensuring that pregnancy does not occur when something is not functioning properly. Stress, dieting, cigarette smoking, alcohol, exposure to radiation, and certain drugs can suppress ovulation. Women who are very overweight may fail to ovulate because their fatty tissues disrupt the hormonal balance in the body by stimulating estrogen production. On the other hand, women who are excessively thin may stop ovulating because their body does not have sufficient fat. Thus, anorexia nervosa, an eating disorder in which the patient loses a great deal of weight, and strenuous athletic training, which can drastically reduce the proportion of body fat, can lead to the cessation of menstruation and ovulation.

Since ovulation is associated with a complex and fine-tuned interaction of several hormones, it can be disrupted by almost any hormonal disturbance. Many endocrine disorders, such as severe diabetes, thyroid abnormalities, underactive adrenal glands, and diseases of the pituitary can disrupt normal menstruation and ovulation.

An elevated level of prolactin, a pituitary hor-

mone that normally suppresses ovulation in nursing women, may cause fertility problems. Lack of ovulation may be suspected if your level of progesterone does not increase appropriately in the second half of your menstrual cycle. Progesterone is released by the corpus luteum and prepares the uterine lining for the implantation of the fertilized egg. Sometimes, you may ovulate but fail to produce progesterone long enough for implantation to take place.

• **Structural Abnormalities.** Defects in the reproductive organs may prevent the union of sperm and egg, or the successful implantation of the fertilized egg. They may also preclude carrying the pregnancy to term.

Cervix—A normal cervix, the narrow neck of the uterus that projects into the vagina, is tightly closed except during labor, when it dilates to allow the passage of a baby. Due to a congenital defect or a trauma that may have occurred during surgery or previous delivery, the cervix may become lax, or incompetent, and thus dilate before it should. Although it does not affect conception, cervical incompetence can lead to the loss of the pregnancy in the second or third trimester or to premature labor and delivery.

Uterus—Uterine fibroids, which are benign growths on the walls of the uterus, are fairly common and usually do not interfere with pregnancy. Occasionally, if fibroids disturb the lining of the uterus or block the Fallopian tubes, they may prevent the fertilized egg from implanting or developing normally. If necessary, fibroids can be surgically removed before (but not during) pregnancy.

Structural problems in the uterus, and sometimes in the cervix and vagina, may occur if a woman was exposed to DES (diethylstilbestrol) while still in the womb. This hormone was sometimes given to women to prevent miscarriage until evidence emerged in the early 1970s that it caused abnormalities of reproductive organs in their daughters.

Fallopian tubes—These thin tubes, through which the egg released by the ovaries travels to the uterus, can easily become obstructed as a result of PID (see Figure 5.3). All infections that develop in the reproductive tract must be rapidly treated to prevent scarring of the tubes and their blockage. Blockage can also be caused by STDs, such as chlamydia and gonorrhea. The damage can be more severe in anyone who was wearing an IUD at the time of the infection. Blockage may also result from adhesions that form after abdominal surgery, particularly if there was an infection.

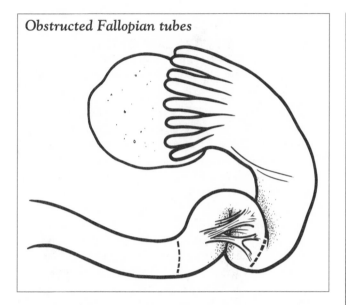

Obstructed Fallopian tubes

Fig. 5.3 *Infections, especially sexually transmitted ones, can leave scar tissue that obstructs the Fallopian tubes.*

Endometriosis—This disorder is characterized by abnormal growth of the uterine lining outside the uterus. It can lead to the formation of scar tissue and adhesions throughout the pelvic cavity, which can in turn cause obstruction in the area of the ovaries and Fallopian tubes. Some doctors believe that in women with endometriosis, fertility may also be affected by biochemical processes triggered by abnormal tissue growth. Endometriosis may be treated with surgery or drugs, or both.

• **An Immune Reaction.** Sometimes, a woman is allergic to her partner's sperm. This happens in a little less than 5 percent of infertile couples. In these cases, the immune system mistakes the sperm for infectious agents and produces antibodies against them. But since normally sperm do not penetrate your tissues, the immune reaction is more likely to be triggered if the lining of your reproductive tract is injured during intercourse.

Some women are allergic to all sperm, while others produce antibodies only against the sperm of a particular partner. The antibodies disable the sperm and prevent them from fertilizing an egg. Some men develop an immune reaction against their own sperm, generally after injury or infection.

When infertility is caused by a woman's immune reaction, the sperm may be washed and placed into her uterus through artificial insemination. Sometimes, the man is advised to use condoms during intercourse to reduce his partner's levels of antibodies

MOST COMMON CAUSES OF INFERTILITY

FEMALE

Endometriosis
Failure to ovulate or other ovulatory disorders
Hostile cervical mucus
Overweight
Tubal scarring or abnormalities
Underweight
Uterine fibroids or malformations

MALE

Ejaculatory disorders
Environmental factors such as exposure to excessive heat or certain toxic chemicals
Epididymitis
Excessive alcohol or other drug use
Impotence
Orchitis
Sperm defects
Underdeveloped, undescended, or injured testicles
Varicocele

BOTH SEXES

Advancing age
Chromosomal and genetic disorders
Hormonal problems (pituitary, thyroid, adrenal disorders)
Immunological incompatibility
Poor timing of intercourse
Sexually transmitted infection
Smoking

to the sperm, and to have sex without a condom only at the time of ovulation.

Major factors that can contribute to a man's infertility are listed in the box "Most Common Causes of Infertility." For example, alcohol, medications, and illicit drugs can reduce both sperm quality and quantity. One small study showed that in men who smoked marijuana daily, sperm production dropped by 35 percent, the proportion of normal sperm decreased, and their motility diminished.

A man's fertility is also affected by his overall health and nutritional status. There is no evidence, however, that a man eating a normal diet can improve the quality and quantity of his sperm by consuming vitamins or other nutritional supplements.

•**Other Problems.** The cervix is lined with mucus, which must be of good quality in order to let the sperm through. Under the influence of infection or hormone abnormalities, the mucus may become hostile to sperm, killing them on contact. Sometimes, the cervix does not produce enough mucus for the smooth passage of sperm, or, conversely, the mucus may be too abundant or too thick for the sperm to penetrate it.

Infection with an organism such as chlamydia and possibly mycoplasma, which are usually sexually transmitted and may be present in the cervix or uterus without causing symptoms, may lead to infertility or early miscarriage. Such infection is usually treated with antibiotics. Another rare cause of infertility is the inflammation of the uterine lining, called chronic endometriosis, which is also treated with antibiotics.

EVALUATION OF THE INFERTILE COUPLE

Although finding the cause of infertility can be a time-consuming and costly process, sometimes it requires only a few simple tests, done progressively, ruling out the most common causes first before going on to the next step. (See box, "When to Seek Help for Infertility.")

In the initial interview, the partners are asked about their respective sexual histories, the presence of genetic and other diseases, and use of medications. The doctor then conducts a physical examination of the couple's reproductive organs and may order blood and urine tests for STDs. More sophisticated tests are ordered later in the course of the workup. These are usually prescribed for the man first because tests for women are generally more invasive and painful.

FERTILITY TESTS FOR MEN Most tests for men involve analysis of the semen. The man is asked to masturbate into a sterile container, or use a special condom during intercourse, and to deliver the semen sample to a doctor's office or laboratory within 30 to 60 minutes. The sample must be kept at room tem-

WHEN TO SEEK HELP FOR INFERTILITY

How soon you should seek professional help with conceiving a child depends largely upon your age. Many physicians believe that a couple in their twenties can wait up to 2 years before consulting a doctor. If the woman is over 30, she should seek help sooner. Some specialists think an infertility workup must start within a year of trying to get pregnant unsuccessfully if you are between 30 and 35, and within 6 months if you are over 35. A couple with specific problems that may affect fertility should consult a physician at the outset. Problems may include irregular periods, pain that suggests endometriosis, or a history of pelvic inflammatory disease. The waiting period may also be shortened if the man has had mumps or a scrotal injury, or has a genital abnormality.

perature. The semen is examined under a microscope to determine the sperm count, the proportion of normal sperm, and their motility. If the results of this examination are abnormal, the test may be repeated because sperm measurements vary greatly as a result of minor illnesses and life events. The semen is also checked for the presence of white blood cells that may signal an infection, and cultures may be taken.

If no infection is found but the sperm are dead or clumping together, the physician may prescribe testing for antisperm antibodies. These tests, which involve taking blood samples from both partners in addition to samples of semen and cervical mucus, are more complicated and expensive, and are usually performed when simpler tests have failed to reveal a diagnosis.

The sperm's penetrating ability may also be tested by placing them in a drop of mucus collected from your cervix during your fertile days. This allows the doctor to evaluate both the sperm and the mucus. The sperm being tested may be compared with semen from a donor known to be fertile.

In some fertility clinics, the ability of sperm to fertilize an egg is tested on the basis of their capacity to penetrate fresh hamster eggs. This test, however, is not completely reliable because it sometimes yields poor penetration results with sperm of men who are nevertheless found to be fertile.

FERTILITY TESTS FOR WOMEN An examination that is routinely performed in the initial fertility workup is the postcoital test, which reveals what happens to sperm in your body. In this test, you have intercourse at home, then go to your doctor's office within 2 to 4 hours. The doctor uses a narrow pipette or a thin plastic tube to collect a few drops of mucus from your cervical canal and then examines it under a microscope to evaluate the quality of the mucus and the presence of active sperm. The timing of this test is crucial: It must be performed 1 to 3 days before ovulation. If it is performed too late or too early in your cycle, results may be poor even in a fertile couple. Also, intercourse must be avoided for a day or two before the test to make sure the man's semen contains an adequate quantity of sperm.

Other fertility tests performed in women evaluate ovulation and the structure of the reproductive organs. The order of the tests may be rearranged if you have a specific known problem, but in general the simpler tests are prescribed first.

OVULATION TESTS

•Basal Body Temperature Charts. A temperature chart is not foolproof, but it is a very simple way of establishing the time of ovulation. (See box, "Keeping a Basal Body Temperature Chart.") Typically, your temperature drops just before ovulation, then rises sharply and remains somewhat elevated until your next menstrual period. A basal temperature chart kept for 2 to 3 months prior to seeing a doctor may provide useful information for the fertility evaluation and treatment. (See Figure 5.4.)

If your periods are regular, you can use the chart to predict the next ovulation and to time intercourse accordingly, but if they are irregular, keeping such a chart may not be very helpful because the most fertile days are immediately before ovulation, not after. Moreover, many women with normal ovulation do not have a clear-cut temperature pattern.

•Home Ovulation Tests. New self-tests for ovulation, which cost about $35 per cycle, are more reliable than the temperature chart. These tests are designed to test your urine for luteinizing hormone, which surges just before ovulation. The kit includes a special dipstick that changes color according to the concentration of the hormone in the urine, which allows you to determine your most fertile days.

•Endometrial Biopsy. In this test, the doctor inserts a small instrument into your uterus through the cervix and removes a tiny sample of the uterine lining. It is then examined to determine whether progesterone has adequately prepared the lining for the implantation of the embryo. If no influence of progesterone is observed, it is certain that ovulation did not occur. The biopsy is performed late in the menstrual cycle. The risk that a biopsy will disturb a

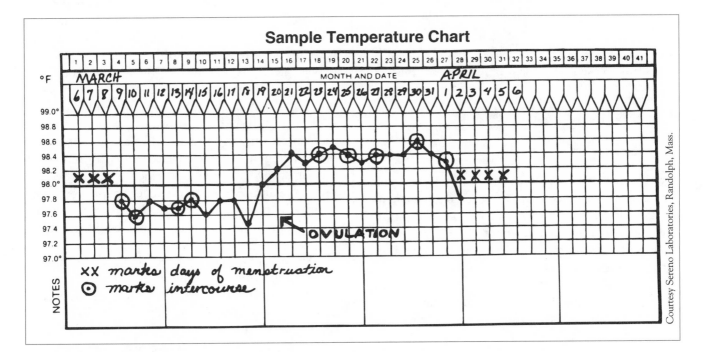

Fig. 5.4 *Charting your temperature and other pertinent information daily makes it easy to see when you are ovulating.*

KEEPING A BASAL BODY TEMPERATURE CHART

Specially calibrated basal thermometers are readily available in drugstores and come with body temperature charts like the one on this page. The following are general instructions for keeping a chart:

1. Insert the date at the top of the column in the space provided. The chart starts on the first day of menstrual flow, not the calendar month.

2. Each morning immediately after awakening and before you get out of bed, place the thermometer under your tongue for at least 2 minutes. Do this every morning except during your period. Be sure not to eat, drink, or smoke before taking your temperature.

3. Accurately record the temperature reading on the graph by placing a dot in the proper box. Indicate days when you have intercourse by circling the dot or placing a down-pointing arrow above it.

4. The first day of menstrual flow (not "spotting") is the start of a cycle. Indicate each day of flow by putting an X in each square indicated on the graph, starting at the extreme left under the first day of the cycle.

5. Note any obvious reasons for temperature variation, such as colds, infection, insomnia, indigestion, etc., on the graph above the reading for that day.

6. Ovulation may be accompanied by a twinge of pain in the lower abdomen. If you notice this, indicate the day it occurred on the graph.

Adapted from "Ovulation Detection," the American Fertility Society, 1991. Used with permission.

---

new pregnancy is very low, but some doctors recommend that it be conducted on the day your temperature drops and a new cycle is about to begin, to make sure you are not pregnant. The procedure is somewhat uncomfortable and may be performed under local anesthesia. It rarely leads to complications, but if you experience abdominal or lower back pain, fever, and excessive bleeding, you may have developed an infection, and you should consult your physician immediately.

• **Hormone Tests.** The fluctuation of the hormones that regulate ovulation and otherwise affect a wom-

an's fertility can be detected through blood tests. Performing such tests on a daily basis is complicated and expensive, but many experts recommend them at the beginning, middle, and end of the menstrual cycle.

TESTS FOR STRUCTURAL PROBLEMS

• **Tubal Insufflation (Rubin) Test.** This test helps determine whether your Fallopian tubes are open. A gas (carbon dioxide) is blown through the cervix into the uterus. If your tubes are normal, the gas will escape through them into your abdomen, but if they are blocked, it will accumulate in your uterus. One drawback of this test is that even when it reveals a blockage, it cannot show the location precisely. Most experts consider the test outdated, and it has been largely replaced by hysterosalpingography.

• **Hysterosalpingography.** In this test, a dye is injected into the uterus and Fallopian tubes, which are then X-rayed to determine structural abnormalities as well as the size and shape of the uterus. The procedure can cause cramping and may be painful if the tubes are blocked. The test is generally conducted in the early part of the cycle, when pregnancy is unlikely. The procedure diagnoses tubal obstruction accurately in about 75 percent of cases. Sometimes this test serves as treatment as well as diagnosis, because the flushing of the dye through the uterus and Fallopian tubes may increase the likelihood of conception in some women. Some experts believe that oil-based dyes are more likely to increase fertility than water-based dyes, although water-based chemicals are preferred for use in those who are prone to pelvic infections. Hysterosalpingography should not be conducted when a pelvic infection is suspected, because it may promote the spread of infectious organisms into the uterus. In women who tend to get such infections, the test should be done after they have undergone a preventive course of antibiotics, or a laparoscopy should be performed instead. (See the Encyclopedia.) Although the level of X-ray exposure during the test is low, hysterosalpingography should not be done if you suspect you may be pregnant.

• **Hysteroscopy.** In this procedure, the doctor inserts a narrow viewing tube through the cervical canal in order to examine the uterus for defects such as polyps, adhesions, or other causes of impaired fertility. Sometimes the instrument is equipped with a device to collect tissue samples for a biopsy. The procedure is usually performed under general anesthesia in the early days of the menstrual cycle.

• **Laparoscopy.** This surgical procedure is performed under general anesthesia and usually comes last in the fertility workup. It allows the physician to view the reproductive organs through a small telescopic instrument, called a laparoscope, that is inserted into the abdomen through a small incision below the navel. A dye injected into the uterus and the Fallopian tubes permits the doctor to evaluate these organs and the extent of blockage if it exists. Laparoscopy provides a great deal of information about the structure and functioning of the reproductive system. It is considered safe, but it does involve the risks associated with general anesthesia, as well as a small risk of damage to internal organs.

TREATMENT FOR INFERTILITY

Once the cause of infertility is established, as it can be in about 90 percent of cases, a variety of treatments are available. Recent technologies have made parenthood possible in cases when it would have been unthinkable only a few years ago. Sometimes, however, infertility cannot be treated even when its cause is known.

When the cause is unknown, a couple are advised to follow simple methods that may increase their chances of achieving pregnancy. (See box, "What You Can Do to Increase Your Chances of Pregnancy.") Together with their doctor, they will decide which tests may need to be repeated and which treatments are worth undertaking. In a small number of cases and after many years of trying, pregnancy occurs without any treatment, a fact that offers hope when all therapies appear ineffective. About 60 percent of couples with unexplained infertility achieve pregnancy within 2½ years of completing a diagnostic fertility workup.

Treatment options for infertile men are fairly limited. Certain drugs may improve sperm count and some anatomical abnormalities may be corrected by surgery. Often, however, infertile men can only be given general advice to avoid potential causes of lowered sperm production, such as excess scrotal heat. They are cautioned not to use saunas and hot tubs, wear tight underpants that hold the testicles close to the body, and work in jobs that expose them to unusual heat. They are also advised to quit smoking, limit alcohol use, and avoid illicit drugs, such as marijuana.

Treatment for women is usually more precise and is described in the following sections. In addition, there are several fertility enhancement technologies that may be helpful when both partners have a fertility problem. Some of these methods, however, are difficult to endure and prohibitively expensive. Moreover, many techniques are still experimental and have a high failure rate. While not being able to have the child you want is by itself extremely painful,

WHAT YOU CAN DO TO INCREASE YOUR CHANCES OF PREGNANCY

• Keep a careful record of your menstrual cycles to establish the earliest day in the cycle that ovulation may occur. Most women who have regular cycles ovulate about 14 days before the beginning of their next period. Thus, if your cycle is 24 days long, ovulation probably occurs around the 10th day, but if it is 40 days long, you are likely to ovulate on the 26th. To establish your ovulation time more accurately, you can also buy a home ovulation test kit.

• Begin intercourse 2 to 3 days before the earliest ovulation day to stimulate sperm production in your partner. However, during the days when you are likely to ovulate, have intercourse regularly but not more often than every 24 to 36 hours because in some situations a man's sperm count may decrease if he has sex too often.

• Do not use lubricants during intercourse, as they may kill sperm or retard their movement. Use saliva if lubrication is necessary.

• Do not douche after intercourse because this may wash some of the sperm out of your vagina.

• For most women, the "missionary" position, in which you lie on your back with the man above and facing you, is the best position for conception. However, if your doctor determines that your uterus is tilted at an unusual angle, you may have to modify the position.

• Put a pillow under your hips during and after intercourse to help the sperm stay deep inside your vagina.

• Your partner should penetrate the vagina as deeply as possible and stop thrusting as he reaches orgasm, so that the semen is deposited close to the opening of the uterus. The first few drops of semen contain the highest concentration of sperm.

• After intercourse, try to lie still on your back with your knees raised for 20 to 30 minutes, to make it easier for the sperm to reach the cervix.

undergoing protracted medical tests and procedures can also be emotionally draining. It may be wise for a couple to consider the pros and cons of each treatment in advance and decide how long they should pursue fertility enhancement if the failure rate remains constant.

The major treatments for infertility that are currently available are described below.

SURGERY Structural problems can often be corrected by surgery. In men, surgery may be required to repair sperm pathways or correct a varicocele. When it is used to reverse vasectomy, 80 percent of the operations are successful and 50 to 65 percent of men are able to become fathers. In women, surgery may be performed to remove uterine fibroids, repair abnormalities in the uterus or cervix, unblock Fallopian tubes (see Figures 5.5–5.7), or control endometriosis. The organs that need to be repaired are often small and delicate, and microsurgical techniques, which involve the use of refined surgical instruments and magnifying lenses, should be employed whenever possible. Lasers are increasingly used in reproductive surgery, but their application is recent and success rates vary, depending on the skill of the surgeon.

HORMONE TREATMENT Hormonal drugs are used to improve fertility in both men and women, although they are given to women much more frequently. Hormones may be prescribed for men who have an endocrine disorder, such as a thyroid deficiency or an adrenal abnormality. Rarely, a man may require injections of gonadotropins, hormones that stimulate testicular function.

Women may also take hormones to treat endocrine diseases or correct hormonal imbalances, but most often they are given hormonal drugs to induce ovulation. The main ovulation-inducing drugs are clomiphene (Clomid); human chorionic gonadotropin, or HCG (Profasi), which is extracted from the human placenta; and human menopausal gonadotropin, or HMG (Pergonal), which is extracted from the urine of post-menopausal women.

In use since the 1960s, clomiphene acts on the brain centers that produce hormones that stimulate the ovaries to start ovulation. The drug is usually taken for 5 days, beginning on the 5th day of the menstrual cycle. Ovulation can occur within 5 days of taking the last clomiphene tablet. Then the couple begin having intercourse every 24 to 36 hours from about the 11th day of the cycle until a day or two after ovulation takes place.

Clomiphene costs $25 to $100 per month. The treatment results in ovulation in about 80 percent of women who have ovaries capable of producing eggs. About 40 percent of all women taking the drug become pregnant, but the success rate increases to 80 percent or more in couples who have no fertility problems other than lack of ovulation. Clomiphene is not associated with birth defects, but it increases the number of multiple births, particularly twins. Twin births occur in 5 to 10 percent of clomiphene pregnancies.

One potential complication of clomiphene is that it may overstimulate the ovaries, leading to the formation of ovarian cysts. You must be checked each month for excessive ovarian stimulation. You should also let your physician know if you develop side effects, such as vision problems. Some women experience headaches, hot flashes, and abdominal pain while taking this or other fertility medications.

If clomiphene fails to induce ovulation, your doctor may prescribe an additional drug, HCG, to stimulate the ovary to release a mature egg. It is usually given as an injection near the time of expected ovulation.

The third hormone, HMG, or Pergonal, is highly potent and may be given if clomiphene and HCG fail. Pergonal is a powerful medication, given by injection, that acts directly on the ovaries and must be administered by a physician skilled in the use and monitoring of the drug. While you are taking the drug, your ovaries are monitored with ultrasound and the estrogen levels in your blood are measured frequently. HCG may also be given to stimulate egg maturation. Ovulation usually occurs approximately 36 hours after the HCG injection.

Of women whose infertility is caused by anovulation (absence of ovulation), about 90 percent or more who are treated with Pergonal ovulate, and 50 to 70 percent achieve pregnancy, although this may take three to four cycles. On the downside, Pergonal treatment requires numerous tests and visits to the doctor, and it is expensive, costing from $1,500 to $3,000 per cycle, including office visits and monitoring. The most common problem of Pergonal treatment is the release of too many eggs. Up to 20 percent of Pergonal pregnancies result in twins, and about 5 percent in triplets. Since a pregnancy that involves multiple fetuses carries risks for both the mother and the babies, most experts recommend avoiding conception if ultrasound reveals that too many eggs are maturing.

Another alternative to Pergonal is treatment with a gonadotropin-releasing hormone (GnRH) pump, a device about the size of a small portable radio that is attached to your body. The pump delivers doses of GnRH—an ovulation-stimulating hormone normally released by the brain—under the skin every 90 minutes through a tiny plastic tube. The idea behind the pump is to stimulate one follicle at a time by delivering the hormone in small amounts, similar to the way it is released in nature. This is useful in treating certain types of infertility problems.

Another hormonal drug used to treat female infertility is bromocriptine (Parlodel), which reduces the levels of the hormone prolactin. In high concentrations, prolactin can suppress ovulation. Parlodel tablets are taken until ovulation resumes, which occurs in at least 80 percent of women, often within 2 months.

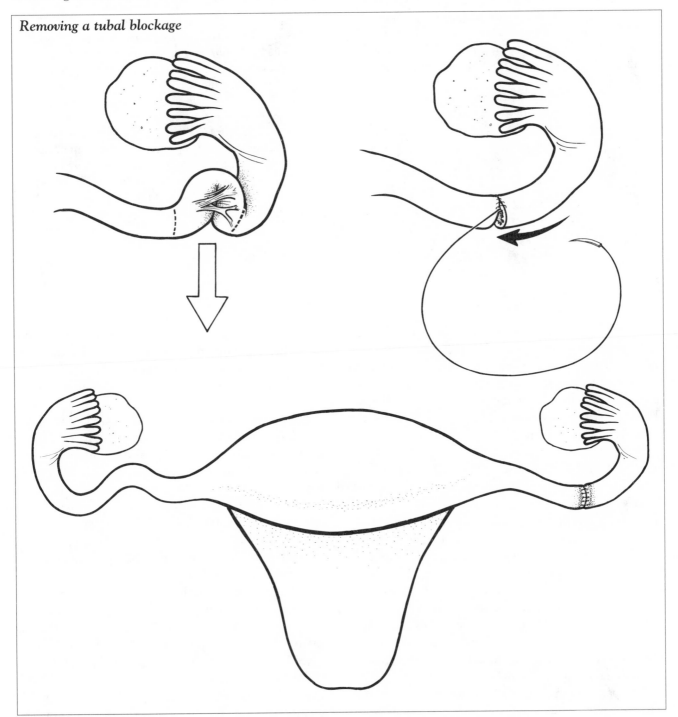

Removing a tubal blockage

Fig. 5.5–5.7 *A small blockage in a Fallopian tube can be excised and the ends of the tubes rejoined to create a clear passage for eggs and sperm.*

WHERE TO SEEK HELP FOR INFERTILITY

Start with your family doctor, your gynecologist, or, for your partner, a urologist. Sometimes the problem can be easily resolved without tests or treatments (for example, by adjusting the timing of intercourse) and you may not need a specialist. If you need an infertility specialist, your primary care doctor can refer you to one. You may also seek names from a department of obstetrics and gynecology at a medical school or teaching hospital, or from:

The American Fertility Society
1209 Montgomery Highway
Birmingham, AL 35216-2809
Tel.: 205-978-5000

RESOLVE
1310 Broadway
Somerville, MA 02144-1731
Tel. (The Help Line, 9 A.M.–4 P.M. EST):
617-623-0744

Both groups provide information, resources, and referrals to doctors nationwide.

When consulting a specialist, make sure he or she spends most of the time treating infertility. Most doctors who specialize in infertility are reproductive endocrinologists or reproductive surgeons. Reproductive endocrinology is a relatively new medical subspecialty; there are currently only some five hundred doctors throughout the United States who are certified by the American Board of Obstetrics and Gynecology's Division of Reproductive Endocrinology.

Reproductive surgery is not recognized officially as a subspecialty. It is best to find a doctor who works as part of a team or in an infertility clinic, as treatment may involve not only gynecologists and urologists but also geneticists or even psychotherapists and nutritionists.

Clomiphene or HCG may also be prescribed if your levels of progesterone in the second part of your menstrual cycle are too low for pregnancy to occur. For the same reason, natural progesterone may be given by injection or vaginal suppositories, although there is disagreement on whether or not this is as effective as clomiphene therapy.

ARTIFICIAL INSEMINATION The oldest and simplest infertility treatment is artificial insemination. In this procedure, a physician uses a syringe to inject sperm into a woman's cervical canal just before or on the day of ovulation. It is possible to perform the insemination at home without the doctor's help, but the success rate is usually lower. Since about half of the sperm would be lost in the cervix, sometimes they are injected directly into the uterus instead to facilitate their journey to the Fallopian tubes. This approach is known as intrauterine insemination, or IUI. Usually, the sperm are separated from the semen and washed before the insemination.

The partner's sperm can be used for artificial insemination in cases where his sperm count is low, only a small proportion of good-quality sperm is produced, overly dense semen hampers the sperm, or he

has retrograde ejaculation or a severe sexual dysfunction that prevents intercourse. If a man is about to undergo a cancer treatment or other procedure that may impair fertility, his sperm may be frozen for future artificial insemination.

If a man's infertility cannot be treated, if he carries a serious genetic abnormality, or if the partners have an Rh incompatibility, artificial insemination with a donor's sperm may be a solution. It is also used when a single woman seeks to conceive a child. Between 10,000 and 20,000 babies conceived with donor sperm are born in the United States every year.

Sperm donors are often students, commonly from medical schools, who may be motivated by a mixture of altruism and financial reward. The donors can be matched to the race, color of eyes and hair, and other physical characteristics of the woman or her partner. One of the major concerns about donor sperm is its safety. Usually, the sperm donors are screened for acquired immune deficiency syndrome (AIDS), gonorrhea, and other sexually transmitted and genetic diseases. However, the strictness of screening varies greatly from one fertility clinic to another, and couples must choose a facility carefully. (See box, "Where to Seek Help for Infertility.") Since antibodies to the virus that causes AIDS can take 3 to 6 months to appear, some experts recommend that donor sperm always be frozen and used only later if the donor blood shows no evidence of AIDS several months after the sperm was collected.

Freezing the sperm does not appear to affect the quality of pregnancy, but it does reduce sperm motility and, as a consequence, the success rate of artificial insemination. With insemination that uses fresh donor semen, about 75 to 85 percent of the women eventually achieve pregnancy, a rate similar to that for normal conception. Often, the procedure must be repeated over several months before conception occurs. Freezing the sperm decreases the chances of success by 10 to 15 percent.

Several emotional and legal issues must be considered before choosing insemination with donor sperm. It should only be undertaken if both partners feel comfortable pursuing this option. Donors usually remain anonymous and are not told who has received their sperm. The husband who agrees that his wife undergo artificial insemination with donor sperm is considered the legal father of the child. There may be situations, however, that raise complex ethical and legal questions, as when a lesbian couple use artificial insemination to achieve pregnancy in one of the partners. In this case, the law does not recognize the woman's partner as a legal parent; thus neither rights nor responsibilities are conferred.

IN VITRO FERTILIZATION

Normally, eggs are fertilized in the Fallopian tubes, but if the tubes are obstructed and surgery cannot restore their normal structure, fertilization will not occur. In this case, eggs can be removed from your ovaries and fertilized with your partner's sperm in a laboratory. Although babies conceived in this manner are popularly known as "test tube babies," fertilization actually occurs in a shallow glass disc called a Petri dish (*in vitro* literally means "in glass"). (See Figure 5.8.) The embryos are then transferred to the uterus. While *in vitro* fertilization (IVF) was originally developed for women with diseased tubes, it is now also used when the woman has endometriosis, or the man has a low sperm count, and in couples with unexplained infertility.

The first IVF baby was born in England in 1978. Today, more than three hundred clinics throughout the United States perform IVF or variations on the procedure. Their success rates vary greatly. Some clinics have never had a successful procedure—one

that resulted in the birth of a baby. Couples considering IVF should take care to choose a reputable facility that provides high-quality care.

According to a survey conducted in 1992 by the American Fertility Society at 245 centers that offer IVF, on average, one cycle of IVF results in the birth of a baby in 16 percent of cases. This assumes successful retrieval of eggs. The rate of pregnancies due to the procedure is higher, but some of the pregnancies result in miscarriages. The fertility society publishes annual reports that cite the success rates of fertility enhancement procedures in different clinics. The reports may be used as a guide to choosing a facility, with one caveat: They cite the success rates reported by the clinics themselves.

The first stage of IVF, fertilizing an egg in a Petri dish, usually succeeds. The stage at which the procedure is most likely to fail is implantation, as many embryos do not attach themselves to the uterine wall and perish in the womb. To increase the chances of success, some doctors try to implant up to three embryos simultaneously. Embryos that are not used can be frozen and saved for later transplantation attempts. The chances of success decrease with age and are believed to drop significantly after the age of 40. Some clinics place limits on the age of the women they accept for IVF. There are also facilities that limit the number of attempts to two to three cycles, while others are willing to perform as many procedures as the couple desires.

The treatment is costly—about $6,000 to $8,000 per cycle. As the success rates continue to rise, IVF is being used increasingly instead of previously standard infertility treatments (such as microsurgery to repair damaged Fallopian tubes).

GIFT

Gamete intrafallopian transfer, or GIFT, first introduced in 1985, is simpler sometimes than IVF but appropriate only for women who have at least one healthy Fallopian tube. In this approach, ripe eggs are removed from the ovaries, mixed with sperm, and immediately injected into one or both Fallopian tubes, so that fertilization can take place in a natural environment rather than in a laboratory dish. Also, GIFT obviates the need for taking care of the embryo in artificial surroundings.

GIFT may be performed when a man has a low sperm count or sperm motility problems, or when a couple have an unexplained difficulty achieving

In vitro fertilization

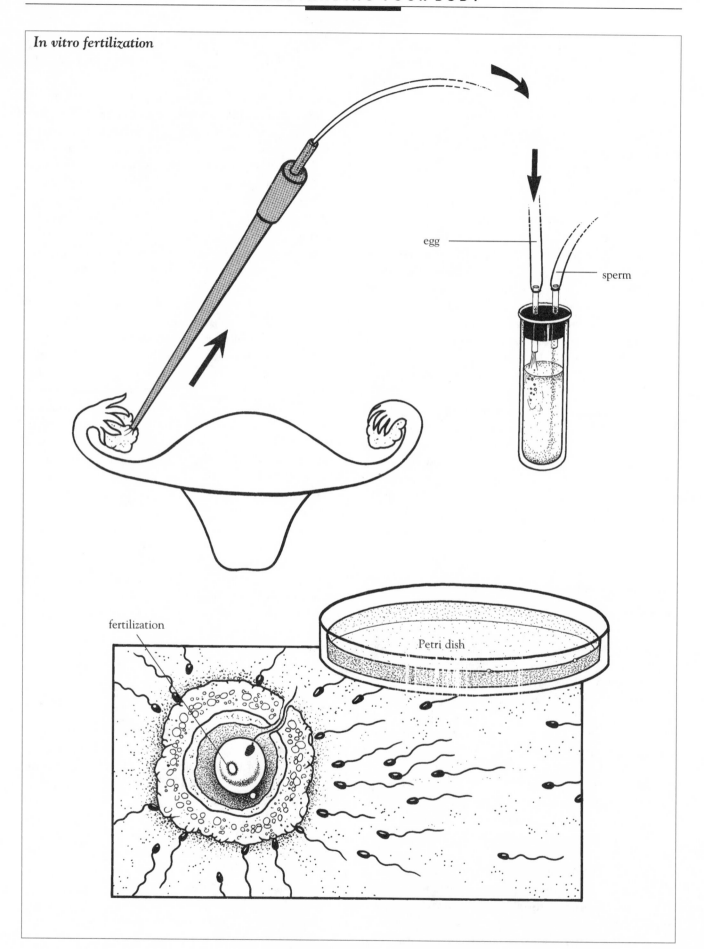

egg

sperm

fertilization

Petri dish

pregnancy. It may be tried after artificial insemination has failed. Several days after GIFT is conducted, ultrasound is usually performed to make sure that the fertilized egg did not become trapped in the Fallopian tube, leading to an ectopic (tubal) pregnancy. The risk of ectopic pregnancy is higher if the tubes are damaged or blocked.

The 1992 figures from the American Fertility Society's survey of 161 facilities that offer GIFT show that where there is successful retrieval of eggs, about 26 percent of the women undergoing one cycle of GIFT will deliver a baby. The procedure costs about $6,000 to $8,000 per cycle.

ZIFT

Zygote intrafallopian transfer, or ZIFT, is a procedure that combines elements of IVF and GIFT. As in IVF, the ovaries are stimulated and several eggs are removed and fertilized with sperm in a Petri dish. Then, rather than being transplanted directly into the uterus as in IVF, the fertilized eggs are placed into the Fallopian tubes. ZIFT can only be performed if the woman has at least one tube that is open and healthy.

ZIFT is preferable to GIFT when there is a doubt about the ability of the sperm to fertilize an egg. Since in ZIFT the fertilization takes place in a test tube, it is possible to expose numerous eggs to the sperm and transplant only the ones that have been fertilized. In GIFT large numbers of eggs cannot be used because fertilization takes place in the Fallopian tubes, and inserting too many eggs would create a risk of a large multiple pregnancy. However, GIFT is easier to endure than ZIFT, since it involves only one procedure in which the eggs are removed and reinserted into the tubes. In ZIFT two procedures must be performed: one to remove the eggs and another one about 2 days later to transplant them into the Fallopian tubes.

The American Fertility Society's survey reports 111 facilities offering ZIFT and, where there is successful retrieval of eggs, a delivery rate of 22 percent for women undergoing one cycle of ZIFT. The pro-

cedure costs about $6,000 to $8,000 per cycle. The success rate of ZIFT is slightly higher than that of IVF because, for reasons that are not fully understood, fertilized eggs placed in Fallopian tubes seem to have a better chance of becoming implanted in the uterus than those placed in the uterus directly.

DONOR EGGS

There are numerous variations on the described methods, depending on the couple's specific problem. If a woman has a healthy uterus but her ovaries cannot produce eggs, a ripened egg may be provided by a donor. The donor is given HCG to stimulate egg production, and several of her mature eggs are removed with a needle. They are fertilized in a Petri dish and transplanted into the uterus of the infertile woman. Many infertile couples prefer that the eggs be donated by someone they know, often a sister. The donor egg technique is available at 107 sites and has a delivery rate of 31 percent.

Egg donation has been a boon for women of childbearing age who wish to become pregnant but who have undergone premature menopause, either naturally, due to radiation therapy, or through surgical removal of their ovaries. However, withdrawal of eggs involves certain risks, such as infection, and some ethicists have expressed reservations about egg donation. For example, in some widely publicized cases in Europe it has been used for postmenopausal women in their late fifties and early sixties who wish to become pregnant. Such a decision must be thought through carefully, taking into consideration not only the health of the prospective mother, but also the practical aspects of child rearing at an advanced age and the ramifications for the child.

It has been speculated that eggs from aborted fetuses might be used for impregnation. Although this is theoretically possible, there are no published reports that the technique has been attempted in humans, and most fertility experts believe that ethical considerations would preclude its use.

Fig. 5.8 *In vitro fertilization involves inserting a thin catheter through a woman's vaginal wall or, less commonly, through the abdominal wall and withdrawing several eggs from her ovary. The eggs are mixed with sperm from her partner, and then placed in a Petri dish until they are fertilized. One or more embryos are then transferred to the uterus for implantation.*

CHAPTER 6

Pregnancy and Childbirth

C hildbirth in the United States has changed dramatically since the late 1960s, and much of the credit for the new attitudes and practices in hospital delivery suites must go to women themselves. The last quarter century has seen the institutionalization of childbirth education and natural childbirth techniques, full participation of fathers or other coaches in the delivery process, the elimination of some routine "prep" practices like pubic shaves, and the availability of birthing rooms and nurse-midwives—all because many women and some doctors have pushed for these innovations.

On the medical side, the development of prenatal testing, ultrasound imaging, and fetal monitoring has increased the chances of having a healthy baby even in a high-risk pregnancy, while the introduction of local and regional anesthesia has made it possible for mothers to minimize pain and still be fully conscious during delivery.

After two decades of mothers and doctors appearing at times to be on opposite sides, the pendulum seems to have swung back to the middle. Pregnant women report no longer being asked if they plan to have "natural childbirth," but rather if they have started their childbirth classes yet. Doctors say that most women no longer reject the idea of pain medication outright, but reserve the right to ask for it without feeling like a failure. Pregnancy is not looked on as a disabling illness, but a part of life that women manage quite well. Although many hospitals have established nurse-midwife programs and birthing centers, the growth of free-standing birthing centers has been static since the mid-1980s. Women seem less interested in alternative birthing positions and chairs and more interested in small comforts and maximum freedom of movement. Medical and technological intervention is being tempered: intermittent monitoring may be used instead of continuous monitoring; routine episiotomy may not be considered necessary; the necessity of many cesarean sections is being questioned; and vaginal birth after a cesarean is encouraged.

In this new atmosphere of enlightenment and co-operation, prospective mothers are encouraged to plan and prepare for their pregnancies, educate themselves about their options, and discuss their preferences with their doctors. If you are one of them, the following sections outline the steps you should take and what you can expect.

PREPREGNANCY PLANNING

The growing emphasis on preventive medical care has prompted many experts to recommend prepregnancy planning and counseling. As soon as you decide to have a child, both you and your partner should assess your health and life-style to see if any changes are necessary to ensure your baby gets the best start possible. It is easier to make changes gradually now before you have to. Moreover, certain substances (such as alcohol and some drugs) should be avoided during pregnancy; since you will probably not realize that you are pregnant until you've missed at least one menstrual period, it is better to avoid these substances while you are trying to conceive.

NUTRITION If you are considering becoming pregnant, it is never too soon to examine your diet. (See box, "Questions to Ask Yourself Before You Become Pregnant.") Recent studies, for example, stress the importance of adequate folic acid intake during pregnancy and even before conception to reduce the risk of neural tube defects (abnormalities of the fetal brain and spinal cord). Green leafy vegetables like spinach, broccoli, and kale are rich in folic acid. Most American women do not eat sufficient amounts of these vegetables to reach recommended pregnancy levels, which are twice the recommended dietary allowance (RDA) for nonpregnant women. In addition to increasing their green vegetable intake, women of childbearing age are advised by many experts to take a multivitamin containing at least 400 micrograms of folic acid as a preventive measure, since most neural tube defects occur early in fetal development, possibly before you know you are pregnant.

EXPOSURE TO TOXIC SUBSTANCES Alerting yourself to chemical and environmental toxins at home and at work can reduce your exposure to these substances. The occupational hazards you are most likely to be exposed to are described in Chapter 17, "Women in the Workplace."

PRESCRIPTION AND NONPRESCRIPTION DRUGS Although drugs known to cause pregnancy complications or danger to the fetus are rare, the fact is that most drugs on the market have not been tested on pregnant women. Anticonvulsant drugs containing phenytoin, the acne drug Accutane, and certain antibiotics, including tetracyclines and chloramphenicol, are associated with birth defects or problems with developing teeth. How a drug will affect you depends on the type of drug, the dosage, and your stage of pregnancy. If you must take medication, check its safety with your doctor before you become pregnant.

Over-the-counter medications should be avoided before and during pregnancy unless they are approved by your doctor. Those considered safe are acetaminophen for headaches, fever, or cold or flu symptoms; Gelusil or Mylanta for heartburn; and Preparation H for hemorrhoids.

THE HEALTH OF THE FATHER Men who use marijuana, cocaine, or alcohol heavily may have infertility problems. There is some evidence that babies of men who drink heavily may be more likely to have low birth weights and possibly heart defects. Although these possible links need further study, it would seem prudent for prospective fathers to stop using illicit drugs and to moderate their alcohol intake. The negative health effects of secondhand smoke on infants and children are well documented, so fathers are also advised to give up smoking by the time their children are born.

WHO WILL DELIVER YOUR BABY?

Early and regular medical care increases your chance of having a healthy baby and may also make your pregnancy easier for you. Even before you become pregnant, you should consider who you want to provide your prenatal care and deliver your baby.

You may have already established a good relationship with your gynecologist and, if your doctor also practices obstetrics, he or she may be the obvious choice. If not, you have several options. The majority of women choose a doctor, either an obstetrician/ gynecologist (ob/gyn), who can continue to provide gynecological care for them, or a family practitioner, who can later attend to the family.

Unless you are considered a high-risk patient, you might choose a nurse-midwife, a registered nurse with advanced training in obstetrics and gynecology. Nurse-midwives may practice independently or be associated with an obstetrician or an obstetrical group or a hospital clinic. Some nurse-midwives also provide routine continuing gynecological care.

Your choice of doctor may also depend on where you want to deliver your baby. (For simplicity, the word "doctor" is used in the rest of this chapter to refer to your maternity caregiver.) In large cities, a doctor may only be affiliated with a single hospital; in smaller cities, he or she may have privileges at several hospitals; in suburban or rural locations, there

QUESTIONS TO ASK YOURSELF BEFORE YOU BECOME PREGNANT

• *Do you take vitamins, especially in large doses?* Certain vitamin dosages may harm a developing fetus. For example, too much vitamin A (derivatives are present in some acne medications) can cause neural tube defects, while megadoses of vitamin D have been linked to fetal heart abnormalities. The safest course of action is to stop taking supplements 3 months before trying to conceive and to consult a health professional about safe alternatives. The one exception is folic acid, which is recommended for all women of childbearing age at a daily dose of 0.4 milligram.

• *Did you take oral contraceptives?* These can deplete the body's stores of iron, folate, and vitamin B_6, which should be rebuilt before you try to become pregnant.

• *Are you a vegetarian?* If so, you may want to consult a nutritionist to help you meet increased pregnancy requirements for iron, protein, calcium, zinc, and vitamin B_6—especially if you don't eat eggs or dairy products.

• *Do you have a history of bulimia or anorexia?* Nutrition is so important during pregnancy that you should discuss this aspect of your health history with your physician.

• *Are you underweight or overweight for your height and build?* Weight gain or loss is best accomplished before you get pregnant.

• *Do you use alcohol, tobacco, or recreational drugs?* Any of these substances can pose a threat to your baby. Alcohol, even in moderate amounts, can cause fetal abnormalities and mental retardation, and recreational drugs have been implicated in a variety of birth defects. Smoking is the single largest preventable cause of low birth weight. Heavy exposure to environmental tobacco smoke is also associated with low birth weight.

• *Do you ingest caffeine through coffee, tea, cola drinks, chocolate, over-the-counter drugs, such as aspirin compounds and cold remedies, or other sources?* Some studies have shown that heavy caffeine consumption may increase the risk of spontaneous abortion. Most experts recommend limiting coffee or other caffeine-containing drinks to one cup a day during pregnancy. Now is the time to start tapering off if you drink more than that.

• *Do you or your partner have any close relatives who have birth defects, are mentally or developmentally retarded, or have health problems that might be inherited?* Seeing a genetic counselor might inform you of prenatal options, such as abortion or fetal surgery, or reassure you about your risk.

• *Do you own a cat or do you eat raw meat on a regular basis?* Toxoplasmosis is a parasitic disease that can be contracted by eating raw meat and by contact with cat feces, among other sources. Serious birth defects, including fetal blindness, can occur if a woman develops this infection in early pregnancy. Wear gloves when changing the litter box, and when gardening, and consider being tested for this disease if you think you are at high risk.

---

may be only one hospital within a reasonable distance of your home. Since maternity services may vary from hospital to hospital, you may wish to choose the hospital first and then ask for a list of its affiliated doctors or certified nurse-midwives. (See section on "Choosing a Delivery Site.")

How a doctor's practice is structured may also affect your choice. If your doctor is in solo practice, for example, you will have a greater opportunity to develop a consistent and personal relationship throughout the months of your pregnancy. By the time you deliver, you will understand each other's personality styles and preferences. On the downside, if for some reason your doctor is unavailable when you go into labor, delivery may be managed by a backup doctor you may not have met.

More and more, ob/gyns are forming group practices. In a small group setting, you may see several doctors on a rotating basis. This ensures that you will know the doctor attending your delivery, but you may not be able to develop a close personal relationship. In a large group practice of perhaps a dozen or more, several doctors may have obstetrical subspecialties, such as infertility or high-risk pregnancy, which can be useful if problems develop. Yet, you may not meet all the members of the group and you may not have a choice of who attends your delivery.

Finally, there are personal considerations. Some women have very strong feelings about how they want their childbirth to be. Fortunately, many doctors and hospitals have responded to women's desires for more natural childbirth and have made significant changes in maternity practice in the past 15 years. Although medical considerations must always override personal considerations, most doctors are willing to accommodate your wishes whenever possible.

If you have a very specific preference, one criterion that matters most, then you should discuss it with your doctor at the first visit. For example, you may want your husband to cut the umbilical cord, or you may want a certain type of pain medication, or you may not want an IV or an episiotomy. Your doctor may be happy to comply with your request, or may point out that it can be met at one hospital but not another, or may be willing to accommodate it under most but not all circumstances. If the latter is the case, he or she should be able to tell you specifically under which conditions you would have to forgo your wishes.

If it is your first pregnancy, the best course is to keep an open mind, realizing that although most deliveries go smoothly, unforeseen situations can develop and you may find yourself reacting differently than you had thought you would.

CHOOSING A DELIVERY SITE

Most American women choose to have their babies in a hospital, where a full range of technological support is usually available if needed and where they have the option of pain medication. For some women, especially first-time mothers, the prospect of childbirth may be anxiety-provoking, and a facility that is equipped to deal with almost any medical emergency offers them reassurance. Women with such medical conditions as diabetes or heart problems are advised to choose a hospital birth regardless of their preferences.

Many hospitals have added birthing rooms where both labor and delivery can take place. These rooms are often equipped with rocking chairs, private showers, and other homelike amenities. Some hospitals have opened entire birthing centers, usually staffed by certified nurse-midwives and backed by one or more staff obstetricians. The nurse-midwives handle all aspects of normal pregnancy, labor, and delivery. If any problems arise, however, they will refer the patient to a physician. This option may appeal to women who want a more natural birth setting but also want the security of a hospital in case of emergency.

Another alternative is the freestanding birth center, a less institutional setting where obstetrical interventions are not routinely used, and family and friends can remain with you when you are in labor. Although virtually all these centers can arrange rapid transport to a hospital if necessary, many experts feel that any time lapse can pose a risk for a mother or baby in distress.

A small proportion of women choose home births, attended by either a doctor or midwife. These women, rarely first-time mothers, prefer to have their babies in the intimacy and privacy of their own homes. Although a home birth may offer greater control over labor and delivery, it poses a small but definite risk of maternal or fetal death or birth asphyxia.

PREPREGNANCY CHECKUP

Even if you have no apparent medical problems, a prepregnancy physical examination is a good idea, if only to assure you that you are fit and healthy and can expect to have a normal pregnancy. Or your doctor may find problems that can be cleared up before you become pregnant, or more serious conditions that may not necessarily preclude pregnancy but need to be monitored and planned for.

A typical prepregnancy physical includes a Pap smear, blood pressure check, and pelvic exam. In addition, your doctor will want to know your age (see box, "Pregnancy After 35") and your menstrual and pregnancy history. Depending on your personal and medical history, the doctor's preferences and, in some cases, local health regulations, other tests may be recommended. These might include:

• urinalysis to check for diabetes, urinary tract infections, or possible kidney problems

• an HIV test

• cervical cultures for sexually transmitted diseases, (STDs) such as gonorrhea and chlamydia

• blood type and screening tests for blood antibodies such as Rh factor

In addition, screening for Tay-Sachs disease is advised if either you or your partner is of Eastern European Jewish descent; for thalassemia if either of you is of southern Mediterranean ancestry; or for sickle-cell trait if both of you are black or Hispanic. (These tests can also be done during pregnancy.)

VACCINATIONS If you do not recall being vaccinated for or having had measles, mumps, or rubella (German measles), a simple blood test can check

PREGNANCY AFTER 35

As more women delay childbearing, older first-time mothers—"elderly primigravidas" in medical parlance—are increasingly common. Nowadays, the health and fitness of many women well past their twenties and thirties create a relatively favorable prognosis for older pregnant women. A woman need not be considered high risk simply because of her age. Still, older women in general are more likely to have high blood pressure, diabetes, or uterine fibroids that develop with advancing age, and these conditions can complicate a pregnancy.

The risks of miscarriage, stillbirth, and other pregnancy-related complications increase gradually after age 30, but they are still relatively low. Some studies indicate that the rate of occurrence of gestational diabetes, pregnancy-induced hypertension, and bleeding is slightly higher in the third trimester for women over 35. The incidence of fetal chromosomal abnormalities increases, although prenatal tests can detect many of them. For example, a 20-year-old mother has about 1 chance in 2,000 of having a baby with Down syndrome, the most common chromosomal abnormality; the risk rises to 1 in 350 at age 35.

Statistically, there is a higher rate of cesarean sections for women over 35, but that may be related to medical problems that develop with age. To assess her risks, an older woman contemplating pregnancy should consider counseling before trying to conceive.

---

your immune status. If you are not immune to any of these, your doctor will probably recommend that you be vaccinated before becoming pregnant. After taking *any* live virus vaccine, you should not try to become pregnant for 3 months to avoid danger to the fetus. Health care workers should also consider being tested for cytomegalovirus (CMV) and hepatitis B, and cat owners for toxoplasmosis.

CHRONIC MEDICAL PROBLEMS If you have a chronic medical condition, such as diabetes, seizure disorders, asthma, multiple sclerosis, systemic lupus erythematosus, high blood pressure, or heart disease, ask your doctor about how your condition or the medications you take may affect your pregnancy. Proper control and monitoring of these conditions reduces the impact of pregnancy on your health and increases the chances of your having a healthy, full-

term baby. Getting diabetes and blood pressure under control before pregnancy is especially important.

Women whose mothers took DES (diethylstilbestrol) during pregnancy may have uterine abnormalities that increase their risk of ectopic (tubal) pregnancies and preterm delivery. A preconception hysterogram (X ray of the uterus) is advised to assess any abnormalities. During pregnancy, monitoring is important, and cerclage (temporary surgical closure of the cervix) or medication may be necessary to prevent preterm labor.

Women with PKU (phenylketonuria), a genetic enzyme deficiency, face an increased risk of spontaneous abortion and birth defects. While dietary restrictions instituted during pregnancy have shown little benefit, dietary changes implemented *before* conception may increase the odds of having a normal infant. Note that routine testing for PKU was not in place until the 1960s. If you remember having been on a restricted diet as a child, you should consider being tested for PKU.

PRENATAL HEALTH CARE

Your first prenatal visit confirms the pregnancy and allows your doctor to take a thorough health, pregnancy, and family history, if this was not done during a prepregnancy planning visit. The pregnancy will most likely be confirmed by a urine test and an internal pelvic exam. Modern urine tests are able to detect pregnancy much sooner after conception than the type that probably told your mother of your existence. Some doctors have their patients come in just for the urine test (results are available within minutes) and then schedule a longer appointment for a first prenatal visit.

A number of tests will be done during the first visit. These usually include: height and weight; blood pressure; urine for sugar, protein, infection, and possible kidney problems; blood tests to check blood group, Rh factor, anemia, rubella, and hepatitis antibodies (if not done previously); pelvic exam; and Pap smear. It may also include tests for gonorrhea, other STDs, or toxoplasmosis.

The pelvic exam will confirm the pregnancy and determine that the uterus is the appropriate size for the due date of the baby, estimated by the date of the missed period. The exam may identify possible structural abnormalities in the vagina or cervix, and give your doctor a sense of whether your pelvis is large enough for a normal delivery, although it is not an absolute indication.

Certain tests will be repeated at every prenatal

visit. These are weight, blood pressure, urinalysis, and a physical exam to check for edema (swelling) and the size and position of the baby. Some doctors perform a pelvic exam at each visit as well. As the pregnancy progresses, the doctor will listen to the fetal heartbeat. (See also section on "Prenatal Testing.")

A typical prenatal visit schedule for a healthy woman whose pregnancy is not considered high risk is once a month until 28 weeks, every second or third week until 36 weeks, and then every week until delivery. In a high-risk case, visits may be scheduled as often as once a week for the duration of the pregnancy. Call your doctor if you have any problems between visits. (See box, "Danger Signs During Pregnancy.")

Note that the average time from conception to delivery is 38 weeks. Because it is difficult to determine the exact date of conception, your doctor will probably date your pregnancy from the first day of your last menstrual period. Since this is typically 2 weeks before conception, your pregnancy can be expected to last 40 weeks. A normal pregnancy, however, can be 1 to 2 weeks longer or shorter. (All references to weeks in this chapter are based on a 40-week pregnancy.)

NUTRITION: EATING FOR TWO

One of the most important things you can do for your unborn baby is to eat well. Odds are that a healthy,

---

DANGER SIGNS DURING PREGNANCY

Call your health care provider immediately if you experience any of the following:

- Vaginal bleeding
- A sudden gush or trickle of waterlike fluid from your vagina (rupture of the amniotic sac)
- A fever of 100°F or higher
- Rapid weight gain or swelling in face and hands
- Severe headache with "double vision," blurred vision, or pinpoint of light
- Absence of noticeable fetal movement for 24 hours after the 6th month
- A sudden increase in thirst no need to urinate
- Severe or steady pain in your upper abdomen
- Severe nausea and vomiting
- Dizziness or fainting
- Burning or painful urination

Adapted from "Healthy Mothers-Healthy Beginnings," President and Fellows of Harvard College, 1992.

---

well-nourished mother will have a healthy baby. A pregnant woman must take care to meet increased daily requirements, of protein, calcium (50 percent more than usual), folic acid, iron (twice as much as usual), and fluids, which are all crucial for the developing fetus. While pregnancy supplements are important, they should not be relied on to supply the majority of nutrients. A detailed discussion of special food needs during pregnancy and suggested food sources can be found in resource books, such as *Eating for Two: The Complete Guide to Nutrition During Pregnancy*, by Mary Abbott Hess, R. D., M. S., and Anne Elise Hunt. A daily food log, at least for a week or so, helps to determine whether your food requirements are being met. It may also be useful to consult a registered dietitian. (See Chapter 9, "Healthful Eating for a Lifetime," for cautions about eating fish during pregnancy and breast-feeding.)

Medical opinion about the amount of weight gain that is most beneficial to mother and fetus has changed over time and remains somewhat controversial. Your mother may have been told to gain as few as 12 pounds, your older sister as many as 35. The American College of Obstetricians and Gynecologists (ACOG) recommends a gain of about 30 pounds for a woman of normal weight carrying a single fetus. A weight gain of less than 20 pounds may require that you have a sonogram to determine if the fetus is developing normally. A new study shows that if you gain more than 40 pounds (unless you are carrying twins), your chance of having a cesarean section doubles.

Many obstetricians recommend a gain of 20 to 30 pounds. If you gain about 25 pounds, you will usually return to your prepregnancy weight without dieting within 6 to 8 weeks after the baby is born. This usually means gaining 3 to 4 pounds during the first trimester and the same amount each month thereafter (see Figures 6.1–6.3). Contrary to what many women believe, this weight gain does not represent pounds and pounds of fat; most of it is accounted for by the baby itself and the changes in your body to accommodate the baby. (See box, "Typical Weight Gain.")

EXERCISE

Women who normally engage in regular aerobic exercise often wonder if they can continue during pregnancy. The answer for most women is definitely yes, as long as they do so in moderation and follow some commonsense guidelines. Even pregnant women who have been sedentary are advised to begin a moderate exercise program, such as brisk walking.

Physical changes in pregnancy

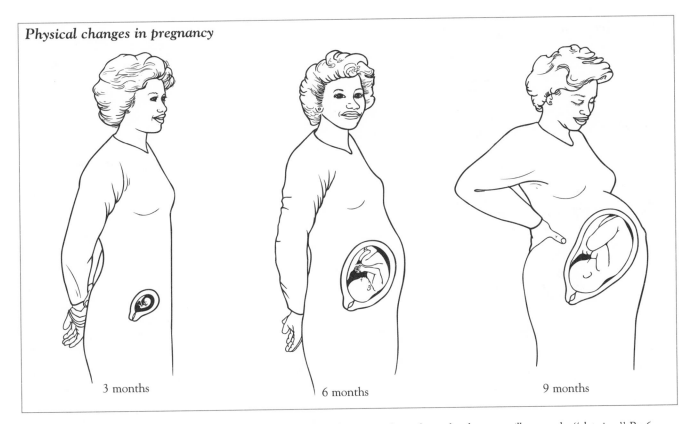

3 months   6 months   9 months

Fig. 6.1–6.3 *At 3 months pregnant, your breasts will have increased in size and may be tender, but you will not yet be "showing." By 6 months, however, your condition will be obvious to all. By 9 months, your baby will take up so much room that your internal organs will be somewhat displaced and your balance may be affected by the change in your center of gravity.*

Although there is no evidence that you will have a healthier baby or an easier labor if you are physically fit, there are some benefits to exercising during pregnancy. Good muscle tone and cardiovascular fitness may make you feel more comfortable and less likely to get out of breath as you carry those extra 20 pounds or so.

Exercise may improve your balance and coordination (which tend to be thrown off as your growing belly shifts your center of gravity), increase your energy levels, and provide a more positive emotional outlook and feeling of well-being. Finally, you may find that continuing to exercise while you are pregnant may make it easier to return to prepregnancy weight and fitness levels later.

Any exercise program should be discussed with your doctor and tailored to your prepregnancy fitness level. Some modifications in routine may be necessary. For example, you should avoid becoming overheated or increasing your heart rate above 140 beats per minute. A cooldown period is suggested after every 15 to 20 minutes of exercise. These precautions are necessary to keep the fetus, which cannot rid itself of excess body heat through perspiration, from becoming overheated. Excessive exercise in the 9th

month may increase the risk of low birth weight, stillbirth, and infant death, and should be avoided.

Sports that pose a danger of falling should not be engaged in during pregnancy. These include horse-

TYPICAL WEIGHT GAIN

Most women gain about 3 to 4 pounds during the first trimester, and about a pound a week during the second and third trimesters. For a gain of 20 to 30 pounds, the weight is typically divided as follows:

Baby	7–8 pounds
Changes in mother's body:	
breast increase	1–2 pounds
increase in blood volume	3–4 pounds
fat and protein stores	5–7 pounds
increase in body fluid	1–2 pounds
expansion of uterus	1–3 pounds
placenta	1–2 pounds
amniotic fluid	1–2 pounds
Total	20–30 pounds

The developing fetus

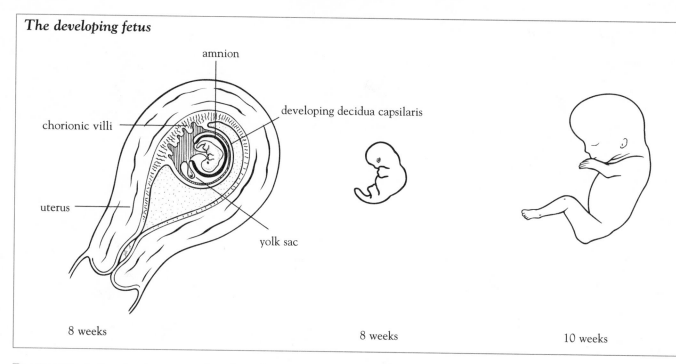

amnion

developing decidua capsilaris

chorionic villi

uterus

yolk sac

8 weeks

8 weeks

10 weeks

Fig. 6.4–6.9 *At 8 weeks of pregnancy, the embryo's heart is beating and the eyes and nostrils become distinct. By the end of week 8, the embryo is about an inch long and its main organs have formed. By week 10, the baby has entered the fetal period and bone growth and ossification begins.*

back riding, rollerblading, downhill skiing, waterskiing, and platform diving. Scuba diving, which in the early months may cause nausea and fatigue and later problems with depth pressure and the constriction of a wet suit, is not recommended. Nor is high-altitude mountain climbing, where insufficient oxygen may stress the fetus.

Sports such as tennis and other racquet sports and cross-country skiing are generally acceptable, as long as you do not overexert yourself, or become overheated or overexposed to the cold. Bicycling is a good choice, but it is wise to switch to a stationary bike toward the end of your pregnancy when balance problems may make falls more likely. Swimming is an excellent choice of exercise, as long as you avoid diving or hot tubs. Walking, hiking, and moderate jogging are also excellent choices.

Besides aerobic exercise, stretching and muscle-toning exercises such as those that strengthen your back and abdominal muscles will help your body adapt to pregnancy. Be careful to avoid jerky, bouncing motions or hyperextending the joints. Relaxin, a hormone that loosens a pregnant woman's joints to prepare the pelvis to expand during labor, also lowers the normal threshold for injury. After the 4th month, you should avoid holding your breath or lying flat on your back, either of which can deprive the fetus of oxygen.

PRENATAL TESTING

Because prenatal tests are not without risk, the American College of Obstetricians and Gynecologists does not routinely recommend them without indication. For women whose age, family history, past pregnancy experiences, or medical condition make a prenatal test advisable, the benefit usually outweighs the risk. It is often important for timing prenatal tests to know how far along a pregnancy has progressed. (See Figures 6.4–6.9.) To help date the pregnancy, you should keep accurate menstrual and, if possible, ovulation records. The most frequently performed prenatal tests are described briefly below. (For more information, see the Encyclopedia.)

SONOGRAM A sonogram can be done to date a pregnancy, determine the cause of maternal bleeding, confirm a multiple birth, or investigate suspicions of fetal abnormalities. It also pinpoints appropriate locations for amniocentesis, verifies the position of the placenta, evaluates fetal well-being when the mother has health problems, and can confirm or rule out an ectopic (tubal) pregnancy.

The procedure, which is painless, uses the ultrasound technique to bounce sound waves off internal structures, creating a visual, albeit blurry, pattern on

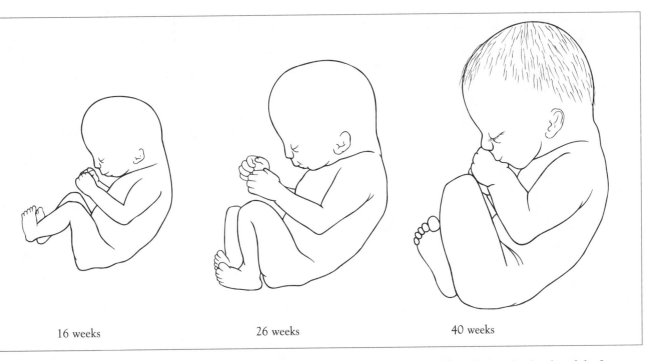

16 weeks   26 weeks   40 weeks

By week 16, the fetus is about 6 inches long, the head is still large in proportion to the body, the facial features are developed, and the fingers and toes are separated. At 26 weeks, the internal sex organs are established and fuzzy hair called lanugo covers the body. By 40 weeks, the baby's skin is pink and smooth, the hair on the head (if there is any) is more than an inch long, and the fingernails are long enough to scratch.

a screen. There are no known risks for mother or fetus.

A sonogram is often done routinely at 20 weeks to check for birth defects, even if none are suspected. A sonogram done at this time will also sometimes diagnose unexpected twins, find that the due date is wrong, or detect a problem with the placenta. When a serious abnormality is picked up at this time, treatment of the condition or termination of the pregnancy may still be options. However, because the incidence of these abnormalities is small, sonograms have to be done on many women to find a few abnormal fetuses, which brings into question the cost-effectiveness of this practice.

AMNIOCENTESIS Amniocentesis is most commonly performed on women over 35, women who previously bore babies with neural tube defects or chromosomal or metabolic abnormalities, and carriers of some X-linked genetic disorders such as hemophilia (which each son has a fifty-fifty chance of inheriting). It is also performed when both parents are carriers of heritable disorders, such as Tay-Sachs disease or sickle-cell disease, or when fetal lung maturity must be assessed pending an early delivery.

The procedure, which is done between the 14th and 17th weeks, uses ultrasound to locate the fetus and placenta. Then the doctor inserts a long, hollow needle through the abdominal wall into the uterus and collects a small amount of amniotic fluid for testing.

Mild cramping is common, and "spotting" may occur. Although complications are rare, there is a slight risk of infection, bleeding, or rupture of the membranes, which may lead to miscarriage in about 1 percent of cases. Women are usually advised to slow their activities for 24 hours after the procedure.

CHORIONIC VILLUS SAMPLING (CVS) Performed much earlier than amniocentesis (between 9 and 12 weeks), CVS entails inserting a thin, flexible plastic catheter into the uterus through the vagina. A sample of cells is suctioned from the villi, the hairlike projections on the chorion, the structure that ultimately forms the placenta. In some cases, because of the position of the uterus or chorion, the cells may be removed by a hollow needle inserted through the abdominal wall. Recent studies indicate a slightly higher miscarriage risk for CVS than for amniocentesis, but this may be because it is done earlier in pregnancy when most miscarriages occur naturally. A small risk of limb defects in the fetus has been associated with CVS, but it is not yet clear if this risk is statistically significant.

LABOR AND DELIVERY

CHILDBIRTH EDUCATION PHILOSOPHIES   There are three main childbirth education philosophies, although many educators combine elements of each. Some women have the misconception that if they take a "natural childbirth" course they will be pressured into forgoing pain medication during labor. This is most assuredly not so; moreover, the courses provide valuable information to expectant mothers and fathers about the changing body during pregnancy and what happens during each step of labor. Knowing what to expect and using the relaxation or distraction techniques taught in these classes can make labor easier and may reduce the need for pain medication.

The Lamaze method is probably the best-known technique in this country. Based on Pavlov's theory of the conditioned reflex, the Lamaze method conditions expectant mothers, through training and practice, to be distracted from the pain of childbirth by special breathing patterns, massage, and external focal points.

The Bradley method started the practice of partner-coached births. The laboring woman reduces pain by focusing inward to relax her body and "get out of the way" of her contracting uterus. Deep abdominal breathing is stressed. The method also emphasizes good diet and exercises to condition muscles for birth, preparing mothers to deliver without medication whenever possible.

The Read method, started by Dr. Grantley Dick-Read in the 1930s, was the first modern "natural childbirth" method. It emphasizes relaxation techniques and understanding of the birth process to break the fear-tension-pain cycle. Dr. Dick-Read's book *Childbirth Without Fear* introduced the then revolutionary idea that with proper education, training, and attitude, a woman with a normal labor can experience childbirth with minimal pain.

THE STAGES OF LABOR

Labor can be divided into three stages, from the earliest contractions through the birth of the baby to the delivery of the placenta. (See box, "The Three Stages of Labor.") The first stage, which is generally the longest and hardest part, can further be divided into early, active, and transition phases. First-stage contractions help the cervix efface (thin out) and dilate (open up) to allow the baby's presenting part (most often the head) to enter the birth canal. (See Figure 6.10.) Dilation is usually measured by internal examination, from 0 to 10 centimeters (cm), or complete dilation.

EARLY SIGNS   Contractions may not be the first sign of impending labor. Some women experience a "show," the passing of the thick, blood-tinged plug of mucus that protects the neck of the uterus during pregnancy. It may precede contractions by hours or up to several days, and it is not necessary to call your doctor when you pass the plug.

Another sign is the rupture of the amniotic membrane, the "bag of waters" that surrounds the baby. You may experience this as a sudden gush or, more likely, a steady trickle. Even if your contractions have not begun, you should call your doctor if your water breaks. You may be asked to come to the hospital or to wait a few more hours. If the amniotic fluid is greenish brown or very bloody rather than clear, call your doctor immediately, as this may indicate some stress to the fetus.

You may experience either of these signs before or after contractions start, but once you feel contractions, labor has officially begun.

EARLY LABOR   Early labor frequently lasts 6 to 8 hours for a first baby, with contractions starting out short (30 to 45 seconds) and irregular (ranging from 2 to 30 minutes apart). During this time, most women would be wise not to go to the hospital. In

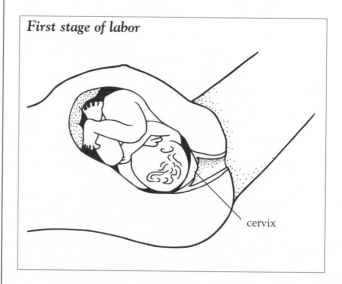

First stage of labor

cervix

Fig. 6.10 *During the first stage of labor, contractions dilate and efface* (thin out) *the cervix.*

fact, you may be sent home again if you are found to be only a few centimeters dilated. The best time to leave for the hospital will depend on your history (your labor will be shorter with a second or subsequent baby), how long it will take to get there, and your doctor's instructions. Usually women are advised to wait until their contractions are regular and 3 to 5 minutes apart, which is considered the beginning of active labor.

Staying home during early labor will give you the most freedom to eat lightly, move around, go to a movie, go for a walk, take a warm bath (if your water has not broken) or shower (if it has), have your partner give you a massage, and rest in the comfort of your own bed. In early labor, you can use gravity to help bring the baby down by walking, sitting backward on a chair facing a pillow, or leaning against a wall or your birthing coach.

ACTIVE LABOR When contractions start coming every 3 to 5 minutes, you have reached active labor and your doctor will probably want you to head for the hospital. When you arrive, you will be examined to see how far your cervix has dilated (usually at least 3 cm at this stage) and effaced (close to 100 percent). Your baby's heart rate will be monitored. This may be done using a special stethoscope called a fetoscope, a Doppler ultrasound monitor, or an electronic fetal monitor. Some hospitals require electronic monitoring, but many of those that do have replaced continuous monitoring with intermittent monitoring except in special circumstances. Once you have been taken to the labor room or birthing room, electronic monitoring will usually be repeated every 15 to 30 minutes until you enter the second stage of labor. (See box, "Electronic Fetal Monitoring.")

Active labor is the time to use the relaxation, breathing, and distraction techniques that are taught in childbirth education classes. Some couples also use massage, visualization, periodic changes in position, acupressure, self-hypnosis, and biofeedback. If these techniques aren't enough to get you through the roughest part of labor, you may want to consider pain relief medication. Modern obstetric medications are generally considered safe, but in general the less used, the better for the baby. Drugs must be administered early enough to be effective during late active labor and transition, but not so early that they wear off too soon. Correct timing also ensures that the baby is not exposed unnecessarily to the drug and that the drug

THE THREE STAGES OF LABOR

Stage I: Effacement and dilation of the cervix to 10 centimeters, or five fingerbreadths. Stage I consists of three phases:

Phase One, Early Labor: Cervix effacing to 100 percent and dilating to 3 centimeters in approximately 6 to 8 hours

Phase Two, Active Labor: Cervix dilating from 3 to 8 centimeters in approximately 3 to 4 hours

Phase Three, Transition: Cervix dilating from 8 to 10 centimeters in approximately 1 hour

Stage II: Birth, with pushing for approximately 1 hour or less (*Note:* Time approximations of stages I and II apply to first babies; subsequent labors usually progress more rapidly.)

Stage III: Expulsion of the placenta, or afterbirth, taking approximately 15 minutes.

Source: *Fritzi Kallop's Birth Book*, Fritzi Farber Kallop, R.N., Vintage Books, N.Y., 1988. Used with permission.

doesn't interfere with the progress of labor. (See box, "Pain Relief Medications.")

Many hospitals require that an intravenous (IV) drip of glucose (sugar water) solution be started during active labor. The glucose provides you with energy. After all, you may not have eaten for many hours, and you are now doing hard work. Another reason for having an IV handy is that it can be used to administer anesthesia should an emergency cesarean section become necessary. Finally, the IV can be used to administer pitocin to help contract the uterus in rare cases when there is heavy bleeding immediately after a vaginal birth. Some women feel that an IV isn't necessary or that it will restrict their ability to walk around. Others find that by this stage they are no longer interested in walking around. If you feel strongly that you do not want an IV, you should discuss this with your doctor well in advance.

• **Pitocin.** If your labor stalls or there is a medical need to speed it up, you may be given pitocin, a synthetic form of oxytocin, the naturally occurring hormone that regulates contractions. Years ago, when pitocin was administered in higher doses than it is today, it gained a reputation for producing strong (and sometimes more painful) contractions. Now a

ELECTRONIC FETAL MONITORING

Fetal heart-rate monitoring assesses the relationship of uterine contractions to the baby's heart rate to determine if there is any stress on the baby during labor. Although this monitoring can be done using a stethoscope or hand-held Doppler ultrasound device, most hospitals today require some type of electronic fetal monitoring.

The most common method is external: Two belts are strapped around your abdomen to hold two small instruments in place. One instrument uses ultrasound to compute the baby's heart rate (pulse), while the other one measures the contractions. This method is less confining and less invasive than internal monitoring and can be used before the amniotic sac has broken. However, it does not yield as much information as internal monitoring.

With internal monitoring, a small electrode is threaded through the vagina and cervix and attached to the baby's scalp to record the heart rate electronically. At the same time, a thin catheter is placed inside the uterus to measure the strength of the contractions. The advantage of the internal monitor is that it can measure the pressure created by the contractions, while the external monitor only records their frequency. Thus, it can give a better indication of the response of the heartbeat to pressure.

Recent improvements in monitoring equipment have made them both more accurate and more comfortable for the mother. Equally important, intermittent monitoring has been found to be just as effective as continuous monitoring in detecting most potential problems for the fetus. The American College of Obstetricians and Gynecologists recommends that monitoring be done every 15 minutes during active labor and every 5 minutes during second-stage labor. Continuous monitoring may be required for a high-risk pregnancy, for example, for preterm labor or if there are medical complications such as diabetes; if epidural anesthesia is given; or if pitocin is being administered.

pump is used to regulate and administer it in small amounts, which simulates the normal progression of labor and contractions. Many physicians prefer to use electronic monitoring while pitocin is being given to ensure that labor follows normal patterns. Pitocin may also be administered to induce labor, that is, to help start contractions if there is a medical reason to do so.

• **Transition.** During the transition phase, the uterus dilates the last few centimeters and switches from the contractions that are meant to open the cervix to 10 cm during the first stage, to the pushing-down variety designed to expel the baby during the second stage. Some women have no symptoms at this time; others experience nausea, vomiting, shivers, and irritability. It is the time of greatest self-doubt when many women feel that they won't be able to make it through labor. A supportive coach and birth team can help overcome these feelings. Fortunately, it usually lasts no more than an hour and the end of it means that baby is ready to be born.

THE SECOND STAGE During this stage, the baby moves down through and out of the birth canal, usually aided by the mother's pushing. (See Figure 6.11.) Contractions lengthen, and in some cases the rest periods between contractions lengthen as well.

Sometimes the cervix is not yet 10 cm dilated, but the mother feels the urge to push. Some attendants advise resisting the urge because the cervix may be bruised if pushing begins too soon. If labor is proceeding without any obstetrical interventions such as pitocin or other medication, others advise that the mother should push if the cervix is soft enough; the pushing urge can be overwhelming and the sensation is not painful. At times, babies are born despite the mother's efforts not to push, because the uterus is pushing down involuntarily.

Depending on the baby's position and how the labor is progressing, alternative positions may be helpful. For example, squatting with support from a partner may be useful if the baby is in the posterior position (facing up). However, squatting may not be possible after an epidural, when the mother's legs are numbed and cannot support her weight. Kneeling or lying on the side with one leg back may also be effective in some labors.

Toward the end of the second stage, the perineum—the area between the vagina and the rectum—will begin to bulge, indicating that the baby's head is beginning to push against it. "Crowning," when the entire circumference of the baby's head is visible, indicates that birth is imminent.

PAIN RELIEF MEDICATIONS

A variety of pain relief medications is available as well as several methods for administering them, although not all are available everywhere. It is impossible to know ahead of time if you will want medication or what type, if it will be appropriate for your particular labor, or if you will be able to have it exactly when you want it. Nevertheless, it is useful to know what your options are. Your doctor can explain their pros and cons, and any potential risks.

The two types of pain medication for labor are analgesics, which dull but don't completely stop pain, and anesthesias, which cause a loss of sensation. The most common analgesic is Demerol, which relaxes you as well as dulls the pain. It is given intravenously or by injection.

Anesthesia is usually identified by the site or region where it is used. It may be injected very locally in the *perineum* just before an episiotomy or while a tear or episiotomy is being repaired. A *pudendal block* also numbs the perineum as well as a wider area around the vagina and rectum. A *paracervical block* is injected into the cervical tissue to numb the pain of the dilating cervix as well as to lessen that of the contractions.

An *epidural block* is administered into the lower back in the space near the spinal cord and numbs the body from the waist down. It is initially given by injection, but a tube may be inserted so that additional small amounts can be given periodically. Although an epidural block deadens pain very effectively, you can still feel certain sensations and you have some muscle control, which allows you to push during labor, albeit not as effectively as without the drug. Epidurals are also commonly used for nonemergency cesarean sections.

A *spinal block* is also injected into the lower back, numbing the body from the waist down. It is injected directly into the spinal fluid, however, and is usually given only once. This type of anesthesia is effective, but it is short-acting, so it is usually given to relieve pain during delivery, especially if forceps or vacuum extraction of the baby must be used. It can also be used for cesarean sections.

General anesthesia is rarely used except for emergency c-sections or other extraordinary circumstances.

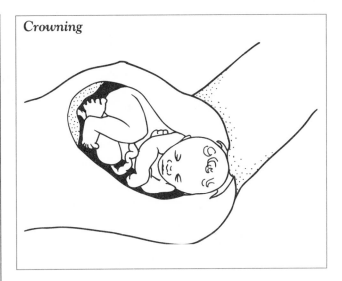

Crowning

Fig. 6.11 *Once the cervix has fully dilated and effaced, contractions, aided by the mother's pushing, will bring the baby down so that the top of the head shows (crowning).*

• **Episiotomy.** This is a surgical incision made in the perineum that enlarges the birth opening. It can shorten the second stage of labor anywhere from 15 to 45 minutes. While there is no evidence to support *routine* episiotomy and ACOG discourages the practice, many first-time mothers may undergo the procedure (it is less likely to be necessary the second time around). The rationale for an episiotomy is that without it, the perineum can tear under the stretching that is necessary to accommodate the baby's head. If so, the tear is likely to be ragged and more difficult to repair than a clean incision. Besides the mother's comfort, there are sometimes medical reasons for an episiotomy. These include fetal distress, when speed is imperative; maternal exhaustion; forceps deliveries; and a large baby that requires an enlarged opening to emerge.

Some women object to the idea of an episiotomy. If you feel strongly about it, you should discuss it with your doctor ahead of time. There are also several things you can do to reduce the chances of experiencing either an episiotomy or perineal tearing. One is to develop well-toned pelvic-floor muscles, the ones that surround the urethra, vagina, and rectum (see box, Chapter 2, "Sexual Health," for exercises to tone these muscles). A leisurely, controlled second stage also allows more time for the vaginal tissues to soften and stretch, so tearing is less likely. Deliberate, panting breaths (taught in childbirth education) help slow down a fast second stage. Some practitioners use perineal massage and warm compresses to ease the tissues' stretching.

•**Birth.** Once the baby's head emerges, it turns spontaneously to one side so that each shoulder can emerge separately (see Figure 6.12). As soon as the shoulders are out, the hard part is over and the rest of the body will emerge quickly, along with any remaining amniotic fluid. The umbilical cord will be clamped and cut.

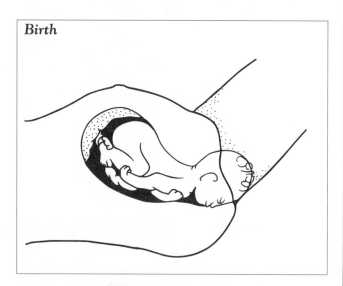

Birth

Fig. 6.12 *With the mother's pushing the baby's head will emerge and turn spontaneously to the side so shoulders can emerge separately.*

THE THIRD STAGE The expulsion of the placenta, or afterbirth, usually occurs between 5 and 45 minutes after the baby is born.

PROBLEMS IN LABOR

PRETERM AND POSTTERM PREGNANCIES Eighty percent of babies are born between the 38th and 42nd week of pregnancy, although only about 5 percent arrive on their expected due dates. About 10 percent of babies are born before the 38th week, and are considered preterm, or premature, while an equal number are born after the 42nd week and are considered postterm, or postmature.

Some of these babies truly arrive early or late, and the rest have been assigned incorrect due dates. The latter most often happens because some menstrual periods are longer or shorter than the standard 28 days, which throws off calculations, since ovulation will be either later or earlier than the norm. Since it becomes harder as the pregnancy progresses to assign the due date accurately, women who do not seek early prenatal care, perhaps because they are unaware that they are pregnant, are more likely to have an inaccurate date.

Advances in neonatal intensive care mean that babies born as early as 25 weeks and weighing as little as 2 pounds have some chance of survival, but the risk of major complications is high. Babies born a month early, on the other hand, have an excellent chance of survival. If you experience preterm labor, call your doctor immediately. It is sometimes possible to avert a preterm delivery if your doctor feels it is advisable.

Compared to preterm pregnancies, those that are postterm, although physically and emotionally hard on the mother, generally pose less of a danger: The baby is usually fully developed and, if necessary, labor can be induced or a cesarean performed. About 95 percent of babies born between 42 and 44 weeks are born safely, according to ACOG. Nevertheless, as the baby approaches full term, the functioning of the placenta may begin to deteriorate and the amount of amniotic fluid may decline. Several tests can help assure that the baby is still developing normally and is not in any distress. Your doctor may begin these tests at 41 to 42 weeks.

PRESENTATION VARIATIONS Babies are usually born head first and face down. The most common variation on this position is the posterior presentation (sometimes called "sunny side up"), in which the back of the baby's head is toward the mother's spine. This usually causes a longer and harder labor.

Breech presentations, in which the baby is born buttocks first, or, rarely, with one or both feet first, comprise 3 to 4 percent of all births (see Figure 6.13). Up to a certain point in development, a baby in the breech position may turn spontaneously. Near delivery, however, there generally isn't enough room for such a big move. A technique called external version, which attempts to rotate the fetus externally to the proper position, is sometimes tried. This is most likely to be successful if the baby is in a frank breech position, is not too large, and is surrounded by sufficient amniotic fluid. A cesarean section is almost always recommended for breech babies, although a small number of doctors will deliver a breech baby vaginally under certain conditions.

A third variation is the transverse lie, in which the baby is in a more or less horizontal position, necessitating a c-section.

Complete breech position

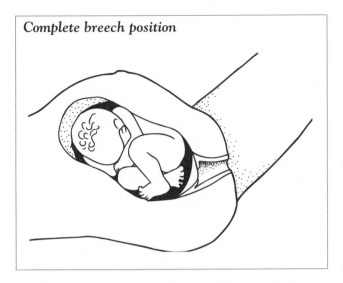

Fig. 6.13 *In a breech birth, the baby's buttocks or feet lie nearest the birth canal and are the first part to "present." The legs may be extended so that the feet are near the head (frank breech) or flexed as they are here (complete breech), or one or both feet may dangle downward (footling breech). Most breech babies are delivered by cesarean section.*

PLACENTAL PROBLEMS In rare instances, the placenta separates from the wall of the uterus (*abruptio placentae*), cutting off the baby's food and oxygen supply and necessitating an emergency cesarean section (see Figure 6.14). Heavy bleeding usually accompanies this condition, and the doctor should be called immediately. If the placenta is only partially separated, a vaginal birth may be possible.

Placenta previa, in which the placenta lies low in the uterus in front of the fetus, partially or completely blocking the exit through the cervix, can also be a serious problem (see Figure 6.15). This condition is also marked by vaginal bleeding, usually during the last 12 weeks of pregnancy, which may require hospitalization. In most cases, a cesarean section will be scheduled before the due date.

MECONIUM The amniotic fluid is normally colorless and odorless. At any time from the first leakage to the last stages of labor, the fluid may sometimes appear to be green or brown. This indicates the presence of meconium, the feces produced by the baby in the uterus. It is a sign of possible stress on the fetus before or during birth and should be reported immediately to the doctor if it happens at home.

CESAREAN SECTION Sometimes it becomes necessary to deliver a baby by cesarean section, that is, by making a surgical incision in the lower abdomen and wall of the uterus to bring the baby out (see Figures

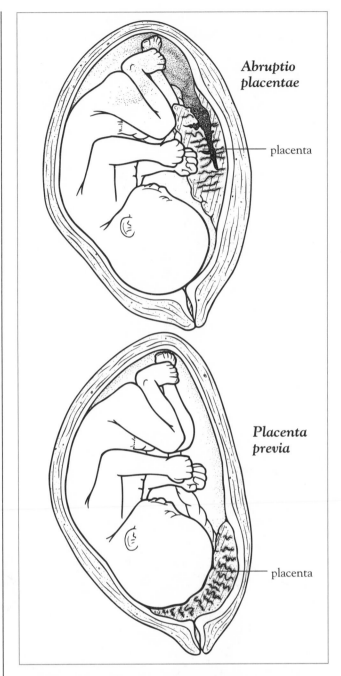

Abruptio placentae

placenta

Placenta previa

placenta

Fig. 6.14–6.15 *The separation of the placenta from the wall of the uterus, known as abruptio placentae or placenta abrupta, may cause severe bleeding, in which case an emergency cesarean section is required. Placenta previa, in which the placenta lies below the fetus in the uterus and blocks its exit through the cervix, requires a cesarean section.*

6.16-6.17). The most common reason for this is cephalopelvic disproportion: a baby that is too large for the mother's pelvis. Other reasons include a baby in a breech or transverse position (see Presentation Variations), problems with the placenta or umbilical cord, stalled labor, fetal distress, or scars on the uterus from previous surgery. A c-section may also be necessary if you have an infection, such as active herpes, that could be transmitted to the baby in the birth canal.

Cesareans may be planned in advance when, for example, it is known that the baby is breech. They must sometimes be done on an emergency basis. Most

commonly, however, they are done after hours of unproductive labor.

Except in emergencies, when the speed of general anesthesia is necessary, a spinal or epidural is the usual method of anesthesia. This allows you to be fully conscious. In most hospitals, the father can be present and both of you will be able to hold the baby shortly after birth.

If a medical complication necessitates a cesarean section, it should be understood that it is best for the baby, even if it means some disappointment for the mother. Women who must deliver by c-section, even while mourning the loss of a fantasy birth, should celebrate the reality: They have a healthy baby.

For a variety of reasons, the cesarean rate has risen to one in four births in the United States, giving many experts concern. Studies show that babies fare just as well in areas where the cesarean rate is under 20 percent as in areas where it reaches 40 percent.

In the past, cesareans were performed using a vertical incision in the uterus. This incision, which posed a risk of rupture during subsequent vaginal deliveries, was the main reason for the old adage "Once a cesarean, always a cesarean." Now the most common incision is a transverse (horizontal) one low in the uterus. (The outer, abdominal incision is usually

Incision for cesarean section

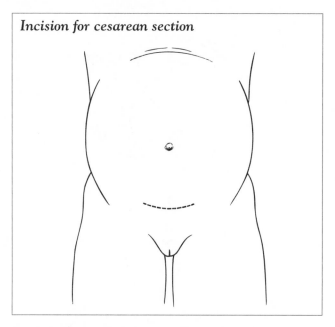

Fig. 6.16 *For a nonemergency cesarean section, the abdominal incision is usually made just above the pubic hairline.*

Cesarean birth

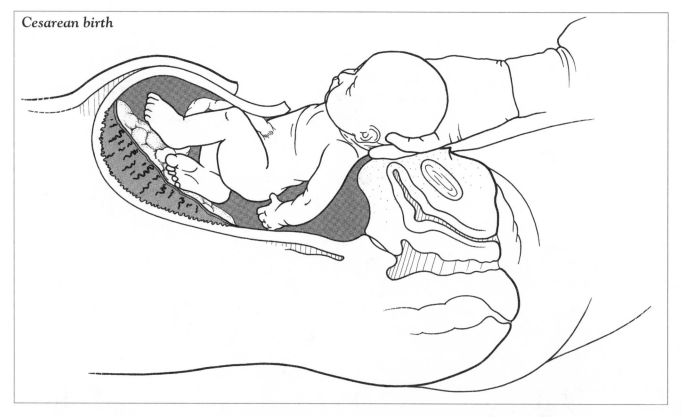

Fig. 6.17 *Cesarean sections like the one shown here account for about one out of every four births in the United States.*

made just above the pubic hairline.) When the transverse uterine incision is used, the risk of uterine rupture in a subsequent pregnancy is low. This has allowed more mothers to deliver subsequent babies vaginally after previous c-sections, a practice which may help bring the overall cesarean rate down again.

(A low transverse *abdominal* scar from a previous cesarean delivery does not guarantee that the *uterine* incision was also low transverse. This can be verified by your obstetrician or a check of the hospital records.)

AFTER DELIVERY

Once the baby is born, he or she is often placed on your abdomen briefly while the umbilical cord is clamped and cut. Then the newborn is taken away briefly to be checked over and attended to. The Apgar test, which rates the baby's color, heart rate, breathing, crying, and muscle tone, is given at 1 minute and 5 minutes after birth. After any excess mucus or amniotic fluid in the nose or mouth is wiped away or suctioned out, the baby is wrapped in a blanket and usually given to the father to hold. In the meantime, you will be examined to be sure that the placenta has been completely expelled, there is no excess bleeding, and the uterus is contracting. If you have had an episiotomy, it will now be stitched up. Then you will be able to hold and bond with your baby.

At some point soon after birth, the baby will be weighed, have footprints taken for record-keeping, and receive silver nitrate or antibiotic eyedrops. The silver nitrate is given to prevent gonorrhea and chlamydial infection of the eyes, in case you have an undiagnosed infection to which the baby was exposed during birth. Some hospitals also give vitamin K to help newborns develop their blood clotting factors.

When you are ready to leave the delivery room and return to your room, the baby will usually go to the nursery for a few hours, to warm up and adjust to the outside world while you rest and adjust to the idea of being a mother.

POSTPARTUM PERIOD

After birth, you will probably have some bleeding for up to 6 weeks as the uterine lining sloughs off. This is normal. As your uterus shrinks back to its prepregnancy size, you may feel afterpains. You may also find that you perspire heavily for several days. Ridding your body of excess fluid helps reduce your blood volume, which doubles during pregnancy. Constipation and difficulty in urinating are other potential problems as your internal organs become readjusted to their normal position.

Pregnancy hormones, which are still present in the postpartum stage, often cause mood swings. Sometimes you may have crying jags and feelings of inadequacy about being a parent, especially if you are a first-time mother. While a degree of postpartum depression is normal after birth, if the so-called baby blues continue for an extended amount of time or become extreme, it could signal serious clinical depression. In that case, professional help is recommended.

Showering is fine as soon as you are able, and tub baths can be resumed after 2 or 3 weeks. Sexual intercourse and exercise should be avoided for at least 2 weeks after a vaginal delivery (4 to 6 weeks after a c-section), although many women may be too tired, and perhaps sore if they have had an episiotomy or tear, to resume sex just yet. Even if you want to conceive again soon, most experts recommend that you wait at least 3 months, so be sure to practice some form of birth control during this period. The same advice holds for breast-feeding mothers. You will be much less fertile while nursing, but it does not offer complete protection. If you have been using a diaphragm, check with your doctor about having a new one fitted, as the size of your vagina may have changed.

Finally, although the postpartum period is officially viewed as 6 weeks, many practitioners advise their patients that it actually lasts at least 18 years, more than enough time to recover from the birth process and experience the joys and problems of being a parent.

CHAPTER 7

Menopause

Once a taboo topic of conversation, menopause is attracting more and more attention as increasing numbers of American women enter middle age. In the first decade of the twenty-first century, more than 21 million baby boomers will enter their fifties and face menopause. At the turn of the twentieth century, many women did not live long enough to experience "the change of life."

Women and doctors agree that far too little is known about the natural workings of menopause and the various health risks associated with it. In recent years, related research has intensified, but for now menopausal women may have a hard time finding definitive answers to all of their questions about their bodies, health, and choices at midlife. Research has yet to quantify, for example, all of the risks and benefits associated with hormone replacement therapy (supplemental estrogen, usually in combination with progestin), which is being prescribed both to alleviate short-term menopausal symptoms, such as hot flashes, and to decrease the risks of such chronic disorders as osteoporosis and heart disease.

Now that women have become more vocal about their individual reactions to menopause, they are learning from each other's experiences by sharing information with friends and even by forming menopause support groups. It has become clear that women react very individually to the changes they are experiencing. Many women hardly notice their symptoms, while others report severe symptoms that interfere daily with their lives. Certain women welcome the end of fertility and the need for contraceptive measures, while others are saddened by no longer being able to have children. In the past, menopausal women were thought to suffer from a variety of psychological symptoms, ranging from depression to anxiety, as a result of decreased hormone levels. More recent research suggests that menopause itself is not associated with an increased risk of emotional problems, but that certain social factors—including children leaving home and the lower status of older women in our culture—may play a greater role in any depression experienced by menopausal women.

Today, the majority of women live a third of their lives after menopause, and these years continue to be active, fulfilling ones. Most find menopause to be more of an inconvenience than a source of regret. The changing concept of menopause is even reflected in advertisements for estrogen replacement therapy in medical journals. Twenty years ago, these ads depicted women as wrinkled and depressed, bemoaning the end of their usefulness in life; now they portray menopausal women as beautiful, youthful, and in charge of their lives.

Because a menopausal woman has many years ahead of her, making wise life-style and medical choices to preserve her health is of prime importance. Although not all choices are clear, there is much that you can do to make your postmenopausal years the best they can be.

DEFINING MENOPAUSE

Technically, the term "menopause" refers to your very last menstrual period, which may not be determined until you have had no subsequent periods for a year. Colloquially, the term has come to mean the transitional phase between your reproductive and nonreproductive lives. This period of time is accurately described as the climacteric. It encompasses the endocrine and psychic changes that accompany the end of the reproductive years. The climacteric is a long process that probably starts in your late twenties or early thirties, when estrogen production in the ovaries begins to taper off, and ends long after you stop menstruating. More specifically, the last few years before and the first year after menopause is called perimenopause. The term "premenopausal" is used to describe menstruating women and "postmenopausal" refers to noncycling women whose ovaries no longer produce much estrogen.

FACTORS THAT DETERMINE THE AGE OF MENOPAUSE

Each baby girl is born with all of her eggs (ovarian follicles), about 400,000 in number, already formed in her ovaries. By the age of 40, women have only between 350 and 28,000 eggs left, and the numbers seem to drop dramatically after that. When you run out of eggs, which mature and are released during each monthly cycle, menopause occurs.

The ovarian follicles are also responsible for producing estrogen and progesterone. Research suggests that menopause is preceded by an accelerated rate of follicle depletion caused by altered neurochemical signals sent to the ovaries from the brain. The follicles also become less responsive to follicle-stimulating hormone (FSH), which prepares the egg for fertilization.

The average age of menopause is 51, while the normal age range is 45 to 55. The age at which you begin menstruating has no influence on when you will stop. Genetic factors may enter into the timing of menopause. That is, the age at which your mother, grandmothers, aunts, or sisters went through menopause is probably a good indication of whether you will enter it early or late.

Perhaps the strongest influence on the onset of menopause is smoking. Smokers experience menopause about 2 years earlier than nonsmokers; heavy smokers may stop menstruating 5 or 10 years before they might normally. Women who have not had children also tend to reach menopause at a younger age. Women who have undergone hysterectomies or who have had their tubes tied (tubal ligation) may enter menopause earlier than usual, possibly because those surgical operations reduce blood flow to the pelvic region. Chemotherapy can also trigger an early menopause.

Menopause before age 40 is called premature ovarian failure, and is usually related either to an inherited tendency to run out of eggs early, an autoimmune disease such as lupus, or a thyroid condition. The advantages of early menopause are no longer having to deal with monthly periods or the risk of becoming pregnant, and being at a decreased risk of ovarian cancer. The disadvantages: no longer being able to have children, increased risks of heart disease and osteoporosis, and vaginal and urinary changes. About 8 percent of women experience early menopause.

About 5 percent of women do not reach menopause until they are older than 53 or even as late as 60. The advantages of late menopause are a younger-looking appearance; prolonged fertility; and a decreased risk of heart disease, osteoporosis, and decreased vaginal and urinary problems. The prime disadvantage is a slightly increased risk of ovarian cancer; doctors may recommend a yearly ovarian exam and ultrasound test for older women who are still premenopausal.

HORMONAL CHANGES In addition to the progressive decrease in estrogen production, there is also a decrease in progesterone levels as you approach menopause. During perimenopause there may be major fluctuations in the levels of these hormones, which can result in heavy or light bleeding, among other symptoms. In an attempt to stimulate the "sluggish" ovaries to get back up to speed, the pituitary gland increases its production of FSH and luteinizing hormone (LH). Higher levels of these hormones are thought to be related to hot flashes. Levels of FSH in the blood are sometimes measured to determine if someone is menopausal.

Before menopause, the follicles in the ovaries produce a type of estrogen called estradiol. As the production of estradiol declines during perimenopause, another form of estrogen, estrone, becomes important. Estrone is converted in body-fat cells from androstenedione, which is produced by the adrenal glands. Thus, a small amount of estrogen continues to be produced after menopause. Women who are overweight and have more stored body fat produce more estrone and as a result tend to have milder menopausal symptoms. Some researchers believe that estrone is more likely to cause cancer than the estradiol that is present before menopause.

Your levels of androgens, the so-called male hormones, also decrease as you approach menopause, which can lower your sex drive, according to some findings. Androgens do not decrease as rapidly as estrogen, so, in effect, they increase proportionately to the levels of this hormone. The reverse hormonal ratio can cause certain symptoms, such as thinning hair, stray facial hairs, or acne, to appear years after menopause.

PHYSICAL SYMPTOMS

Some of the symptoms of menopause appear early as you approach this stage and your hormone levels are in flux. Since doctors usually don't "diagnose" menopause until at least 6 months (and as long as a year) after your last period, you can be menopausal for months without realizing it.

IRREGULAR PERIODS During perimenopause, generally when you are in your midforties, your periods begin to change in length, flow, or frequency. Initially, they may be heavier and more frequent, and then later become lighter and farther apart. Some women, however, may not experience any menstrual changes. In a month when you do not ovulate, you will have low levels of progesterone and you may have only "spotting" or very light bleeding. If the irregularities are bothersome, or your doctor suspects that the uterine lining is not being shed completely during menstruation, he or she may prescribe a synthetic progestin to regulate your cycle.

Women approaching menopause can still become pregnant. In fact, when perimenopausal women miss their first period, they often assume they are pregnant. To compound this misconception, older women are more likely than younger women to have a false-positive result on a home pregnancy test. It is important to use an effective method of birth control for at least 6 months after your last period. While doctors formerly advised against using birth control pills after age 35, low-dose oral contraceptives are now believed to be safe for some healthy, nonsmoking women through menopause. Newly developed IUDs may be ideal for women who have completed their families and want a birth control method that involves minimal bother. Sterilization remains the method of choice of most married couples in this country.

HOT FLASHES These uncomfortable and often embarrassing waves of heat are considered the most annoying aspect of menopause. Hot flashes are estimated to occur in 85 percent of all women, and most end within 3 to 5 years, although between one quarter and one half of sufferers report that they persist longer. Most women experience warmth and mild discomfort, but 15 to 25 percent have severe and/or frequent (sometimes every hour) episodes that may interfere with sleep and contribute to fatigue, irritability, anxiety, depression, or memory problems. Nocturnal flashes, commonly called night sweats, are responsible for most of the menopausal insomnia.

Called vasomotor flushes or vasomotor instability by doctors, hot flashes are the result of a malfunction in the brain's temperature-control center, the hypothalamus. Flashes can be triggered at any time by a variety of activities that affect temperature, such as exercise, stress, entering a cool or warm room, or sleeping under a warm blanket.

A hot flash begins when the temperature center wrongly perceives that the body is too cool and sends out signals to constrict blood vessels in the skin, thus reducing the flow of warm blood to the surface, where the warmth can be lost to the surrounding air. This vasoconstriction redirects the warm blood to the vital inner organs. Then, because the body really wasn't cold, it responds by dilating the blood vessels again in order to cool down. The result is an increase in blood flow to the surface of the upper body, which produces a flush.

What causes this temperature-control malfunction is not completely understood, but it is thought to be related to lower levels of estrogen and related higher levels of FSH and LH. The part of the brain that regulates body temperature is near the area that controls release of the hormones.

The vasomotor symptoms generally include a feeling of intense heat in the face, neck, and chest, which may spread to other parts of the body, and sweating, which is often followed by chills and a clammy or itchy sensation (the result of a drop in skin and internal temperatures). About half of women have a visibly reddish flush on the face, neck, and chest, and some experience headaches, dizziness, or palpitations. In some women, the flashes are preceded by a chill or an aura, by which they recognize that a flash is about to occur. (See box, "Handling Hot Flashes.") Flashes last from a few seconds to a half hour, but most are about 5 minutes long. Although someone experiencing a hot flash may feel as if everyone in the room is staring at her, other people are often unaware that anything is happening.

PALPITATIONS Caused by the same vasomotor instability as hot flashes, irregular heartbeats—or feeling as if your heart were "skipping a beat"—have been reported. Although these palpitations may be frightening, they are harmless. If they are very bothersome, your doctor may prescribe a beta-blocker, a drug often used to treat heart disease and high blood pressure.

PAINFUL SEX Since estrogen maintains the tissues in the vagina and uterus, decreased estrogen levels can lead to vaginal shrinkage and dryness (see Figure 7.1), which can cause pain during and after intercourse (dyspareunia) in at least half of all women over 50. Vaginal secretions also become less acidic, often causing burning and itching (vaginitis). Contrary to popular belief, there are no fluid-secreting glands in the vagina; most moisture is absorbed from blood vessels in the vaginal walls, and after meno-

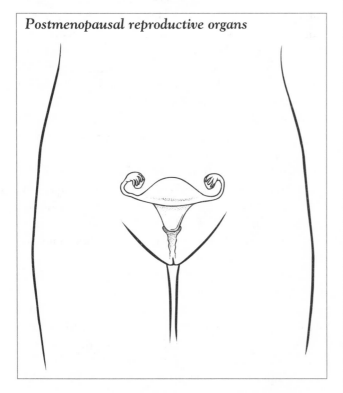

Postmenopausal reproductive organs

Fig. 7.1 *Declining levels of estrogen at menopause cause changes in the reproductive organs: The uterus becomes smaller and the tissue lining the vagina shrinks and becomes thinner.*

HANDLING HOT FLASHES

Hot flashes can be stopped by taking estrogen, and many women choose to take hormone replacement therapy specifically to put an end to them. Some women who cannot take estrogen may get some relief from taking only progestin. Doctors may also prescribe a beta-blocker like propranolol (Inderal, used to treat heart disease), or Bellergal-S, a combination of phenobarbital, ergotamine, and belladona alkaloids, which the FDA has approved for hot flashes. Clonidine, a high blood pressure drug, can help reduce flashes, although other blood pressure medications (as well as niacin, a B vitamin often prescribed for high cholesterol levels) may actually make them worse. Many of the drugs taken for hot flashes eventually become less effective over time.

Ways to deal with hot flashes that do not involve drugs:

- Dress in layers of light, natural-fiber clothing that can be removed and put back on easily.

- Have a cold drink.

- Carry a pretty fan with you and don't be shy about using it.

- Place a cool washcloth on your forehead, wrists, or temples.

- Stand by an open window (if it's cool outside).

- Keep rooms at a cool temperature. (If you and your partner argue about whether to leave the window open at night, getting an electric blanket with dual controls may solve the problem.

- Sleep with light blankets.

- Take a lukewarm shower if you can.

- Note when flashes occur (such as in months when you don't menstruate or when you wear a heavy sweater), so you can be better prepared for them.

- Eat foods rich in vitamin E, such as wheat and rice germs, legumes, corn, almonds, and vegetable oils (wheat germ, corn, soybean). Egg yolks contain vitamin E, but should be eaten in moderation because of their high cholesterol content. Consult with your doctor about taking a vitamin E supplement; many physicians recommend starting with 25 milligrams (mg) a day, and gradually increasing the dose to no higher than 400 or 800 mg.

- Cut back on caffeine, alcohol, spicy food, hot soup and drinks, and large meals, all of which can trigger hot flashes.

pause there is less blood flow to or through the vagina. Research suggests, however, that having sex and/or orgasms regularly helps reduce vaginal symptoms. A long-lasting vaginal moisturizer (Replens), a lubricant (K-Y jelly) or an estrogen cream, as well as estrogen replacement therapy, can help make intercourse more comfortable.

URINARY PROBLEMS Estrogen is also responsible for keeping tissues in the urinary tract healthy. In some women, declining estrogen levels can cause urinary tract infections, with burning, itching, and painful urination. Lowered estrogen can also contribute to stress incontinence (see section on "Other Gynecological Conditions"), or urine leakage during exercise or while laughing, coughing, or sneezing.

WEIGHT GAIN When women get older, they may gain a few pounds a year, thanks to less exercise and/or a slower metabolism, although this is not necessarily related to menopause itself. Older women tend to gain weight around the abdomen; unfortunately, excess abdominal weight seems to increase cholesterol and blood glucose levels and thus the risk of heart attack. Exercising regularly and eating in moderation can help control your weight.

BLOATING Menopausal women often complain of bloating and intestinal gas, similar to the fluid retention and swelling experienced premenstrually or in early pregnancy. Premenstrual bloating is caused by a rise in progesterone levels, but it is not known why menopausal women experience the same symptoms. Wearing loose-waisted clothing and avoiding foods that provoke gassiness may help.

PSYCHOLOGICAL SYMPTOMS

Perhaps the biggest myth surrounding menopause is that this "change of life" goes hand in hand with depression, anxiety, and feelings of worthlessness. False assumptions; outdated, poorly designed studies; and bias against women (particularly older ones) are responsible for the prevalence of this myth. The physiological cause for mood and behavioral changes during menopause—like those of premenstrual syndrome—remains unknown.

That is not to deny that some women do experience mood swings, depression, anxiety, and even memory loss at this time of life. Some of these symptoms may be due to hormonal shifts, but research

suggests that they are probably related to other life events, such as children leaving home, strains in interpersonal relationships, divorce, a decline in personal health or in a mate's health, or illness or death of parents. The Massachusetts Women's Health Study, conducted by the New England Research Institute and published in 1991, found that 70 percent of the 7,500 women surveyed reported a sense of relief or neutral feelings about the end of their menstrual periods. Although the study discovered a slightly higher rate of depression among postmenopausal women, it was largely in reaction to unpleasant physical symptoms, such as hot flashes and sleep loss, and was only temporary. Women who were depressed after menopause were more likely to have suffered from depression before menopause, or to have derived their feelings of self-esteem and purpose in life from being able to bear children.

Some women report having less sexual desire during and after menopause, and this may also have something to do with hormone swings as well as with the fact that sex may be more uncomfortable than it used to be. It is natural not to want to have sex if it hurts, and vaginal dryness can be a significant issue for many couples. As one doctor put it: Stress usually doesn't cause pain during sex, but the pain can certainly cause stress.

Women may be hesitant to talk to their partners about painful sexual intercourse or other troublesome symptoms. However, the Wyeth-Ayerst pharmaceutical company commissioned a study of 2,000 men and women ages 45 to 65 and found that most men wished their mates would talk to them more about their menopausal symptoms. And the women surveyed in the study underestimated men's comfort level in discussing the topic. For example, two thirds of men surveyed said they were "very comfortable" with the topic and 8 out 10 said it would be useful to know more, but 1 in 4 could not name any symptoms or conditions linked to menopause.

Estrogen replacement therapy is thought to increase sexual desire as well as to lessen various mood changes or depression. Some women who suffer these problems, however, find that estrogen alone is not enough. Recent research from Emory University School of Medicine in Atlanta and Baylor College of Medicine in Houston suggests that administering a combination of androgens and estrogen results in a greater improvement in sexual desire and helps alleviate other psychological symptoms. Although the higher-dose androgen products used in the past sometimes produced excess facial hair and a deepened voice, the dosage usually prescribed today is much lower and these problems are rare.

SURGICAL MENOPAUSE

Hysterectomy, the removal of the uterus, is the second most frequently performed operation in this country, accounting for more than 650,000 procedures every year. (Only cesarean sections are more common.) At present rates, 37 percent of all women will have had a hysterectomy by age 60; the rate in American women is four times that of women in other industrialized nations. Although removing the uterus alone brings an end to menstrual periods, cyclical hormone production continues. Statistically, women who have had hysterectomies do reach menopause somewhat earlier than women who have not had them. This may be due to a change in the blood flow to the ovaries after hysterectomy.

A hysterectomy may be partial (removal of the uterus only, leaving the cervix) or total (uterus and cervix). Also, it has become increasingly common for doctors to remove both ovaries and the Fallopian tubes. This procedure is called hysterectomy with bilateral salpingo-oophorectomy.

The rationale for the removal of the Fallopian tubes and ovaries at the time of hysterectomy has been that it eliminates the risk of developing ovarian cancer, which increases with age. Removing both ovaries triggers immediate ("artificial") menopause, and carries a significantly higher risk of menopausal symptoms, such as hot flashes, as well as osteoporosis and heart disease. Leaving the ovaries in place allows a natural production of hormones until the time of menopause. If you need to have a hysterectomy, you should discuss with your physician the pros and cons of removing or keeping your ovaries. Many doctors rely on an age cutoff, removing the ovaries if you are over age 45, for example. Women who have had hysterectomies are particularly good candidates for hormone replacement therapy because they can benefit from the estrogen without the threat of uterine cancer.

Although hysterectomies were once performed as a means of birth control, now the primary reasons for them are: 30 percent, uterine fibroids; 19 percent, endometriosis; 16 percent, prolapse ("dropping") of the uterus; 10 percent, uterine cancer; and 6 percent, hyperplasia, a precancerous condition.

Claiming that doctors who perform hysterectomies are often motivated by profit, some consumer and women's health advocates have led an effort to curtail the number of procedures performed each year. Regardless of whether you suspect your doctor's motives, if he or she recommends a hysterectomy, you should seek a second opinion. For example, women who have fibroids that cause excessive bleeding are being encouraged to discuss having a myomectomy, in which just the fibroids are removed and the uterus is left intact. (See earlier section on the physiological conditions associated with menopause.) Endometriosis may be treated by less radical surgery or by medication in many cases.

MENOPAUSE-RELATED DISORDERS

Several chronic diseases are considered to be related to menopause. Although they are partially linked to the overall aging process, most of them have a hormonal component: Reduced levels of estrogen accelerate disease risks that wouldn't be as high if a woman had late menopause or were on hormone replacement therapy. Unfortunately, the benefit of using hormone replacement therapy to reduce disease risk is not clear-cut in all cases. It may reduce the risk of some diseases, while simultaneously increasing the risk of others.

CORONARY HEART DISEASE Although your family history of cardiovascular disease (including heart attack and stroke) plays a big role in your risk of developing it, several large studies, including the Nurses' Health Study, have found that a lack of estrogen doubles the risk of having a heart attack. This is largely due to the shift in the ratio of "good" to "bad" cholesterol levels after menopause. Estrogen causes a rise in the beneficial high-density lipoprotein (HDL) cholesterol and a decrease in the harmful low-density lipoproteins (LDL), which explains why premenopausal women have a very low rate of heart disease. After menopause, however, the HDL levels drop and the LDL levels rise, with the result that women's risk climbs and eventually approximates that of men. Estrogen also causes the arteries to dilate, which eases blood flow, although progestin causes them to constrict somewhat. Estrogen replacement therapy cuts in half the risk of heart disease, the number one cause of death in women.

OSTEOPOROSIS This disease, characterized by fragile bones that are prone to fractures, is fast becoming a major public health problem. According to the National Osteoporosis Foundation, one third of women over age 50 will have a vertebral fracture, which can cause a loss of height and stooped posture ("dowager's hump"); the risk of hip fracture is equal to the combined risks of breast, uterine, and ovarian cancers—hip fractures lead to 50,000 deaths each year. Being postmenopausal is just one risk factor for osteoporosis, but it is probably the most important one. (See box, "Are You Bound for Brittle Bones?")

Although the relationship between female hormones and bone strength is not completely understood, it is generally believed that estrogen assures that new bone is built faster than old bone is broken down. In addition, it preserves skeletal stores of calcium by enhancing the absorption and utilization of dietary calcium. Women reach their peak bone mass between ages 25 and 35, but after menopause there is a sudden decline in bone density. It is assumed that low bone density increases the likelihood that bones will break, but this has not been proved absolutely. Certainly, a woman with osteoporosis who falls down is more likely to fracture her hip than a 20-year-old who falls. Estrogen replacement therapy has been approved by the Food and Drug Administration (FDA) specifically for the purpose of reducing the risk of osteoporosis.

BREAST CANCER The risk of breast cancer increases with age, although cancers in premenopausal women tend to spread more quickly and are more likely to be hereditary than cancers in postmenopausal women. Whether hormone replacement therapy increases the risk remains controversial. The Nurses' Health Study found that women currently using estrogen had a 33 percent higher risk of breast cancer than nonusers or past users. Most studies have not found an increased risk associated with short-term use (less than 15 years), although some have shown that the risk rises with increasing length of use, or with dosages greater than 1.25 milligrams a day. It is believed that estrogen promotes the growth of certain cancerous tumors (ones with estrogen receptors on them), but it is not clear if the doses given to menopausal women are high enough to have an impact on this growth or if estrogen can initiate cancerous mutations in cells. Interestingly, though, research suggests that women taking estrogen who develop breast cancer have a better survival rate than women not on estrogen, possibly because they are under closer medical supervision. The role of progestin will remain uncertain until the conclusion of research studies currently under way.

ENDOMETRIAL (UTERINE) CANCER Cancer of the lining of the uterus (endometrium) usually strikes women over 50. Although a history of infertility or lack of ovulation increases risk, estrogen replacement therapy without progestin has been found to augment it at least fivefold. (Previous studies of higher doses found that it increased risk as much as twentyfold.) Precancerous changes (hyperplasia) are even more common. Estrogen promotes a thickening of the uterine lining, which can cause cancerous changes if

ARE YOU BOUND FOR BRITTLE BONES?

Your doctor can use various scanning techniques, such as single- or dual-photon absorptiometry, dual-energy X-ray absorptiometry, CAT scan or radiographic absorptiometry, to measure your bone density and assess your risk of osteoporosis.

These risk factors increase your chances of developing the disease:

• Caucasian or Asian heritage

• A thin, small-boned frame

• Older relatives (especially women) with broken bones or stooped posture

• Natural or surgical menopause before age 45

• Advanced age

• Estrogen deficiency as a result of premenopausal amenorrhea (no menstrual periods)

• A low-calcium diet

• A sedentary life-style with little or no exercise

• Cigarette smoking

• Excessive use of alcohol

• Prolonged use of certain medications, including thyroid hormone, glucocorticoids (antiinflammatory drugs used to treat asthma, arthritis, and certain cancers), and antiseizure medicines

Adapted from "Stand Up to Osteoporosis," National Osteoporosis Foundation, 1993. Used with permission.

there is no progestin to balance the estrogen and thin the uterine lining. Therefore, women who have not had hysterectomies are generally prescribed progestin along with estrogen. Some doctors feel that periodic endometrial biopsies in women taking estrogen alone can detect cancers in an early stage so that hysterectomies can be done prior to the spread of the disease.

OVARIAN CANCER Although there are tragic stories of young women such as Gilda Radner dying from this usually silently spreading cancer, it is most common in women over 60. Early menopause reduces the risk of ovarian cancer, and late menopause may increase it slightly. Hormone replacement therapy is not thought to have an effect on your chances of developing ovarian cancer.

GALLBLADDER DISEASE The risk of developing gallstones, most common in women over 40, is increased by supplemental estrogen use. It is estimated that 131 out of 100,000 cases of gallbladder disease are related to taking estrogen. Research has found that estrogen raises your chances of developing gallstones, even after you have stopped taking the hormone.

OTHER GYNECOLOGICAL CONDITIONS Decreased hormonal levels in menopause may cause pelvic relaxation, the gradual weakening of pubococcygeal (PC) muscles that support the bladder, rectum, and uterus. Without the proper support, these organs can begin to press against the vaginal walls or protrude into the vagina itself, conditions called, respectively, cystocele, rectocele, and uterine prolapse (see the Encyclopedia). Women who have had many children or difficult deliveries, or are genetically predisposed to these conditions, are more prone to develop them. Symptoms may include frequent urination, vaginal or lower abdominal pressure, lower back pain, or a general feeling that something is falling out.

Strengthening the PC muscles by performing simple exercises (see Chapter 2, "Sexual Health") can help prevent or alleviate some of these problems. The exercises, sometimes called Kegel exercises, can also be useful in alleviating another common postmenopausal condition—urinary stress incontinence—the involuntary leakage of urine during exercise, coughing, or sneezing. (See the Encyclopedia.)

HORMONE REPLACEMENT THERAPY

HISTORY Hormone replacement therapy and medical opinions about it have changed with the times. The popularity of estrogen replacement therapy surged in the 1960s, thanks largely to one man, Dr. R. A. Wilson, who praised the lifelong use of the hormone as the way for women to stay "feminine forever." He wrote in both medical and lay publications, saying that, based on his experience, estrogen prevented "hypertension, arteriosclerosis, flabby breast, dowager's hump and atrophic genitals." Studies (in men!) suggested that doses of estrogen ten to fifteen times higher than those given to menopausal women reduced the risk of heart disease. But further research and studies of the effects of birth control pills indicated that estrogen might actually increase heart disease risk.

In the 1970s, estrogen fell further out of favor. Women who smoked and took birth control pills were found to have many times the risk of heart attacks and strokes than nonsmokers not on the pills. Doctors also discovered that postmenopausal women taking estrogen were developing more uterine cancer. As a result of these reports, many women stopped taking postmenopausal estrogen replacement therapy and birth control pills, and pharmaceutical companies began developing safer, lower-dose products. Today, the amount of estrogen you receive supplementally after menopause is only about 20 percent of the amount you produce premenopausally.

Postmenopausal women were still taking estrogen in the early 1980s, although doctors prescribed the lowest dose for the shortest length of time possible. During the eighties three major research findings led to the increased use of hormone replacement therapy: First, estrogen use helps prevent bone loss and fractures in the years after menopause. Second, estrogen helps protect women against cardiovascular disease, and third, taking progestin along with estrogen reduces the risk of endometrial cancer.

In the 1990s, the focus is on identifying subgroups of women who would benefit most and least from hormone therapy. The risks and benefits of estrogen and progestin (for women with a family history of breast cancer or heart disease, for example) and the effectiveness of various dosage regimens are being examined. Experts increasingly believe that hormone therapy will be beneficial for most women because heart disease is the number one cause of death among women, and because many of the tissues in the female body are nourished by estrogen. The final word will probably come with the conclusion of major research studies, including the Postmenopausal Estrogen and Progestin Interventions (PEPI), which are currently under way.

OPPOSED AND UNOPPOSED ESTROGEN Doctors use these terms to describe hormone therapy with and without progestin. Estrogen used alone is called unopposed, while combination therapy is called opposed estrogen. Because estrogen, despite its beneficial effects, tends to increase the risk of endometrial cancer, most women who have a uterus also take progestin, which tends to counteract this risk. Some physicians believe that taking unopposed estrogen is safe as long you have regular endometrial biopsies. Unfortunately, most of the reported side effects of hormone therapy—breast tenderness, bloating, edema, abdominal cramps, weight gain, anxiety, irritability, and depression, as well as monthly bleeding—are associated with progestin use, leading some women to forego their progestin pills.

HORMONE THERAPY EFFECTS

•**Heart Disease and Cholesterol Levels.** Estrogen taken orally maintains the beneficial ratio of HDLs to LDLs, and seems to prevent the increase in heart disease risk that accompanies menopause. In contrast, it also may raise the body's levels of triglycerides, another form of fat in the blood, which may in turn raise heart disease risk. Some doctors believe that progestin may limit the benefits of estrogen on the heart, and they advocate using the lowest dose of progestin possible. Research has yet to determine the validity of this theory.

•**Osteoporosis.** Estrogen prevents the rapid bone loss associated with the first several years of menopause. Going off estrogen, however, causes subsequent bone loss. Progestin is not thought to have an impact on bone strength.

•**Breast Cancer.** Using estrogen may increase the risk of breast cancer, particularly if taken for more than 15 years. It is not known if progestin causes the risk to increase, although some researchers suspect that it may.

•**Sexuality.** Estrogen keeps the vaginal tissues healthy and maintains premenopausal lubrication to make intercourse more comfortable. Some women report that estrogen therapy increases their sexual desire. The addition of progestin in the regimen causes many women to "menstruate," which may interfere with sexual intercourse some days of the month, just as it may premenopausally. If cyclic bleeding is a problem, ask your physician if you can switch to a daily estrogen-progestin routine that will not cause bleeding.

•**Urinary Tract.** Estrogen reduces the likelihood of urinary tract infections or incontinence associated with age and menopause.

•**Skin.** Estrogen helps maintain the elasticity, moisture, and thickness of the skin.

•**Memory and Emotions.** Many women report that estrogen increases (or stabilizes) moods and improves memory. Unfortunately, progestin often causes mood swings reminiscent of premenstrual syndrome.

•**Alzheimer's Disease.** There is some preliminary evidence that a steady supply of estrogen helps protect against Alzheimer's disease and other forms of dementia. This may explain why women, who lose most of their estrogen supply after menopause, suffer from Alzheimer's more frequently than men, in whom the male hormone testosterone, which does not diminish much with age, is converted to estrogen in the brain.

FORMS OF REPLACEMENT ESTROGEN The primary forms of replacement estrogen are pills, a transdermal ("through the skin") patch, creams, and, although not generally used, by injection. There are about twenty products on the market that are approved to treat hot flashes, but only two, Premarin pills and the Estraderm patch, have been approved specifically to prevent osteoporosis. The FDA is currently considering whether to allow pharmaceutical companies to promote the relationship of estrogen products to reducing heart disease risk. Hormonal products of the future are expected to expand in quantity and variety and may, for example, include progestin patches and androgen gels.

Three classes of estrogens are used for replacement therapy: Conjugated, natural, and synthetic. Premarin (the name comes from PREgnant MARe urINe), the only conjugated estrogen on the market, is most generally prescribed and was in fact the most often dispensed drug in the United States in 1993. Estratest, another brand of pill, combines androgens with estrogen.

Estraderm, the estrogen patch, is made with a synthetic form of estradiol, the type of estrogen normally produced by the ovaries. The clear patch is worn on the abdomen or buttocks, and it is changed twice a week. (See Figure 7.2.) The most frequently reported side effect, in up to 30 percent of users, is skin irritation at the patch site.

The primary difference between the patch and the pills is that the estrogen delivered by the patch is absorbed directly into the bloodstream, not filtered through the liver as oral estrogens are. As a result, the patch may not have the same beneficial effect on heart disease and cholesterol, nor does it raise triglyceride levels, which are manufactured in the liver. Recent research, however, suggests that transdermal estrogen may also increase HDL levels, but it takes 12 to 24 weeks to do so, compared with 4 to 8 weeks for oral estrogen. Oral estrogen may be prescribed for women with low HDLs or a family history of heart disease; transdermal estrogen may be given to women with high triglyceride levels or liver disease.

Some women may choose to use vaginal estrogen creams, which mostly relieve local symptoms of estrogen deficiency, such as dryness or irritation. They are not thought to be potent enough to reduce the risk of osteoporosis or coronary heart disease. Estrogen injections, as well as estrogen-androgen injections, which also go directly into the bloodstream, must be administered by a doctor every 3 to 4 weeks.

Although the FDA has not officially approved progestins for use in hormone therapy, the most widely used form of progestin is synthetic medroxy-progesterone, and the most common brand is Provera. A natural progesterone that has been "micronized" (broken into tiny particles and coated so it can pass through the stomach without being inactivated) is not yet approved for use in the United States. Some experts believe the natural form may have fewer side effects.

• **Regimens.** There are a variety of ways in which women can take estrogen and progestin over the course of each month. The FDA has not approved any particular regimen, and so it is up to individual doctors to advise their patients. Estrogens are taken all month or with a break of a few days at the end of the month. For cyclic estrogen-progestin, there are several regimens. The two most followed are:

• estrogen and progestin together for the first 10 to 12 days (after which bleeding occurs), then estrogen alone for the rest of the month)

• estrogen for the first 25 days of the month, with progestin added on days 14 to 25 or days 16 to 25; bleeding follows in the last days of the month

Because it can eliminate monthly bleeding, continuous low-dose estrogen combined with progestin is becoming increasingly popular, although more

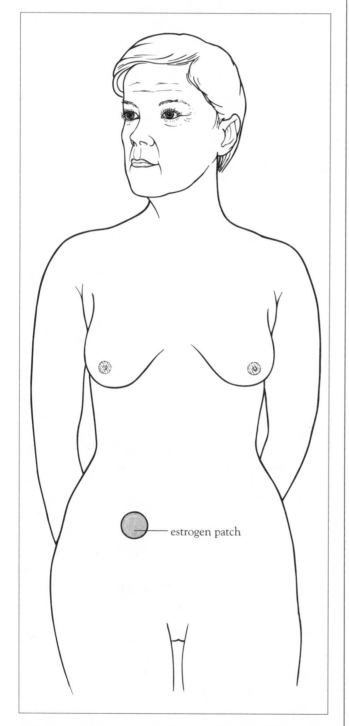

estrogen patch

Fig. 7.2 *Symptoms of menopause vary considerably among women and may be mild or severe. Replacement hormones, taken orally or delivered via a patch as shown here, are helpful in relieving such symptoms as hot flashes and vaginal dryness.*

symptoms of depression have been reported than for other regimens. The PEPI trials are comparing all these regimens.

Recent research from the University of Southern California School of Medicine suggests another possibility: taking estrogen daily and using a progesterone-releasing IUD. In a small study, researchers found that this combined therapy eliminated monthly bleeding after 6 months, had as beneficial an effect on cholesterol as estrogen alone, and caused no side effects.

• **When to Start and Stop.** Timing of hormone replacement is another area of controversy. The sooner you start taking hormones, the sooner you can reduce your risk of osteoporosis and heart disease. Despite the desire to alleviate symptoms such as hot flashes, many doctors think women should wait until a full year after their last period before taking hormones. Others believe that 6 months is an adequate cutoff; taking hormones any earlier than that, when it is quite possible that menopause has not yet occurred, can complicate your hormonal levels and bleeding patterns. Women with certain medical conditions, such as fibroids and endometriosis, benefit from waiting for more than a year before starting hormone therapy.

There are no specific guidelines on how long you should continue to take hormones. Many doctors think that women should take them indefinitely. Although most bone loss occurs in the first 5 years after menopause, women who stop taking estrogen quickly lose all the bone mass they have conserved. Continuous use maintains your lowered risk of developing cardiovascular disease. Perhaps most controversial is the association with breast cancer: Some studies suggest that hormones only increase the risk if they are used for longer than 15 years.

• **Cost.** Replacement hormones cost $15 to $20 a month, depending on the type used. Vaginal hormone creams cost less.

• **Contraindications.** The most generally accepted contraindications are a history of breast cancer, stroke, recent heart attack, endometrial cancer, liver, pancreatic or gallbladder disease, blood clotting problems, or undiagnosed vaginal bleeding. Many doctors also consider the following to be contraindications: smoking, severe fibrocystic breast disease, inherited high cholesterol, hypertension, and endometriosis. Doctors are divided over whether a family history of breast cancer contraindicates hormone replacement therapy.

The rules are changing, however, and now hormone therapy is sometimes given to women who have had breast cancer, thought to be the number one contraindication. Studies involving women who have had breast cancer are being conducted now, but results are not expected for several years.

• **Making the Decision.** The advantages of hormone replacement in reducing the risk of several major diseases are clear, and the potential side effects are well documented. What is not as clear is the instances in which women should not use estrogen. Until more definitive studies are available, experts advise that you and your doctor evaluate your personal or family history of various diseases when weighing the pros and cons of hormone therapy.

OTHER TREATMENTS FOR OSTEOPOROSIS Many drugs are being developed to treat osteoporosis. The most recent one approved by the FDA is Miacalcin, an injectable, synthetic form of salmon calcitonin. Calcitonin is a hormone (found in humans but more potent in salmon) that regulates the level of calcium in the blood. It has been found to slow bone loss in the vertebrae by inhibiting the normal breakdown, or resorption, of bone. Calcitonin is currently being tested in nasal-spray form.

A HEALTHY LIFE-STYLE There is much that you can do both before and after menopause to help reduce your risk of disease. While lifelong attention to a healthy diet and regular exercise may put the menopausal women of the future at an advantage, if you are facing menopause now, it is not too late to start.

• **Diet.** Eating right can help reduce your risk of osteoporosis and heart disease. A diet rich in calcium (1,000 milligrams [mg] a day for premenopausal women and postmenopausal women taking estrogen; 1,500 mg a day for postmenopausal women who are not taking estrogen) and, if necessary, calcium supplements can help bolster bones. (See box, "Calcium Supplements.") Combining calcium with estrogen and exercise enhances the hormone's beneficial effect on your bones. Eating a diet that is low in fat, especially saturated fat, and cholesterol and high in grains, fruits, and vegetables can help keep cholesterol levels in the recommended range, and possibly reduce the risk of breast cancer.

Research suggests that certain dietary choices can reduce the incidence of hot flashes. Japanese women have far fewer than American women, and some researchers theorize that it has to do with low levels of

CALCIUM SUPPLEMENTS

Ask your doctor if your diet includes enough calcium or if you should take calcium supplements. Reading the labels of these supplements can be confusing because the total number of milligrams (mg) in a pill is not the same as the amount of calcium in it. Supplements contain various calcium compounds or salts (such as calcium carbonate or calcium phosphate), and the amount of elemental, or actual, calcium in each pill varies from brand to brand. A tablet might contain 1250 mg of calcium carbonate, for example, but only 500 mg of elemental calcium.

Not all calcium supplements dissolve adequately enough to be absorbed by your stomach. To test your supplement, place it in a glass of vinegar at room temperature, stirring occasionally for 30 minutes. If the tablet hasn't disintegrated, it won't in your stomach either.

Other tips:

• Do not take bone meal or dolomite calcium supplements, which may contain lead or other toxic metals.

• Do not take more than 500 mg at one time.

• Take calcium carbonate supplements with meals.

• Talk to your doctor or pharmacist about potential interactions between calcium and prescription or nonprescription medications you are taking.

• Increased calcium may in some women raise the risk of kidney stones; talk to your doctor before taking supplements if you have a personal or family history of them.

• If you are taking iron supplements, do not take them at the same time, as they can interfere with calcium absorption.

estrogen in the nonanimal foods—for example, tofu—that comprise much of the Japanese diet.

• **Exercise.** Weight-bearing exercise (walking, running, and aerobic dance, but not swimming or biking), which stresses and thus strengthens the bones, has been found to reduce the risk of osteoporosis, although it probably will not have a significant effect in women not taking estrogen.

It is important to exercise both the upper and lower body. Weight training, combined with aerobic exercise, is a good way to ensure that the entire body gets a good workout. Regular (three times a week) aerobic exercise, even at moderate levels, also conditions the heart, keeps total cholesterol levels low and HDLs high, and controls weight, diabetes, and blood pressure.

Exercises that strengthen back and abdominal muscles, maintain flexibility, and improve balance can help prevent falls, a primary cause of debilitating fractures.

• **Smoking.** The Framingham Heart Study and other research have shown that smoking not only increases the risk of heart disease and stroke but also that of osteoporosis and hip fractures, counteracting the beneficial effects of estrogen on the bones. One reason for this may be that smoking accelerates menopause (by as much as 5 to 10 years in heavy smokers).

• **Alcohol.** Although heavy drinking is clearly bad for the health, and may make bone-breaking falls more likely, moderate drinking has pros and cons: It seems to reduce heart disease risk by having a positive effect on cholesterol levels, but it may increase the risks of breast cancer and osteoporosis.

• **Stress.** Trying to do too many things at once and to be everything to everyone is a problem for women throughout adulthood. Research suggests, however, that excess stress can worsen both the psychological and physical symptoms of menopause, such as vaginal dryness.

The Aging Process

At the turn of the last century, women were considered to be in their prime in their thirties—the pinnacle before the decline into brief old age. The development of many new vaccines, drugs, and surgical techniques, plus a better understanding of the role of poor nutrition and other lifestyle factors in the development of disease, have changed that picture dramatically. Since 1900, the percentage of people in the United States who are 65 and older has more than tripled. As a new century approaches, many people consider their fifties to be the prime of life.

For many women, this age is a time of new beginnings. If they have been raising a family, they may now have more time to spend on themselves, go back to school, take up sports, or change careers. They may feel more competent and confident in their abilities and accomplishments. They may have more discretionary income for travel or new hobbies. With care, they can enjoy this new freedom for several decades more.

Learning to recognize the normal effects of growing older can be somehow comforting. It allows you to distinguish conditions that may warrant medical attention from those that affect nearly everyone. You can plan for these normal changes, compensate for

those that you cannot avoid, and accept the fact that you may not be able to do everything in the same way or as quickly as you once did.

A positive attitude, a commitment to lifelong learning, and continued physical activity can go a long way toward staving off the mental and physical changes that come with the calendar. Slowing down may be inevitable, but giving up is not. In short, you can still lead a productive life, enjoy sexual fulfillment, and make vital contributions, no matter how many candles light your birthday cake.

WHAT IS AGING?

By the time most of us begin to worry about growing old, the aging process has been in effect for decades. In fact, some organ systems start to decline during adolescence. These changes, however, are generally imperceptible; it is not until bothersome symptoms occur later in life that we start to fear what has been going on all along. However, that need not interfere with our enjoyment of life and the benefits of being older. Although a positive attitude is not an insurance policy against disease—everyone knows a sprightly soul who is plagued with the worst difficulties aging can bestow—it is preferable to the fear that paralyzes some people who may never actually experience serious problems.

The parameters defining youth, middle age, and old age are vague because there are no standard measurements. While there is a general order of progression, aging does not occur in the same way at the same rate in any two people. From a purely mathematical point of view, if we designate 75 as the average life span, then middle age begins at 25; yet few 25-year-old women worry about their aging bodies.

So when do we become old? A 36-year-old poet feels young when her work is included in a young poets' anthology, but feels past her prime when she discusses pregnancy with her physician. A 55-year-old woman who may feel youthful in the presence of her parents, finds herself facing grandmotherhood at the same time. What one person feels at 39, another may feel at 54.

Women tend to examine their mother's pathway through middle and old age, expecting to follow the same course. Depending on the mother's physical and mental health, this can be disheartening or encouraging, but it should not be assumed.

Some of the changes of aging are subtle. For example, the speed of nerve conduction decreases by only about 1 percent every 3 to 4 years between ages 30 and 80. Others, wrinkles, "liver spots" on the hands, increased fat deposits on the upper arms, are more noticeable but certainly not debilitating except perhaps to the ego. Still others, such as a decline in eyesight and hearing, can have profound effects on the quality of our lives.

In the absence of disease, the function of individual organs tends to decrease only gradually. Where complex processes involving more than one organ system are concerned, however, the decline can be more pronounced. For example, although muscle strength declines slowly and very little, muscle coordination, which involves the nervous system as well, alters much more noticeably. Many of the normal changes associated with aging do not seriously affect our ability to live our lives, but they can decrease the ability of our organ systems to cope with stresses brought on by injury or disease. Many an older woman has been heard to lament that she can still do everything she used to do, but she needs more time to recover.

This chapter examines the physical and psychological changes that aging brings as well as various disorders that become more prevalent as we grow older.

EARLY ADULTHOOD

PHYSICAL CHANGES During early adulthood—roughly ages 25 to 44—the physical changes associated with normal aging usually have little effect on daily life. It is true that speed, strength, and agility peak between ages 18 and 29, which explains why most professional athletes are considered "over the hill" in their thirties. For most of us, however, the minor loss in these abilities goes unnoticed. For instance, around age 45 we begin to lose muscle strength at a rate of about 1.5 percent a year, but that small difference does not affect our ability to open a jar or hold on to a bag of groceries.

• **The Eyes.** Noticeable changes in vision are common during early adulthood. Even before middle age, the lens of the eye starts to become less elastic, so that it may become more difficult to focus when looking at things at different distances or in different amounts of light. By age 40, this reduced elasticity will cause most people whose vision is normal to have some difficulty focusing on close objects, a condition known as presbyopia (farsightedness). People who start out in life with vision problems often find that they become more pronounced in early and middle age. Vision loss at this age can often be corrected with reading glasses, bifocals or trifocals, or bifocal contact lenses.

PSYCHOLOGICAL CHANGES For some women, the psychological aspects of growing older begin early. In their twenties and thirties, they may revel in their increasing competence and independence. Or they may struggle with the questions of timing career, marriage, and parenthood. If they devote their twenties to a career, will they find someone to marry and have children with before their time is up? If they settle down and have children right away, will they have a career to return to?

The ticking of the biological clock may be a source of anguish for some women in early adulthood. The realization that having a family is no longer a given may be one of the most difficult to face. Foregoing motherhood because you are not married or because you believe your career will be compromised can be the most far-reaching life decision you will make. Deciding to have a child later in life may be just as stressful, especially if infertility, single parenthood, or marital problems become factors in your decision.

New opportunities for women and the expectations that accompany these options can bring stress coping strategies for adapting to new circumstances. The wisdom that comes with maturity makes it easier to accept some of these changes with equanimity. Menopause is the most notable physical—and for some, mental—adjustment. For many women, the freedom it brings from the necessity for birth control is most welcome. (See Chapter 7, "Menopause.")

Some women notice significant changes that result from normal wear and tear, or complain that they tire more easily. Others *feel* much as they did in their early thirties, but wrinkles, gray hair, and the redistribution of body fat may have changed the way they look. Our youth-oriented society often exerts pressure on us to maintain the illusion of being young and physically attractive by covering up signs of maturity. Acknowledging the different kind of beauty that comes with middle and old age may be difficult, but it may also be the least troublesome way of dealing with the changes.

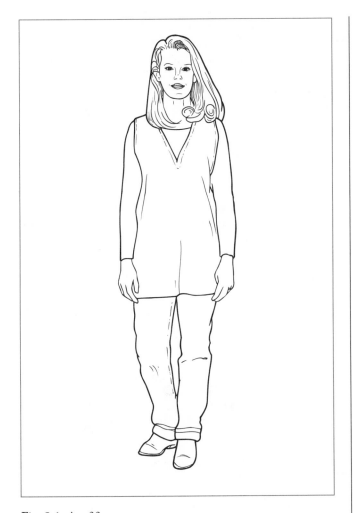

Fig. 8.1 *Age 30*

as well as success. Most women are able to cope by finding a comfortable compromise among the forces that shape their lives. Some experience temporary feelings of depression when life's misfortunes seem overwhelming, and they may benefit from short-term therapy. Others may suffer more profound problems, and in some cases may be genetically predisposed to mental illness. Psychiatric problems that tend to manifest themselves among women in young adulthood include agoraphobia (fear of being in open, crowded, or public places) and other phobias, eating disorders, schizophrenia, major depression, and obsessive-compulsive disorders. Talk therapy, behavior modification, medication, or a combination of these treatments, may help these women live more normal lives.

MIDDLE ADULTHOOD

PHYSICAL CHANGES Middle age, approximately ages 45 to 64, can be a time of extreme change. Fortunately, by this time, many women have honed their

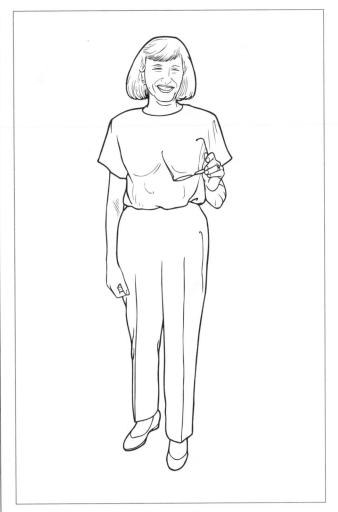

Fig. 8.2 *Age 50*

• **The Skin.** The first signs of aging may show up in the skin. Wrinkles, the results of lost elasticity, occur first across the brow and around the mouth (laugh lines). Eventually the creases around the eyes and nose and on the cheeks become more noticeable, and the skin around the neck loosens. Age spots ("liver spots") appear on the hands as the pigment-producing skin cells become concentrated in small areas.

Three factors affect how much you will wrinkle as you age: heredity, sun exposure, and smoking. Although you can do nothing about the first, quitting smoking, avoiding sun exposure as much as possible, and using sunscreens when you can't can help limit these hallmarks of the passing years.

Age-spot lighteners and most wrinkle creams have only temporary effects. Retin-A cream can have a positive effect on wrinkles, but only if used continuously. Cosmetic surgery can restore a youthful appearance, but it is not a decision to be made lightly. A change in attitude may be healthier and certainly less expensive. (See Chapter 15, "Body Care.")

• **Bones, Joints, and Muscles.** In normal aging, a major change in the bones is an accelerated loss of calcium, which can eventually lead to osteoporosis in old age. The risk of osteoporosis can be lowered somewhat by getting adequate amounts of dietary calcium (with supplements if necessary) and engaging in regular weight-bearing exercise such as walking, step aerobics, or aerobic dance.

Lack of use is the primary reason why so many people lose muscular function. Although coordination and flexibility decrease slightly, you can maintain and even increase strength well into old age through regular exercise. (See Chapter 10, "Keeping Fit.")

The best way to maintain muscular function is to keep moving. Walk around the neighborhood or join a mall-walking group or an exercise class. Be realistic about your current physical condition and skills. Ease into exercise by first warming up at a lower intensity. Cool down afterward by slowing down gradually, and then do some stretching.

A joint disease that appears in some people in their thirties and forties is rheumatoid arthritis, which afflicts more than 7 million people and about three times as many women as men. One of the more disabling types of arthritis, it produces severe inflammation of the joints—most often the knees, hands, feet, and ankles—and may also produce weight loss, general weakness, and have some effect on other organs, such as the heart or lungs. Its causes are not completely understood, but it may be the result of a genetic predisposition to the disease or an autoimmune response to a virus. (For more information, see the Encyclopedia.)

• **Hearing.** By age 65, about one third of all people experience some hearing loss, which usually starts with difficulty in hearing high-pitched tones. The most common diagnosis is presbycusis, which means age-related hearing loss. It is important, however, to have your ears examined because in some cases, there may simply be some wax buildup in the ear canal, which is easily remedied.

Age-related hearing loss, though common, does not necessarily cause problems in everyday activities. With irreversible hearing loss, however, hearing aids

TIPS FOR PEOPLE WITH HEARING LOSS

• Ask people to get your attention before speaking, by tapping your arm or standing in front of you.

• Be sure that you are facing the speaker.

• Stand no more than about 3 feet from the speaker and be sure the room is adequately lit so you can see lip movement and facial expression. Even if you have not been formally trained in lip reading, you can pick up a lot from watching the speaker's face.

• Try to control background noise. Turn off radios or appliances or move to another room.

• Ask people to enunciate and speak loudly without shouting.

• If you do not understand what someone is saying, ask him or her to repeat the information using different words.

• Be sure you understand important information completely. Do not be afraid to ask for clarification.

• If you join a group of people, ask them to tell you what they are talking about instead of trying to figure it out yourself.

• When you are in a group, try to face as many people as possible. Sit at the head or the foot of a table or on a chair rather than a couch.

and special training in lip reading may help. There are many types of hearing aids, so it is wise to consult an audiologist or physician before selecting one. (See box, "Tips for People with Hearing Loss.")

• **The Eyes.** Vision continues to decline in most people during middle age. Farsightedness becomes more pronounced, and adjusting to different light levels and to glare may take more time. More light is necessary to see well, and the field of vision may decrease slightly. It is important to exercise caution in, for example, driving, especially at night.

Glaucoma, excessively high pressure in the eye that causes damage to the retinal nerve cells and optic nerve, is often diagnosed in middle age. By damaging the nerve cells, glaucoma can cause "tunnel vision" as the visual field decreases. Since glaucoma often has no symptoms in its early stages, the American Academy of Ophthalmology recommends a screening every 2 to 4 years, starting at age 40 and every 1 to 2 years after age 65. Untreated glaucoma is the leading cause of blindness in older people.

DIABETES Type II, or non-insulin-dependent, diabetes is most common in people over 40 and affects more women than men. It often occurs in overweight individuals and can usually be controlled by weight reduction, dietary changes, and oral medication. People with diabetes are predisposed to other disorders affecting the feet, eyes, heart, and blood vessels, necessitating careful monitoring by a physician.

CANCER Cancer claims one out of five lives in the United States, and it is usually during middle and later adulthood that many of us mourn the death from cancer of a close friend or relative. Early diagnosis is the most important factor in the successful treatment of most cancers. In fact, some types of cancer, such as that of the cervix, are routinely cured when diagnosed at the very earliest (usually precancerous) stages. In many cases, regular screenings and self-exams can lead to early detection of breast, colorectal, cervical, and skin cancers. (For more information, see Chapter 14, "Breast Care," and the Encyclopedia.)

HEART AND BLOOD VESSELS The heart is a remarkably strong pump that, under normal circumstances, can perform quite adequately well into old age. Nevertheless, the heart muscle eventually begins to thicken and the arteries may become narrowed, leading to one of several disorders that make cardiovascular disease the nation's number one killer of both men and women. (See box, "Heart Attack—

Signals and Action.") Younger men are affected far more often than younger women, but after menopause women begin to catch up. For example, only 12 percent of women aged 35 to 44 have cholesterol levels considered high; that figure jumps to 25 percent among women aged 45 to 54, and 40 percent between 55 and 64. According to the American Heart Association, one in seven women aged 45 to 64 has some form of heart or blood vessel disease; the ratio soars to one in three after age 65. More than half of all women over age 65 have high blood pressure, or hypertension.

Estrogen is believed to help protect younger women against heart disease, and for this reason, many doctors recommend estrogen replacement therapy after menopause. (See Chapter 7, "Menopause.")

Cardiovascular disorders that occur with aging include angina pectoris (chest pain), high blood pressure, congestive heart failure, heart attack, and stroke. (For more information about specific disorders, see the Encyclopedia.)

REPRODUCTIVE AND URINARY SYSTEMS The most profound change your body undergoes comes during menopause, but most women weather this transition quite well. Menopause affects both the reproductive system and the urinary system. Because estrogen helps keep the tissue in the vaginal and urinary tracts healthy, declining levels of this hormone may increase the chances of certain vaginal and urinary problems.

For example, vaginal dryness and the loss of elasticity of vaginal tissue may produce itching and burning and may make intercourse painful. A long-lasting vaginal moisturizer or estrogen-containing vaginal cream can help the itching and burning. Taking extra time to be sure you are fully aroused and using a lubricant such as K-Y jelly or Replens will usually alleviate any discomfort during intercourse. Estrogen replacement therapy may preclude these problems in many cases.

Although the lubrication process usually takes longer, sexual functioning remains undiminished for most women as they age. In fact, regular orgasms, whether through intercourse or masturbation, appear to help keep the vaginal tissue from atrophying.

Urinary tract infections, characterized by burning, itching, and painful urination, also become more prevalent and may necessitate taking antibiotics, especially for recurrent episodes.

A condition called stress incontinence, in which weakened pelvic muscles cause some urine to leak

HEART ATTACK—SIGNALS AND ACTION

Know the warning signals of a heart attack:
Uncomfortable pressure, fullness, squeezing or pain in the center of the chest that lasts more than a few minutes.

• Pain spreading to the shoulders, neck, or arms.

• Chest discomfort with lightheadedness, fainting, sweating, nausea, or shortness of breath.

Not all of these warning signs occur in every heart attack. If some start to occur, however, don't wait. Get help immediately. Delay can be deadly!

Know what to do in an emergency:
Find out which area hospitals have 24-hour emergency cardiac care.

• Know (in advance) which hospital or medical facility is nearest your home and office, and tell your family and friends to call this facility in an emergency.

• Keep a list of emergency rescue service numbers next to the telephone and in your pocket, wallet or purse.

• If you have chest discomfort that lasts more than a few minutes, call the emergency rescue service.

• If you can get to a hospital faster by going yourself and not waiting for an ambulance, have someone drive you there. Don't try to drive yourself.

Be a Heart Saver:

• If you're with someone experiencing the signs of a heart attack—and the warning signs last more than a few minutes—act immediately.

• Expect a "denial." It's normal for someone with chest discomfort to deny the possibility of something as serious as a heart attack. But don't take "no" for an answer. Insist on taking prompt action.

• Call the emergency service, or

• Get to the nearest hospital emergency room that offers 24-hour emergency cardiac care.

• Give CPR (mouth-to-mouth breathing and chest compression) if it's necessary and you're properly trained.

Source: American Heart Association, *1994 Heart and Stroke Facts.*

when you cough or strain, is also age related. Stress incontinence occurs most frequently in women whose bladder support muscles have been injured during childbirth; decreased estrogen levels at menopause are also thought to contribute. (For specific disorders, see the Encyclopedia.) Kegel exercises can strengthen pelvic muscles and help prevent or alleviate incontinence. (See box, Chapter 2, "Sexual Health.")

PSYCHOLOGICAL CHANGES For women who have children, middle adulthood usually means redistributing their time and energy as the children become more independent. This freedom can be a positive force in your life: You can look forward to finding yourself again and enjoying other family members, a career, or neglected hobbies. If you have spent your life establishing a career, now is the time to take satisfaction in your achievements and find more time for other enjoyable ventures.

As career and family issues become less pressing, different concerns may now come to the fore. For instance, as your children leave, you may feel you have less purpose in life or you may fear spending your old age alone. Now is the time to reestablish your relationship with your partner, to rediscover the joy of being just a couple.

If it's nurturing you miss, volunteer work provides a myriad of opportunities for you to contribute. Many schools and hospitals rely on volunteers to tutor or act as foster grandparents to ill or abandoned babies. Even if you have no parenting experience, you are very welcome at many social service agencies that need mentors for the adolescents they serve.

Going back to school, whether in a degree program or to take a course in art or music, can not only be stimulating but it is a wonderful way to make new friends. A number of colleges have started programs just for older adults, but don't discount the exhilaration you may get from mixing with college-age students.

Consider your hobbies and interests when you want to widen your social circle. Garden clubs, theater groups, political organizations, and churches and synagogues offer a way to meet people with whom you will immediately have something in common. Many women who wouldn't dream of going to a bar or striking up a conversation on the street feel comfortable chatting with a stranger in a museum or at a concert or university lecture.

LATER ADULTHOOD

Despite the fears of many people, there is no benchmark against which we are all considered "old." Although some would say old age begins at 65, because this coincides with retirement for so many of us, it might be better to consider this event as merely a transition to a different type of productivity. It is unfortunate that our society seems intent on writing off those who are capable of great contributions well into their later years. It is especially important for women, who may be just coming into their own, to struggle against this stereotype and continue to place themselves in challenging roles.

While later adulthood may bring on troublesome physical symptoms, caution and common sense can help safeguard against some of the most frequent hazards. For instance, a 75-year-old woman who falls in the bathtub can easily fracture her hip, but installing grab bars on the wall and nonslip pads in the bottom of the tub will reduce that possibility considerably. Life does not have to change drastically—only the way in which we approach it.

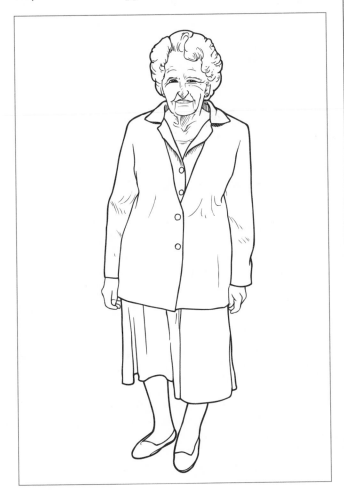

Fig. 8.3 *Age 80*

PHYSICAL CHANGES Inevitable physical transformations occur, but they need not create hardships. Hair usually becomes thinner, coarser, and more completely gray or white; skin texture changes and becomes less elastic; and the senses are less sharp, but there are ways of compensating for these changes if any seem problematic. Glasses correct vision and hearing aids help restore hearing. You can turn up the volume on the radio and television and add stronger spices to foods. Good nutrition and exercise keep physical and mental reserves high, and quitting bad habits, such as smoking, excessive drinking, and harmful sun exposure, creates a sense of accomplishment and well-being while cutting the losses already incurred.

BONES, JOINTS, AND MUSCLES Stiff joints are more common (but not inevitable) as your body ages. Stiffness may be especially noticeable in the morning and can be eased with a warm shower and flexibility exercises. (See Chapter 10, "Keeping Fit.") Far more serious are osteoporosis and various types of arthritis.

•**Osteoporosis.** Half of women over age 50 will suffer a fracture as a result of osteoporosis, a disorder in which loss of calcium from the bones and resultant fractures can lead to severe disability and even death. Women suffer from fractures of the hip more often than men. In both men and women, compression fractures in the spine cause it to shorten and curve, resulting in loss of height.

Prevention of osteoporosis is one of the strongest arguments for taking estrogen replacement therapy; indeed, osteoporosis is mainly seen in women after menopause who are estrogen deficient. (See Chapter 7, "Menopause.") Calcium supplements do not increase bone mass at this age, but they seem to slow or stop bone loss, thus helping prevent future fractures. Calcitonin or etidronate may be taken in conjunction with calcium, but the doses must be strictly supervised by a physician to avoid toxic reactions. Although there is no cure for osteoporosis, early treatment can forestall some of its worst symptoms.

•**Arthritis.** This umbrella term covers more than one hundred conditions that affect the joints. They are all characterized by some degree of pain, swelling, and stiffness. Osteoarthritis, which is much more common than the more serious rheumatoid arthritis, is a "wear and tear" disease caused by a lifetime of movement. Joint pain is caused by the breakdown of cartilage, the rubbery shock absorber that surrounds and protects bone ends, enabling free movement of joints. Weight-bearing joints—hips, knees, and spine—are most often affected, as are the joints of the fingers. Areas that have been chronically stressed often show the first signs. For example, knitters may have problems with fingers; runners, with knees; and tennis players, with elbows. Some people seem to be genetically predisposed to arthritis, but almost everyone gets osteoarthritis eventually, though the symptoms may be mild. Aspirin or other nonprescription medications usually relieve mild discomfort, and exercise helps maintain joint mobility. In more severe cases, prescription antiinflammatory drugs, physical therapy, heat treatments, and resting splints can restore pain-free activity. Steroid injections may be used judiciously, but oral steroids are virtually never warranted. For badly damaged joints, joint replacement may be necessary.

THE DIGESTIVE SYSTEM As we age, it takes longer for food to pass through our intestines. In some people, this may lead to constipation. It is not a problem unless pain and discomfort are present. Eating, exercise, and elimination habits may have more to do with constipation than age does. The cultivation of regular elimination habits is important because feces that remain in the colon for too long may become hard and difficult to pass. "Regular" does not necessarily mean daily, however. Normal elimination patterns can range from three or four times a day to twice a week. Slowly increasing the amount of fiber in your diet (adding more fruits, vegetables, and whole grains, or using fiber supplements), getting regular exercise, drinking more water, and learning to control stress should improve bowel function for most people. Resist regular use of laxatives and call a doctor if constipation persists for more than a week.

Other conditions, such as ulcers, diverticular disease, and cancers of the digestive tract occur more frequently with age. Women are more prone to gallbladder disease than men.

THE EYES A continuing decline in vision is so common with age that few people over 65 can do without glasses at least some of the time. Complete loss of eyesight is, perhaps, what people fear most, yet many go for years without an eye examination, the first step in protecting eyesight. Regular checkups are especially important for glaucoma (see earlier section on "The Eyes") as well as for two conditions, cataracts and macular degeneration, that affect more people in later adulthood.

• **Cataracts.** In this condition, the lens of the eye becomes cloudy. What begins as a small spot soon grows until vision becomes more and more misty.

About 75 percent of cataracts occur with aging. Although surgery is the only treatment, it is successful in 90 to 95 percent of all cases.

• **Macular Degeneration.** This is a deterioration of part of the retina, the causes of which are not well understood. It occurs in about 10 percent of all people aged 65 to 74 and nearly 30 percent of people over 75. Women are more often affected than men. A large blind spot develops in the middle of the field of vision, which may make activities like driving and reading difficult. Magnifying glasses can help, and most people retain enough vision to care for themselves. Laser treatment can sometimes halt the progression of the disorder, but there is no cure for it.

OTHER PHYSICAL PROBLEMS

• **Influenza, Pneumonia, and Other Infectious Diseases.** As the immune system declines, even small infections are harder to fight off, and many people find that they don't "bounce back" as quickly as they once did. You can decrease the chances of contracting infectious diseases by getting sufficient rest, eating a nutritious diet, exercising, taking extra care when traveling abroad, and generally taking measures to avoid exposure to infection. For people over 65, physicians sometimes recommend vaccinations to protect against influenza and certain types of pneumonia.

• **Temperature Sensitivity.** The body becomes less sensitive to temperature changes, causing older people to be more susceptible to hypothermia, persistent low body temperature. While young adults often notice when the room temperature decreases by as little as 1 degree, elderly people may be unable to discern that the temperature has fallen by 4 or 5 degrees. Hypothermia is a serious condition that can be fatal. The symptoms are apathy, confusion, and lethargy, followed by a loss of consciousness. A person with hypothermia should be wrapped in a blanket to prevent heat loss while his or her surroundings are gradually warmed.

• **Itching.** The skin becomes drier with age, making itching a common annoyance, especially in winter when the air is dry. Since bathing removes the oil that traps water and hydrates the skin, keep baths and showers to a minimum. Limit your bath to 15 minutes. Use a mild soap, followed by a moisturizer, to help control the itching. An air humidifier is also useful. Itching that does not respond to these measures deserves examination, as it may be caused by liver, kidney, or thyroid disorders, among others.

• **The Lungs.** Except in the case of cigarette smokers, age-related changes in the lungs do not necessarily reduce your ability to perform normal activities. Your lungs may work less efficiently and become more stiff with time, decreasing the ability to clear air passages of mucus, but chronic lung conditions such as emphysema (chronic obstructive pulmonary disease, or COPD) and bronchitis occur primarily in smokers. While these diseases have traditionally affected men more than women, as greater numbers of women continue to smoke, their rates of COPD and bronchitis will probably also rise.

THE NERVOUS SYSTEM Mental impairment is often considered inevitable, but the nervous system becomes only slightly less efficient, causing minor difficulty with memory and decreased balance and coordination. Most people do not succumb to more serious disorders, such as Alzheimer's disease or stroke. In the United States, about 15 percent of all people over 65 have some degree of intellectual impairment, half of it traceable to Alzheimer's disease; approximately a quarter, to stroke; and the remainder, to many other conditions. Because women tend to live longer than men, they may have a higher chance of losing some mental function.

Occasional forgetfulness should not be considered any more serious in a 70-year-old than it is in a 30-year-old. In fact, studies comparing people at these ages have shown that it takes the 70-year-old a quarter of a second longer to identify a familiar object, but this is rarely noticeable in everyday activities. (See box, "Memory Changes That Come with Age.") Older people may be less likely to rely on memory aids, however. Using certain techniques to remember important information may at least reduce the anxiety associated with occasional memory lapses. Jotting down important ideas right away, using "prompters" to help remember names, dates, and other facts, and making outlines to organize one's thoughts are just a few ways of making life a little easier.

Alzheimer's disease is estimated to affect 4 million Americans. Its cause is unknown, and as yet there is no cure, although it is currently one of the top research priorities in the United States. The symptoms of Alzheimer's disease include *severe* memory loss, disorientation, decline in ability to perform routine tasks, loss of language skills, and personality changes. Eventually its victims, who are more likely to be female, become completely dependent on caregivers. There are more than one hundred other conditions—some treatable or even curable—that cause dementialike symptoms often mistaken for signs of

MEMORY CHANGES THAT COME WITH AGE

Normal changes include:

• *Slowed thinking processes:* This may be particularly apparent when dealing with new problems or a problem requiring an immediate reaction.

• *Reduced attention span:* Many people find they have difficulty paying attention and ignoring distractions in the environment.

• *Decreased use of memory strategies:* Older people do not make as much use of associations and pictorial cues as younger people do, even though they may have an increased need for them.

• *Longer learning time:* This is especially true when an older person is confronted with new information.

Areas of the memory that do *not* usually change include:

• *Immediate or short-term memory:* For example, remembering the name of someone to whom you were just introduced will not become any harder—or any easier.

• *World knowledge or semantic memory:* You will still remember familiar information such as who is president, your children's birthdays, and how to get to the bank or supermarket. World knowledge is actually likely to increase with age.

• *Susceptibility to interference:* Newly learned information in a specific area competes with original information, making it hard, for example, to break old habits. This characteristic is present in both old and young people.

• *Ability to retain well-learned information:* The old forget no faster than the young.

• *Ability to search for stored information:* Older people may take longer to come up with the information, but the search technique does not change with age. Searching occurs automatically as well as with conscious effort.

Adapted from *The 40+ Guide to Health*, Consumer Reports Books, Yonkers, N.Y., 1993.

Alzheimer's disease. Only by a thorough medical evaluation can these conditions, which range from malnutrition to drug interactions, be identified.

Severe depression requiring treatment affects approximately 10 to 15 percent of older Americans, according to the National Institute of Mental Health. Clinical depression involves more than just "feeling down." It is thought to be the result of biochemical changes in the body and its symptoms may be so severe that they mimic dementia. (See Table 8.1, "Major Differences Between Depression and Dementia.") The cause of severe depression is often unknown, but it is sometimes triggered by a loss, such as the death of a family member. Diagnosis can be tricky—there is no foolproof way to confirm it—but treatment with medication often provides complete relief.

PSYCHOLOGICAL CHANGES Later adulthood, usually a time of retirement and some relief from family and other responsibilities, should also be the time to enjoy life. However, this requires advance planning. Women caught up in raising families or building careers may not think about how they will fill their aging years until they are upon them. Even more than men, because of their longer life spans, women must consider how they will manage in their later years.

Attitude is a key to enjoying the entire span of life, and the old saw about being only as old as you feel holds a lot of truth. Age does not significantly affect learning skills. Taking a class in a new subject may be no more difficult, and possibly more rewarding, than it was in high school. Expanding your horizons and those of your fellow students can be extremely satisfying.

Because women live longer than men, they are more likely to be the surviving spouse. In 1990, about 36 percent of women aged 65 to 74 were widowed, compared to only about 10 percent of their male counterparts. Women are less apt to remarry than men, perhaps because they are more independent and there are fewer men around to marry. Widowhood, even when it is expected, can be the most difficult time of your life. It is important to tap all sources of support and reestablish a social life. The best way to cope is to stay active and make new connections: Join groups that fit your interests, take in a roommate, start conversations with people you would like to make friends with, or go back to school.

The most profound psychological event in later adulthood is the acceptance (or denial) of your own mortality. Death can be an extremely frightening prospect, and dealing with it in a healthy way may be difficult at best. It is important to look back upon life without succumbing to regret. Often there is still time to compensate for any perceived inadequacies. If you want closer relationships with family members, now is the time to start. If fulfillment through work is important, make an effort. People do accomplish all of these things well into old age. Do not be afraid to try.

TABLE 8.1
MAJOR DIFFERENCES BETWEEN DEPRESSION AND DEMENTIA

DEPRESSION	DEMENTIA	DEPRESSION	DEMENTIA
Comes on in a short period of time with full-blown symptoms. Medical attention is sought soon after onset.	Usually comes on gradually, and patient and family may not be aware of symptoms, or will not seek help until later.	Ability to attend to task and concentrate is generally good.	Ability to attend to task and concentrate is generally poor.
Patient can describe decline in function in great detail; may state how bad memory is or how confused he or she feels.	Patient is vague in describing symptoms; denies problems with memory or feelings of confusion.	Prior history of depressive episodes in patient or family.	No prior history of depressive episodes.
Patient appears depressed.	Patient has mood swings, shows little emotion or may be depressed.	Patient able to answer most questions of orientation and general knowledge such as age, date, address, current President's name.	Patient cannot answer most questions regarding orientation or general knowledge.
Variable performance on test items of similar difficulty. Impaired social relations early in course of illness; insecure around others.	Consistent performance on test items of similar difficulty. Impaired social relations later in course of illness; demanding around others.	Able to cook for self, dress, do household chores. Able to find way home.	Unable to perform activities of daily living without difficulty. Gets lost in own community or neighborhood.
Patient shows little motivation in completing tasks on performance tests; however, objective performance is better than own accounts of decline.	Patient tries hard to complete task, at least in early stages; objective performance is worse than own accounts of decline.		

Source: *The 40+ Guide to Health*, Consumer Reports Books, Yonkers, N.Y., 1993.

PART

III

Taking Care of Your Body

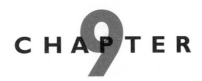

Healthful Eating for a Lifetime

I t's axiomatic that good nutrition is the foundation of good health. Over a lifetime, a proper diet provides energy, maintains the body's growth and functioning, and helps reduce the risk of some chronic diseases. What is less clear is what constitutes a "proper" diet. Although a number of major health authorities agree on the basic tenets of good nutrition, self-proclaimed nutrition experts and purveyors of so-called health foods continue to push their panaceas. And each report of new research, even when it comes from a reputable source, seems to confuse the issue even more.

Throughout most of history, the greatest nutritional challenge was simply getting enough to eat. In developed nations today, the main problem is likely to be *over*nutrition. Add to this a lack of exercise and the result is obesity and its related health problems, such as diabetes and heart disease.

Still, nutritional deficiencies may remain a risk for many people, especially women, whose needs in this area are more complex than those of men. Most women, being physically smaller than men, require fewer calories. As a result, they may also get fewer vitamins and minerals. Pregnancy, nursing, menopause, and weight-loss efforts can all take their toll on your nutritional status.

Variety, balance, and moderation are the watchwords of good eating and a good diet. You can make healthful changes in your diet, such as reducing fat and calories or increasing fiber, without elaborate menu plans or strict limitations. There is no need to give up favorite foods completely. Dietitians point out that there are no "bad foods," only bad diets. And a good diet should allow you to enjoy food, not worry about it!

The information in this chapter is directed primarily toward adult women who are in good health. Individuals who have certain medical conditions, such as high blood pressure, coronary heart disease, gastrointestinal disorders, diabetes, or kidney problems, or who take certain types of medication, such as chemotherapy or some antidepressants, may have special dietary requirements and need more detailed advice. If you are one of these, your doctor is the first person to ask for individualized guidance. Many physicians, however, lack the time and detailed training to offer satisfactory nutritional counseling. Therefore, you may wish to consult a registered dietitian (R.D.). Ask your doctor or local hospital for a referral.

BASICS OF GOOD NUTRITION

Scientists still don't know exactly what constitutes the "perfect" human diet, and some controversies and fine tuning are sure to go on for years. However, the following guidelines, based on decades of careful research, have been devised by the American Cancer Society, American Dietetic Association, American Heart Association, National Cancer Institute, National Heart, Lung, and Blood Institute, U.S. Department of Agriculture, Centers for Disease Control and Prevention, and U.S. Department of Health and Human Services.

1. Eat a nutritionally adequate diet based on a variety of foods. There are more than forty nutrients essential to good health. How do you know you're getting enough of them? The best way is to keep your bases covered: Eat a wide variety of foods, and none to excess.

Today's model for a healthy diet is a pyramid of five food groups. (See Figure 9.1.) Bread, cereals, and other grain products, the pyramid's foundation, should form the basis of most meals—from six to eleven servings a day, depending on the total number of calories that is appropriate for you (see box, "Calculating Calorie Needs"). Next come fruits and vegetables, which should account for five or more servings daily. The next level on the pyramid, dairy and meat products, should be limited to two or three servings of each. At the top of the pyramid are fats, oils, and sweets—everything from salad dressing to candy bars. There's no "requirement" for these rich

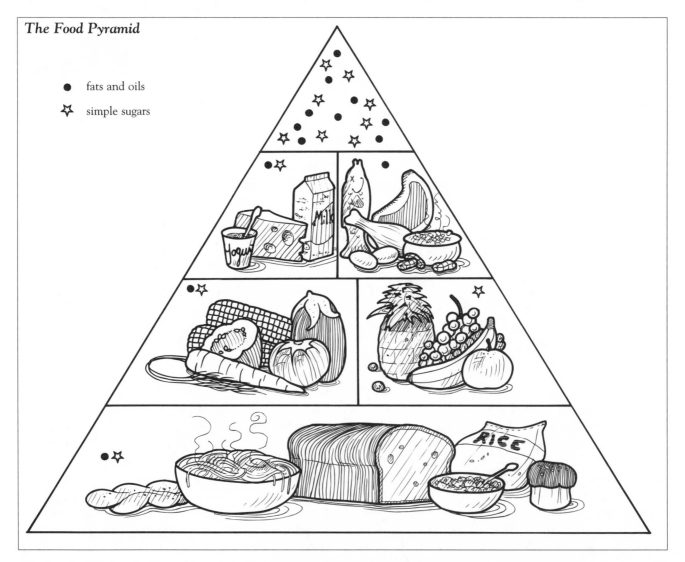

The Food Pyramid

● fats and oils

✪ simple sugars

Fig. 9.1 *The relative importance of the five food groups is easily discernible from the new Food Pyramid developed by the U.S. Department of Agriculture to illustrate that breads, cereals, and grains should be the foundation of our diet, while simple sugars, fats, and oils, at the top of the pyramid, should be used sparingly.*

foods, so eat them sparingly, especially if you are trying to restrict your intake of calories.

At first glance, the pyramid plan may seem to call for eating a surprising quantity of food. However, the plan presents a range of recommended daily servings for all adults. Smaller and less active women, who need fewer calories, should choose from the lower end of the range. Note also that the definition of a "serving" may be quite small. For instance, each of the following equals one serving from the grains group: one slice of bread; half a bun, bagel, or English muffin; one ounce of dry cereal; or half a cup of cooked cereal, rice, or pasta. (See box, "Examples of Serving Sizes.")

2. Choose a diet low in fat, especially saturated fat, and cholesterol. Small amounts of fat and cholesterol are necessary to the functioning of the human body. However, the typical American diet delivers them in excess, mainly through fatty meats, rich desserts, whole-milk dairy products, and high-fat snack foods.

Cholesterol and fat are not the same thing, and not all fats are alike. Here are some guidelines:

Fat. A high-fat diet promotes obesity because fat has more calories, ounce for ounce, than protein or carbohydrates. It may be linked to the development of certain types of cancer. And fat—especially saturated fat—raises the level of cholesterol in the blood, which in turn contributes to atherosclerosis and diseases of the heart and blood vessels.

Ideally, fat should account for no more than 30 percent of all calories in the diet. (For adults, especially those at high risk of heart disease, an even lower fat intake is recommended, although it may be harder to achieve.)

Total dietary fat should be split, roughly equally, among the three main types of fat: polyunsaturated, monounsaturated, and saturated.

Polyunsaturated fats, which are liquid at room temperature, are predominant in safflower, soybean, sunflower, and corn oils. These fats lower the levels of LDL (the "bad" cholesterol) in the blood, but some studies suggest that they may also lower HDL (the "good" cholesterol) in some individuals.

Monounsaturated fats, also liquid at room temperature, are predominant in rapeseed (canola) oil and olive oil. These oils lower LDL cholesterol but do not affect HDL.

Saturated fats are solid at room temperature. High concentrations are found in butterfat, coconut and palm oils, and hydrogenated vegetable oil as well as in meats. They have a greater effect on raising blood levels of cholesterol than dietary cholesterol itself. Replace these fats with those that are less saturated whenever possible, as in cooking.

Cholesterol. All human and animal tissue contains a waxy substance known as cholesterol. Cholesterol in the diet can raise the cholesterol level in the bloodstream (from which it is ultimately deposited on the inner walls of arteries), although not to

EXAMPLES OF SERVING SIZES

FOOD GROUP	RECOMMENDED DAILY SERVINGS	TYPICAL SERVINGS
Bread, cereals, rice, pasta	6–11	1 slice bread ½ bun, bagel, or English muffin 1 oz dry ready-to-eat cereal ½ cup cooked cereal, rice, or pasta
Vegetables	3–5	1 cup raw leafy greens ½ cup other vegetables ¾ cup vegetable juice
Fruits	2–4	1 medium apple, orange, or banana ½ cup small or diced fruit ¾ cup fruit juice
Milk, yogurt, cheese	2–3	1 cup milk or yogurt 1½ oz cheese
Meats, poultry, fish, dry beans and peas, eggs	2–3	3 oz lean, cooked meat (portion about the size of a deck of cards) ½ cup cooked beans 1 egg

the same degree in all people. Limit your consumption of dietary cholesterol—found in all meat, poultry, fish, and dairy products—to no more than 300 milligrams (mg) a day.

There is no need, however, to count cholesterol obsessively or give up eating meat and dairy products. Some foods containing saturated fat and cholesterol, such as meat, poultry, milk, cheese, and eggs, are also valuable sources of protein and other nutrients. Choose low-fat versions of these products when possible, and compensate for smaller portions by eating more complex carbohydrates. Skim or trim all visible fat, and use fats and oils sparingly in cooking.

Many high-fat foods are also high in dietary cholesterol, but not all. Be wary of food labels that announce "No cholesterol." The food may still contain high amounts of saturated fat—for example, palm kernel oil—and are not really "heart healthy" after all.

What do the numbers mean? Calories from fat should constitute no more than 30 percent of the total calories you consume, but how can you tell if you're on the mark? One simple method is to set yourself a daily fat "allowance" based on your calorie needs. (See box, "Keeping Tabs on Dietary Fat.") For convenience, determine your fat allowance in grams of fat, a unit of weight used in food labeling. Then keep tabs on your fat intake by checking the nutrition labels of foods (or, if foods are unlabeled, by looking up their fat content on food tables).

Once you are familiar with the fat content of the foods you eat regularly, making smart choices will become second nature. For example, if you need about 1,800 calories a day (typical for a moderately active woman), you should consume no more than 60 grams of fat per day. Knowing your daily fat quotient helps make it easier to select foods. If you have a choice between an ice cream cone, with 22 grams of fat, and frozen yogurt, with 2 grams of fat, you may choose the ice cream cone, but your selections for the rest of the day will have to be very low in fat if you wish to stick to your goal.

Remember that these guidelines apply to the overall diet, not to each individual food or meal. If you indulge in a high-fat or high-calorie meal, do not punish or starve yourself afterward; just make careful food selections in the next few days.

3. Maintain a healthy body weight. Body weight is the result of two factors: how many calories you consume, and how many you expend ("burn") in exercise. If your weight is appropriate for your height, then your calorie intake is about right for your activity level. If not, then at least one side of the equation must be adjusted: You need to exercise more, consume fewer calories, or both.

Obesity is a major risk factor for heart disease, adult-onset diabetes, high blood pressure, elevated levels of blood cholesterol and blood sugar, and other health problems. Excess weight is especially risky if it is located around the midsection (an "apple" shape) rather than around the hips and thighs (a "pear" shape). A woman whose waist measurement is greater than her hip measurement seems to have a greater risk of developing coronary heart disease, stroke, diabetes mellitus, hypertension, breast cancer, endometrial cancer, and gallbladder disease than one whose proportions are the reverse.

If the weight range listed for your height in the height-weight table suggests that you need to lose weight, the best advice is to set reasonable goals and achieve them through gradual changes in eating habits and modest increases in aerobic exercise. (See section on "Weight Control for Life.")

4. Choose a diet rich in vegetables, fruits, and grain products. In a traditional American dinner, meat is the main course, and grains and vegetables are side dishes. A healthier pattern is just the opposite: meals based on complex carbohydrates (starches) such as rice, pasta, grains, and bread, with generous servings of fruits and vegetables—and rel-

KEEPING TABS ON DIETARY FAT

Fat should make up no more than 30 percent of the total calories in your diet. For a diet of about 1,800 calories a day (what an average woman needs), that works out as follows: 30 percent of 1,800 calories equals 540 calories from fat per day. How much fat is that? One gram of fat contains 9 calories, and 540 calories divided by 9 equals 60 grams of fat.

DAILY CALORIE INTAKE	MAXIMUM FAT INTAKE PER DAY	
	IN CALORIES	IN GRAMS
1,000	300	33
1,200	360	40
1,400	420	47
1,600	480	53
1,800	540	60
2,000	600	67

APPROPRIATE WEIGHT IN YOUTH AND MIDDLE AGE

This height-weight table was published in 1990 as part of the federal government's *Dietary Guidelines for Americans*. Keep in mind:

RISK FACTORS MATTER. Excess weight is a more pressing concern if you also have certain medical conditions, such as high blood pressure, high blood cholesterol, and diabetes, which may improve with weight loss. Ask your doctor.

WEIGHT DISTRIBUTION MATTERS. Extra pounds located around the middle are associated with greater health risk than fat located around the hips and thighs.

HEIGHT (WITHOUT SHOES)	WEIGHT (WITHOUT CLOTHES)	
	Age 19–34	Age 35+
5'0"	97–128	108–138
5'1"	101–132	111–143
5'2"	104–137	115–148
5'3"	107–141	119–152
5'4"	111–146	122–157
5'5"	114–150	126–162
5'6"	118–155	130–167
5'7"	121–160	134–172
5'8"	125–164	138–178
5'9"	129–169	142–183
5'10"	132–174	146–188
5'11"	136–179	151–194
6'0"	140–184	155–199
6'1"	144–189	159–205

FIBER: SOME GOOD FOOD SOURCES

WHOLE GRAIN PRODUCTS: cereals, whole wheat breads and crackers, brown or wild rice, buckwheat groats (kasha), bulgur wheat, popcorn, oatmeal, wheat germ

BEANS AND LEGUMES: navy, kidney, pinto, or lima beans; green or black-eyed peas; lentils

FRUITS: citrus fruits; apples, peaches, and plums (skins intact); raspberries; prunes; figs

VEGETABLES: broccoli, carrots, okra, Brussels sprouts, cabbage (and virtually all other vegetables)

atively smaller portions of meat, poultry, fish, or other protein.

Complex carbohydrates tend to be high in dietary fiber and rich in a wide variety of nutrients. (See box, "Fiber: Some Good Food Sources.") And, despite what many of us have been taught, they are *not* high in calories unless prepared with butter, cream sauces, or cheese toppings.

To include more complex carbohydrates in your diet, try main-dish casseroles or salads based on grains, pasta, beans, and legumes. For snacks, keep plenty of plain, air-popped popcorn, fresh fruit, and raw vegetables on hand. Choose low-fat preparations of complex carbohydrates. For example, instead of french-fried potatoes, have a baked potato topped with freshly ground black pepper, salsa, nonfat yogurt, or low-fat sour cream.

5. Use salt and sodium in moderation. Sodium is a major element in table salt and many other food additives. The human body requires a small amount of it to function properly, but most Americans consume much more than they need. In some people with hypertension, cutting back on sodium may help reduce blood pressure; in others, this may have little effect. It is still unclear whether a low-sodium diet will help *prevent* high blood pressure.

Experts recommend limiting sodium to 3,000 mgs a day (the equivalent of 1½ teaspoons of table salt), or even less if you already have high blood pressure. Most people can reduce their sodium intake with no sense of deprivation. The key is to make the changes gradually. Over time, your taste for salty foods will lessen. Try leaving the saltshaker off the table, and purchase low-sodium alternatives to salty snacks. In cooking replace salt with herbs, spices, and a little citrus juice or grated peel. Whenever possible, choose fresh foods over canned, processed, or packaged versions.

A very low-salt diet may be more difficult to follow because many foods, such as commercial baked goods and canned vegetables, contain "hidden" sodium. Strict sodium reduction may not even be necessary, since not everyone with hypertension is sensitive to sodium's effects on blood pressure. Have your blood pressure checked at recommended intervals (see Chapter 15, "Body Care") and, if it *is* too high, consult your doctor before cutting down on salt drastically.

6. If you drink alcohol, do so in moderation. Alcoholic beverages, with virtually no nutritional value, are the ultimate "empty calories." Given the addictive potential of alcohol, and the major health problems associated with heavy consumption—from high blood pressure to liver damage and accidental injuries—it is clear why moderation in drinking is so important.

For some people, the right amount of alcohol is *no* alcohol. Those who should abstain completely include children and adolescents, pregnant women, anyone planning to drive a vehicle or operate dangerous machinery, persons taking certain medications that may compound the effects of alcohol, and anyone with a personal or family history of alcohol addiction.

For women, "moderate" drinking means having no more than one drink a day, and for men, no more than two. (The difference is based mainly on body size and on the fact that women don't metabolize alcohol as well as men.) One drink equals 12 ounces of regular beer, 5 ounces of wine, or 1 ½ ounces of distilled spirits (80 proof).

Considerable evidence suggests that a moderate alcohol intake may actually reduce the risk of heart disease because it raises the level of HDL (the "good" cholesterol) in the blood and possibly because of alcohol's impact on blood clotting.

The relationship between alcohol and heart disease has caught the public's attention via the so-called French paradox—the finding that while the French eat about the same amount of fat as Americans do, their death rates from coronary heart disease are lower. Some researchers believe that the higher rate of red wine consumption in France accounts for the difference (although research studies here have attributed similar effects to white wine, any type of alcohol, and even pineapple juice!).

In fact, there are several differences in eating habits between the two countries. The French tend to drink their wine regularly and with meals. They also take their main meal at noon; eat more fruits and vegetables, less red meat, and fewer snacks; and get most of their fat from goose fat and olive oil, both of which are high in monounsaturated fats. With so many possible confounding factors, it is difficult to credit red wine alone. Until there is stronger evidence, teetotalers are not advised to take up drinking for their hearts' sake. Although truly moderate drinking will probably do no harm, if you don't drink, the best advice remains: Don't start.

7. Use sugar only in moderation. A glance at a processed food package will confirm that there are many varieties of sugars—not just the white cane type that fills the sugar bowl, but honey, molasses, fructose, corn syrup, and other natural and processed sugars (many of which end in "ose"). They all give a sweet taste, bulk, and texture to foods.

Sugar is not a "poison," as some food faddists have claimed. However, it does provide a concentrated source of nutrient-poor calories, and that poses a potential problem for people watching their weight. Sugar also contributes to tooth decay. (Both natural and processed sugars promote dental cavities, and so do starches, which break down into sugars in the acid environment of the mouth.)

Anyone who has a weight problem is well advised to curtail concentrated sources of sugar, including sweetened soft drinks and candy. Natural sweets like dried fruit are also high in calories, although they have greater nutritional value and some fiber content.

What about artificial sweeteners such as aspartame and saccharine? In theory, they should help cut calories and control weight. In reality, the use of artificial sweeteners does not necessarily lead to weight loss. Perhaps it is because consuming low-calorie products such as diet soft drinks encourages some people to overindulge in other foods. You do not have to avoid artificially sweetened foods and beverages, provided they don't take the place of needed nutrients. Just don't count on them as a weight-loss panacea.

THE ROLE OF VITAMINS AND MINERALS

Vitamins are organic compounds in food that are vital for such diverse bodily functions as building and repairing cells, controlling metabolism, and aiding digestion and blood clotting. A vitamin deficiency produces distinctive symptoms of disease (for example, scurvy in deficiencies of vitamin C). Most foods contain at least small amounts of several of the thirteen vitamins known to be essential to human nutrition, but no food, unless it has been fortified in processing, provides enough of them all. Minerals are inorganic substances, and at least a dozen (some in minute, or trace, amounts) are also essential for good health.

Vitamins and minerals are found naturally in a vast number of foods. And food, not pills, is still their best source. Average, healthy American women who eat a reasonably varied diet will get an adequate supply of both. True vitamin deficiency is rare in this country.

There are three instances when women should take supplemental vitamins: when trying to conceive, during pregnancy, and when breast-feeding. (See Chapter 6, "Pregnancy and Childbirth.") Others who may need a vitamin supplement include heavy smokers, heavy drinkers, strict vegetarians (vegans), those on very restrictive weight-loss diets, people with disorders that prevent them from absorbing certain nutrients from foods, and those on chemotherapy and certain medications.

Although there is no reason to advocate vitamin supplements for healthy women, there is also no evidence that a supplement that provides 100 percent of the Recommended Dietary Allowance (RDA) for each vitamin and mineral will do any harm (except perhaps to the wallet). Doses considerably above this level are another story. Various claims have been made for the preventive or therapeutic effects of taking large amounts, or megadoses, of various vitamins and minerals, but the scientific proof for these claims is slim. Some vitamins and minerals can be taken in amounts far exceeding the body's requirements with no ill effects; others are toxic in high doses or, at the very least, can interfere with the absorption and utilization of other vitamins and minerals. Do not take high doses of any nutritional supplement without your doctor's approval.

Two minerals of particular concern to women are calcium and iron, but simply taking supplements of these nutrients without considering the complexities of their metabolism can raise more problems than it solves.

CALCIUM Vital to forming and maintaining strong bones and teeth, calcium also helps regulate other key bodily processes, such as heart and muscle function. Adequate dietary calcium may also help reduce the risk of high blood pressure. But perhaps the best-known role for calcium is in helping to prevent osteoporosis, the bone-thinning condition that afflicts older people, particularly women after menopause, and makes them prone to serious fractures. (See the Encyclopedia.)

Bone tissue is a dynamic substance that acts as a calcium storehouse for the rest of the body. Because the key period for building bone density is between ages 11 and 25; it is most important to have an adequate intake of dietary calcium, along with weight-bearing exercise, during this time. Later in life, bone density tends to decline, prompted by the hormonal changes of menopause and, in many women, by a lack of activity. Some research suggests that high calcium intake during the years after menopause may help deter osteoporosis, but not as successfully as taking steps early in life to ensure maximum bone density.

Many young women believe that all calcium-containing foods are high in fat and calories. Triple-cream cheese may be best saved for special occasions, but you do not have to skimp on dairy products, the chief dietary source of calcium, to control calories. Instead, choose milk, yogurt, cheese, sour cream, and ice cream in low-fat or nonfat versions.

If you have a lactose intolerance, a condition that makes it hard to digest milk and other dairy products high in lactose (milk sugar), these are some new enzyme products that make these foods more digestible. You may also be able to tolerate aged cheeses like Cheddar, Parmesan, and Swiss, which contain only very small amounts of lactose, and yogurt with active cultures, which produce the lactase enzyme that aids in the digestion of lactose.

If you don't like drinking milk, you can get calcium by using liquid or dry skim milk in cocoa, casseroles, soups, quick breads, and puddings. Other relatively low-fat food sources include water-packed sardines and salmon when eaten with their soft bones. (See box, "Calcium: Selected Good Food Sources.")

How much calcium do you need? According to the RDA, adults 25 and older should get at least 800 mg of calcium a day, or the amount in about three servings of a calcium-rich food. For females aged 11 to 24 and those who are pregnant or breast-feeding, the RDA is even higher—1,200 mg, or the amount found in about four calcium-rich food portions (for example, four cups of skim milk).

Many women consume only about half this amount. If you find it hard to get adequate calcium from food on a regular basis, it may be a good idea to take supplements. Ask your doctor first. A very high calcium intake may cause other problems, such as reduced iron absorption. People at risk for developing kidney stones should heed their physician's advice about calcium consumption. Further, not all calcium supplements are created equal. Bone meal and dolomite may contain high levels of lead.

IRON Insufficient iron is one of the few common nutritional deficiencies in our well-nourished country.

CALCIUM: SELECTED GOOD FOOD SOURCES

The recommended daily allowance for calcium is 800 milligrams (mg) for women over age 24 and girls under 11, and 1,200 mg for women aged 11 to 24.

FOOD	SERVING	CALCIUM (MG)
Milk	8 oz	
skim		302
low-fat (1%)		300
low-fat (2%)		297
whole		291
Yogurt	8 oz	
plain, nonfat		452
plain, low-fat		415
fruit, low-fat		345
Cheese		
ricotta, part-skim	4 oz	337
Parmesan, hard	1 oz	336
Swiss	1 oz	272
Monterey Jack	1 oz	212
mozzarella, part-skim	1 oz	207
Cheddar	1 oz	204
Muenster	1 oz	203
American	1 oz	174
cottage, low-fat (2%)	4 oz	77
Ice milk, vanilla, soft-serve	1 cup	276
Fish		
sardines, canned in oil, with bones	3½ oz	382
salmon, canned, with bones	3½ oz	226
Beans		
bean curd (tofu)	3½ oz	105
white beans, canned	½ cup	96
pinto, canned	½ cup	44
garbanzo (chick-peas), canned	½ cup	39
red kidney, canned	½ cup	31
Vegetables		
turnip greens, cooked	½ cup	99
kale, cooked	½ cup	90
mustard greens	½ cup	75
okra, cooked	8 pods	54
chard, cooked	½ cup	51
fennel, raw	3½ oz	43
Corn tortilla	1 medium	44

Iron deficiency occurs most often in growing children and adolescents, women before menopause (especially those who menstruate heavily), and pregnant women, whose blood volume increases markedly as the fetus grows. Even so, only about 3 percent of women are iron deficient.

Iron is a key player in the transport of oxygen within red blood cells, and a serious lack of this mineral can result in iron-deficiency anemia. Good dietary sources of iron are lean red meat, poultry, fish, and enriched breads and cereals. Some vegetables also contain significant amounts of iron, but in a form that is not as readily absorbed by the body. Foods high in vitamin C, such as fruits and vegetables, help the body absorb iron, while coffee, tea, and high-fiber foods, among others, can interfere with its absorption.

Although iron supplements are available in many formulations without a prescription, you should check with your physician before taking them. Too much iron can be toxic and may interfere with the absorption of some antibiotics; also, too much iron in the body may be a risk factor for heart attack.

WEIGHT CONTROL FOR LIFE

Millions of Americans are overweight, and they spend billions of dollars to remedy the situation, often relying on quick weight-loss schemes that seldom deliver permanent results. Unfortunately, there are no miracle diets, but weight control is possible without constant deprivation. In fact, a "crash" approach to weight loss is not only likely to fail, but may have adverse health effects.

TIPPING THE SCALES Scientists' understanding of obesity is still evolving. Authorities disagree on many issues, including the cause of weight gain. For years it was presumed that overweight people just ate excessively, or were lazy and didn't burn enough calories. Now there is evidence that a tendency to be overweight may be inherited; that this tendency may be related to inborn metabolic rate (the body's "idling speed"); and that overweight people may actually consume the same number of calories as lean people, or even fewer.

WHY DIETS DON'T WORK From the number of diet books on the market, it's clear that many people never stop hoping that sheer willpower, coupled with a drastic change in eating patterns, will melt pounds away forever. Whether the diet regimen is based on a liquid supplement, a single food (say, grapefruit), or has a celebrity endorsement, the same pitfalls exist. When calories are severely restricted, the body reacts as if it were being starved, and metabolism slows down accordingly. This makes it even harder to lose weight, even with eating less food. Physical discomforts such as hunger and lightheadedness sap morale, and the inconvenience of eating tiny or highly selective meals makes it hard to stay the course. Most important, no one can eat in this unnatural manner forever, and when the dieter returns to normal eating, the pounds are likely to come right back on, a phenomenon called "yo-yo dieting."

Yo-yo dieting may carry risks of its own. Rapid weight loss can cause the body to shed muscle tissue rather than fat, and can result in dangerous heart rhythm irregularities. Preliminary evidence suggests that yo-yo dieters tend to gain back more weight as fat than as lean body mass (muscle), and they regain those pounds around the abdomen. Over time, yo-yo dieting may also increase the risk of heart disease and death, and may be more dangerous than a stable weight that is a few pounds too heavy.

The caution against yo-yo dieting is not meant to suggest that overweight people give up and stay obese, but, rather, that they accept more modest weight-reduction goals. Some obesity experts suggest that the greatest benefit to health may come from losing only 5 to 10 pounds and keeping them off permanently—even if you remain overweight.

THE RIGHT WAY The only effective way to lose excess weight, and keep it off, is to make gradual, *permanent* changes in your eating habits *and* to exercise. Set reasonable goals: Adjust your daily intake of calories to lose no more than a pound or two each week. (See box, "Calculating Calorie Needs.") Adapt new dietary habits that you can live with and enjoy. (See box, "Weight-Loss Tips.")

The best way to cut down on calories without drastic cuts in portion size is to replace high-fat, calorie-dense foods (potato chips, cheese, nuts, and chocolate) with low-fat, complex carbohydrate foods (unbuttered, air-popped popcorn or fresh fruits and vegetables). It seems that this is also the most effective way to lose weight. Diet experts once believed that all calories were created equal. Now there is overwhelming evidence that excess calories from fat are more likely to end up as fat on the body than an equal number of excess calories from carbohydrates or proteins. A lower fat intake, combined with a gradual increase in activity level, will lead to slow but steady weight loss.

One of the most successful methods for making permanent changes in your eating habits is to keep a food diary. In this diary, keep track of what you eat and how much, when, and why (when hungry, nervous, bored, to be sociable or polite), and how you feel afterward (satisfied, stuffed, tired, angry). Rate your actual hunger on a scale of 1 to 5. Keep the diary for at least a week to see weekday and weekend eating patterns before you attempt any changes. Then use it to analyze your relationship to food.

The purpose of the diary is not to police what you eat (although this may happen). Rather, it is to help you design a way of eating that works for you. For example, if you find that you eat between meals, you can plan for this by saving a piece of fruit, a roll, or some yogurt from each meal to have as a snack. If you tend to eat when you are bored or under stress, you can make up a list of alternative activities to engage in when the urge arises. If your pattern is to delay lunch and then make up for it by overeating, adjust your mealtimes so you eat more regularly, or keep low-calorie snacks on hand when you know lunch or dinner will be late. If you skip breakfast because traditional breakfast food or early-morning eating doesn't appeal to you, plan to eat a midmorning meal or an unconventional breakfast (plain pizza, a mug of soup, a fruit and yogurt shake). If your downfall is snacking in front of the TV, keep your fingers busy knitting or doing needlework instead.

WEIGHT-LOSS PROGRAMS Commercial weight-loss programs help people lose weight, but there is less evidence that people are able to keep it off over the long haul. However, if other efforts haven't worked, a well-run and medically sound program may be helpful, especially if you do best in a structured setting.

Some programs are run by hospitals that have medical oversight, and may include their own line of

WEIGHT-LOSS TIPS

- Plan all of your meals beforehand—at least a day at a time, and preferably a week ahead. This will help you choose a variety of foods and keep you from resorting to old habits at the last minute.

- Never shop for groceries on an empty stomach.

- An occasional taste during cooking may be necessary, but if you find you constantly nibble, try chewing sugarless gum instead.

- Dish out portions in the kitchen, rather than bringing serving dishes to the table. Immediately refrigerate leftovers; freeze them after dinner.

- Take time to enjoy your meals; eat slowly, be conscious of what you are eating, and relax. Do not eat in front of the TV, standing in the kitchen, in the car, on the run, or while reading.

- Eat only at the kitchen or dining room table to limit the number of places (such as the bedroom or den) that you associate with food.

- Do not be tempted to finish what your children leave on their plates. Save it for after-school snacks.

- Brush your teeth or chew sugarless gum right after eating to keep your mind off the taste of the food.

- Cut down on the "empty" calories in alcoholic beverages.

- Drink lots of water or seltzer. Add a wedge of lemon or lime to make even plain water a treat.

- Stock plenty of low-fat, high-fiber snacks, and take them with you to work as an alternative to the candy machine.

- Store snack foods out of sight—in translucent containers, on high shelves, behind closet doors.

- If you go on food binges, know what your "trigger" foods are. If you cannot open a bag of cookies or chips without finishing it, do not keep these foods in the house. If ice cream is irresistible, buy a single scoop, or a lunchbox bag of chips, or a single cookie.

- If you do binge, do not try to make up for it by starving. Just resolve to keep eating sensibly as often as possible.

- Plan ahead before eating out and at parties, too. Know what you are going to order before you arrive at a restaurant. If you are not familiar with the menu, call ahead. For parties, decide ahead of time how many hors d'oeuvres you will eat and pace yourself. See what else is available before you take the first item that is passed. If you must drink, have a wine spritzer. Do not arrive famished. Eat a piece of fruit, a plain roll, or a cup of yogurt first.

- Expect to hit a temporary weight-loss plateau—most people do. Congratulate yourself on what you have lost so far. Check your measurements instead of the scale. You may find, especially if you are exercising regularly, that you have replaced fat with muscle, which weighs more. If the plateau continues for more than 2 or 3 weeks, you may need to adjust your calorie or exercise level to compensate for the new needs of a lighter body. Try reducing your daily calorie intake by 100, or add fifteen minutes to your exercise routine.

---

liquid meal substitute along with intensive behavioral modification. (While still controversial, these liquid diets are not the dangerous liquid-protein regimens that caused several deaths in past years.) These programs are only appropriate for adults who are 30 to 50 percent overweight.

Other programs may offer a range of nutrition counseling, behavior modification, small support groups, and exercise programs, and they, too, may market a line of prepared foods or supplements. Be wary of any program that pressures you to buy these foods or supplements, or that emphasizes quick, short-term weight loss rather than permanent changes in eating behavior and increased exercise.

Before you join any weight-loss program, consult your physician, and find out all you can about the proposed regimen. Experts at *Good Housekeeping* recommend that the program you choose meet minimum criteria. It should provide:

- at least 1,200 calories daily (for women), unless there is strict medical supervision

- a nutritionally balanced diet that includes all the major food groups with at least 50 percent of calories from carbohydrates, 15 to 20 percent from protein, and 20 to 30 percent from fat

- sensible weight loss of no more than 1 to 2 pounds a week

• behavior-modification classes and a program that will help you maintain your goal weight

HOW TO BURN MORE CALORIES Exercise is the other half of the weight-loss equation. In theory, it is possible to lose weight merely by being more active, even without a change in caloric intake. In practice, it may be hard to make significant progress through exercise alone, at least not without fairly athletic levels of exertion. The combination of dietary modification and increased, moderate exercise (such as a brisk daily walk) will definitely result in steady weight loss. Exercising also ensures that more of the weight you lose comes from fat tissue. The same amount of weight that is lost through dieting alone results in the loss of more muscle tissue and less fat tissue than when diet and exercise are combined.

Sedentary women with many pounds to lose can take heart in knowing that they will burn more calories when they perform weight-bearing exercise, such as walking, than their slimmer sisters—their extra weight means that it takes more calories just to move their bodies.

Exercising aids weight loss in another way: It increases your body's muscle mass, which increases your basal metabolic rate (the rate at which the body burns calories for basic functions). This means that you will burn more calories 24 hours a day than someone who weighs the same as you but has more fat tissue and less muscle tissue. (See Chapter 10, "Keeping Fit.")

DESPERATE MEASURES There is no shortage of shortcuts to a slimmer body, but most of them are unsuccessful in the long run or carry a significant health risk.

• **Drugs.** Appetite-suppressant drugs are available by prescription and over the counter, but none is without side effects, some potentially serious. Even without side effects, the pills cannot be used indefinitely. Since they don't promote any real dietary changes, you end up returning to the eating habits that caused you to gain weight in the first place.

• **Devices.** Sweatpants, massage machines, creams, and other gimmicks marketed to "melt fat" simply don't work. Systems claiming to get rid of "cellulite" are also a rip-off. Cellulite is nothing more than ordinary body fat that appears dimpled as a result of the structure of the underlying tissue. Only weight loss will get rid of this fat.

• **Surgery.** Various techniques, such as stapling the stomach to make it smaller or inflating a small balloon in the stomach, have been attempted in cases of life-threatening obesity where rapid weight loss was considered worth the risk. Serious complications can be associated with any of these procedures, as well as with liposuction, a far more frequently performed plastic surgery that involves suctioning or "vacuuming" out fatty tissue.

DIET AND DISEASE PREVENTION

There is growing evidence that a good diet does more than prevent diseases of nutritional deficiency. It may help protect the body against coronary heart disease, high blood pressure, diabetes, and certain forms of cancer. Beware, however, of exaggerated claims for so-called healing foods, individual vitamins, and miracle diets. It takes a well-informed consumer to separate myths from facts about some of these highly publicized foods and nutrients. Following are some of the major sources of confusion.

FIBER: OAT BRAN AND BEYOND One of the big nutritional stories of the last decade was fiber, the portion of plant foods that the human body can't digest.

CALCULATING CALORIE NEEDS

1. Find your appropriate weight on Table 9.3

2. Figure your energy requirement by multiplying your appropriate weight by your activity level. If you are:

Sedentary	multiply by	13
Active	multiply by	15
Very active	multiply by	17

_____
(Appropriate Body Weight) × (Activity Level)

= _____ Calories/Day

3. If you weigh more than your appropriate weight, add calories; if less, subtract.

_____ − 500 = _____ To LOSE 1
(Calories from item 2 above)   pound a week

_____ + 500 = _____ To GAIN 1
                                 pound a week

4. Set your daily goal: _____ Calories

Once an unglamorous substance known only to combat constipation, fiber is now recognized as a possible agent for lowering the risk of coronary heart disease and some forms of cancer, and for controlling diabetes.

There are two types of food fiber. One is *insoluble*, or roughage, found in fruit and vegetable skins and the outer coating (or bran) of wheat kernels. The other is *soluble*, consisting of substances that dissolve and thicken in water. Concentrated sources of soluble fiber include oat bran, beans, citrus fruits, and broccoli.

Fiber regulates the passage of food through the digestive tract: Soluble fiber slows it down, insoluble fiber speeds it up. Both types of fiber absorb water and assist regular elimination by softening and enlarging the stool. A high-fiber diet can also help prevent or relieve diverticulosis (inflammation-prone pouches in the colon wall) and hemorrhoids.

Studies of various population groups have indicated there is a definite connection between high intake of insoluble fiber and low rates of colon cancer. For people trying to control their weight, high-fiber foods can contribute a feeling of fullness without excessive calories, as long as they are not prepared with excess sugar or fat.

Consuming significant levels of soluble fiber, meanwhile, has been shown to help reduce the level of cholesterol in the bloodstream and may help people with diabetes to keep their blood sugar on a more even keel. The amounts used in some studies, however, are far higher than some people would be comfortable eating.

Experts recommend consuming 20 to 35 grams of fiber a day; the average American consumes 12 grams. To get more fiber in the diet, start slowly, and increase your fluid intake accordingly. A sudden increase in fiber, especially if you do not drink enough water, can lead to intestinal discomfort. Try to eat a good source of fiber at every meal. Substitute high-fiber foods (unpeeled fruits, whole-grain bread, popcorn) for low-fiber foods (fruit juice, white bread, potato chips). To make sure your diet includes both soluble and insoluble fiber, choose a variety of foods. (See box, "Fiber: Some Good Food Sources.")

Commercial fiber supplements should be used only for occasional constipation unless your doctor or dietitian advises otherwise. While supplements may provide a concentrated source of fiber, they do not deliver the broad range of nutrients, or the eating pleasure, of naturally high-fiber foods.

FISH AND FISH OILS Fish, except for the ubiquitous canned tuna, is underappreciated and underutilized in the American diet. Not only is fish an excellent source of vitamins and protein, it is also low in fat. A growing body of evidence suggests that certain types of fish may help prevent heart and blood vessel disease. Some studies have shown that people who eat moderate amounts of any kind of fish have lower rates of death from heart disease than people who eat no fish, regardless of other risk factors.

Oily, coldwater fish, such as salmon, tuna, mackerel, and herring, while low in fat compared with many cuts of red meat, are high in a polyunsaturated fat called omega-3 fatty acids. It has been noted that people who consume a lot of this type of fish—for example, Greenland Eskimos—have lower rates of heart disease. Scientists postulate that omega-3 oils, which are present in all types of fish and shellfish, may help prevent blood clotting, which can trigger a heart attack in narrowed coronary arteries. However, fish that are high in these oils also contain somewhat higher levels of total fat than warm-water and fresh-water fish.

The best recommendation is to eat a variety of grilled, poached, or steamed fish and shellfish, preferably three times a week. Canned tuna and salmon (packed in water, not oil) are fine, especially if high-quality fresh seafood is unavailable. Go easy on seafood salads made with heavy, creamy dressings or mayonnaise; breaded or deep-fried fish; and fish with buttery sauces.

Like fiber, fish oil is available in supplement form, but these capsules are not recommended without a physician's approval. Some supplements may be high in calories or cholesterol, and may not be safe for those taking aspirin or blood-thinning medications. Moreover, it is still not clear whether it is the omega-3 oil or some other substance in fish that makes it beneficial.

Some women are concerned about eating fish and shellfish during pregnancy. In general, fish is safe and an excellent source of protein for mothers and their fetuses. Flounder, sole, and catfish are examples of fish that can be eaten without restriction. Notable exceptions are fish likely to be high in methylmercury and polychlorinated biphenyls (PCBs). Mercury tends to accumulate in fish with long life spans, such as fresh tuna, swordfish, and shark. These should be limited to no more than once a month during pregnancy and breast-feeding. Canned tuna has been found to be low in mercury and can be eaten several times a week.

Although PCBs have been banned, residual levels are still found in some freshwater lakes and rivers and in ocean bays and harbors. If PCBs are present, salmon, lake whitefish, and other fatty fish are likely to be contaminated and should be eaten sparingly, if at all, during pregnancy and breast-feeding.

Eating raw fish or shellfish always poses the possibility of viral or bacterial contamination, and this practice should be avoided at any time, but especially during pregnancy and breast-feeding. Steaming shellfish and cooking fish until it is opaque and begins to flake renders it safe to eat.

If you eat recreationally caught fish, heed local contamination warnings that are posted at water's edge, published in local newspapers, or distributed with sportfishing licenses, or check with your state department of natural resources or local department of public health.

ANTIOXIDANT VITAMINS AND BETA-CAROTENE

Recent research in more than 87,000 female nurses, as well as studies in men, has shown that people who regularly consume foods that are high in beta-carotene and other carotenoids, vitamins C and E, and in some cases, vitamin E supplements, have a lower risk of heart disease and stroke than those who do not. Other studies suggest that eating fruits and vegetables rich in these vitamins, known as antioxidants, may also reduce the risk of cancer.

It seems that antioxidants help control the damage caused by chemicals called free oxygen radicals, which are a by-product of the body's normal metabolic processes, but are also found in cigarette smoke, polluted air, and rancid food. Free radicals may weaken body cells' defenses against carcinogens (cancer-causing substances) and they may also promote cardiovascular disease by converting LDL cholesterol into a form that clogs arteries.

Beta-carotene is found in carrots, sweet potatoes, cantaloupe, and other dark yellow and orange fruits, as well as in broccoli, spinach, and other green leafy vegetables. Vitamin E is found in some vegetable oils, seeds, nuts, green leafy vegetables, liver, certain cereal grains, and egg yolks. Good sources of vitamin C include red and green peppers, broccoli, Brussels sprouts, cauliflower, strawberries, and oranges.

Most nutrition experts are not ready to suggest taking supplements of antioxidant vitamins. Current evidence is not sufficient to prove that it is the vitamins themselves and not some other substances that are truly protective. For now, the best advice is still to eat a wide variety of fruits and vegetables, and be sure to get at least five servings a day.

SPECIAL SITUATIONS The basics of proper nutrition are the same from childhood to old age, but physiological and life-style changes can shift the emphasis considerably.

• **Adolescence.** Around puberty, a girl begins to need more of two important minerals: iron (to replace that lost through menstruation) and calcium (to build bone mass). During this time of rapid growth, she also needs more calories than she will as an adult.

The teen years are not known for sensible eating, however. Girls may alternate between junk-food overeating and ill-considered efforts to lose weight. During this period they are at special risk for eating disorders.

The best approach for parents is to set a proper example, make low-fat, nutritious, and appealing foods readily available, and be willing to talk about diet fads and worries without sounding judgmental. Short-term food jags or binges won't do any permanent harm; but if an adolescent girl is seriously over- or underweight, a doctor's advice should be sought.

• **Pregnancy and Breast-Feeding.** Pregnant women need higher levels of all vital nutrients (especially iron and calcium) to keep up with their bodies' rapid changes. Many doctors recommend taking prenatal vitamin supplements, especially if morning sickness makes it temporarily hard to eat enough food for adequate nutrition. Ask your doctor for specific recommendations.

In particular, folic acid supplementation may help prevent birth defects of the neural tube (the developing spinal cord). Because these birth defects occur in the first month of pregnancy, women need to get protective amounts of folic acid even before they realize that they are pregnant. For this reason, the U.S. Public Health Service now recommends that all women of childbearing age consume 0.4 mg of folic acid daily. Good dietary sources of folic acid include leafy dark green vegetables, citrus fruits and juices, bread, dried beans, and fortified breakfast cereals.

Women who breast-feed continue to need a higher calorie intake with a focus on nutrient-dense foods. (See Chapter 6, "Pregnancy and Childbirth.")

• **Nutrition and Older Women.** Before menopause, women are less likely than men to develop heart disease, but after menopause they tend to lose this edge. Women in middle age and beyond are also more apt to be overweight and to develop Type II (non-insulin-dependent) diabetes. All these factors make it prudent to follow a low-fat diet in later life.

Calcium is still vital to older women, and may help offset some of the effects of osteoporosis.

The nutritional needs of the elderly have been poorly researched, and much is still unknown. However, it is well established that older people of both sexes are at increased risk for borderline nutritional status, for several reasons. A more sedentary life usually means a lower calorie intake, which narrows the "safety margins" for good nutrition. Many older people live alone or on fixed incomes, and may feel disinclined to purchase or prepare meals as carefully as when their families were at home. Medical condi-

tions like arthritis, poor vision, or memory loss can make it difficult to prepare meals and dental problems can interfere with proper chewing. In addition, many older people take one or more types of medication, whose side effects can affect appetite or digestion (including causing dry mouth).

Older people who find it a challenge to stay well nourished should look into mealtime programs at senior or community centers, or consider sharing meals informally with neighbors or family members. In this oldest age group, it is less important to restrict fat and cholesterol; the main thing is to enjoy a diet that is as varied, convenient, and affordable as possible.

CHAPTER 10

Keeping Fit

Most women know that they should make exercise a regular part of their lives, and many do. More than six million American women, ranging in age from the teens to the seventies, jog regularly to keep fit. Some thirty million women walk for exercise. Nevertheless, 1992 figures indicate that more than half the population is relatively inactive, and that fewer than 10 percent of all Americans over 18 exercise regularly and vigorously.

Perhaps women have been discouraged by the "no pain, no gain" attitude of exercise enthusiasts, or by the exercise prescriptions given them by doctors. Perhaps they have felt that becoming fit and healthy means training for a 10-kilometer run. Indeed, that was the message until very recently. Today, however, it is accepted that you do not have to exercise rigorously to reap the health benefits of physical activity. Many ordinary activities—weeding the garden, walking briskly, taking the stairs rather than the elevator—increase your odds of living a long, healthy life.

The American Heart Association sums up the new approach by saying that "even modest levels of exercise can be helpful, if done regularly and long-term." The federal Centers for Disease Control and Prevention, the American College of Sports Medicine, and other groups joined together in 1993 to recommend that every American adult engage in thirty minutes or more of moderate activity, such as brisk walking (3 to 4 miles an hour), at least 5 days a week.

The greatest gain comes from not being categorized as "sedentary," rather than from seeking the fitness level of the dedicated athlete. A major 8-year study performed at the Institute for Aerobics Research and the Cooper Clinic in Texas suggests that sedentary individuals can substantially reduce their risk of death from heart disease and cancer by walking briskly for half an hour a day.

DEFINING FITNESS

Fitness can be defined as the ability to exercise or carry on daily activities without undue distress or fatigue, as well as being able to respond effectively when extra exertion is called for. Fitness has three major components: stamina, strength, and flexibility. Many experts consider a fourth component of total fitness to be control of body fat or maintenance of a reasonable fat-to-muscle ratio. For women, body fat should account for no more than 30 percent of total weight. (See Chapter 1, "The Female Body.")

In terms of daily activities, fitness is the ability to climb stairs without breathlessness or aching legs (stamina), to carry heavy bags of groceries without difficulty (strength), and to stoop and bend with ease (flexibility). Physical skills such as coordination and balance, which are important to success in various sports, are not essential to general fitness.

At the turn of the century, housework and laundry were done by hand and going shopping meant walking. Today, our jobs and our daily lives place relatively few physical demands on us. We have to look actively for ways to keep fit. We have to exercise.

THE MANY BENEFITS OF EXERCISE

Exercise leads to fitness and also, in a wider sense, to good health. Exercise makes the body trimmer, the bones stronger, the joints more flexible, the digestion and elimination more efficient, and sleep more satisfying. For many it staves off depression and anxiety. It promotes a more positive self-image and better powers of concentration.

Even moderate exercise helps prevent heart and blood vessel disease by strengthening the heart muscle and increasing its blood output. It lowers blood pressure and total blood cholesterol while increasing the levels of high-density lipoproteins (HDL) in the bloodstream. The American Heart Association has recently concluded that lack of exercise is a major risk factor for coronary heart disease, along with cigarette smoking, high blood pressure, and high blood cholesterol levels.

Exercise helps ward off adult-onset diabetes and helps control insulin-dependent diabetes. It can help prevent the pain and loss of joint mobility that can accompany osteoarthritis. Moreover, many of the body changes that traditionally accompany aging—increased body fat, decreased muscle and bone mass, shallower breathing, poorer circulation, depressed neuromuscular function, decreased flexibility—may be slowed or in some cases totally avoided by exercising regularly. And it is never too late to start: Stud-

ies suggest that even frail elderly women can increase their strength, muscle mass, and mobility by following a gentle resistance-training regimen.

Athletic women, especially those who started exercising as girls, are less likely than sedentary women to develop breast cancer. The reason for this seems to be that women who are active begin menstruating at a later age. They also have a smaller percentage of body fat—and it is theorized that fatty tissue releases cancer-promoting hormones. Many athletic women also have less premenstrual tension and shorter periods.

Exercise is an essential part of any weight-loss and weight-maintenance program. It counters overweight in two ways: It increases your caloric use (see box, "Exercise and Calories") and it conserves and even increases your body's lean tissue (muscle), which in turn increases your metabolic rate. Because muscle tissue requires more energy than fat tissue, you will burn more calories than someone of the same weight who has more fat tissue and less muscle tissue. It's not surprising that exercise devotees who have lost weight find it easier to maintain the loss than non-exercisers.

A plus is exercise euphoria, the much-talked-about "runner's high." After about 30 minutes of vigorous exercise, the body begins to produce opiatelike hormones, called beta-endorphins, which both deaden pain and bring a feeling of happiness and tranquillity. These calming aftereffects last for an hour or more. Experts have noted that conditioned athletes produce more beta-endorphins more quickly than people who are not as fit.

Women who exercise not only gain fitness and increase their chances of living a long and healthy life, they also feel good about themselves. A University of Pittsburgh study of healthy, "moderately active" middle-age women bears this out. The participants in the study were asked to give their reasons for exercising. The top reason given was to achieve or maintain fitness (28 percent); the second was just to "feel good" (21 percent); the third was to lose or maintain weight (15 percent).

A BALANCED PROGRAM

A balanced exercise program has three components, corresponding to the three main fitness components: aerobic exercise for stamina and calorie burning, resistance or weight training for strength, and stretching exercises for flexibility. (See box, "Guidelines for Developing an Exercise Routine.")

GUIDELINES FOR DEVELOPING AN EXERCISE ROUTINE

- Include activities that will develop all three major components of fitness: endurance, strength, and flexibility.

- Exercise regularly in order to gain maximum benefit. Three sessions a week are the minimum for cardiovascular fitness. For weight loss, five to seven sessions a week may be necessary.

- Include at least 5 minutes of warm-up and another 5 minutes or more for cooling down.

- Start off slowly, to avoid injury and soreness.

AEROBIC EXERCISE Aerobic exercise is any form of physical activity that uses large muscle groups (for example, those of the legs and the arms) in continuous repetitive action to raise the heart rate and increase the body's demands for oxygen. "Continuous" is the key word: Long-distance running is aerobic; sprinting isn't.

Regular aerobic exercise conditions the cardiovascular system—that is, it improves the efficiency of the heart, the blood vessels, and the lungs. A strengthened heart muscle can pump more blood with each beat. It can rest longer between beats, both during exercise and at rest. Blood vessels that are stronger and more elastic offer less resistance to the flow of blood and thus help lower the blood pressure.

Cardiovascular conditioning occurs when you exercise hard and long enough to raise your heartbeat for significant periods at regular intervals. According to the American College of Sports Medicine, this means exercising three to five times a week, at least twenty minutes each time, with your heart beating at a rate that is between 60 and 90 percent of its maximum rate (known as the target zone). You estimate your maximum heart rate by subtracting your age in years from 220. For example, if you are 40 years old, your estimated maximum heart rate is 180 beats a minute and your target zone is between 108 and 163 beats a minute. (See box, "Target Zones.")

The maximum-heart-rate formula holds true for most forms of exercise. New research, however, shows that it should be adjusted for swimming and other primarily upper body exercises. The maximum heart rate for swimming is about 13 beats per minute lower than for running. To adjust the formula for swimming, subtract your age from 220, then subtract 13 from your answer to get your maximum heart rate. As with other exercises, multiply the rate by 60 percent, then 90 percent, to get your target zone.

Exercise at less than 60 percent of maximum provides little conditioning; exercise at more than 90 percent is quite strenuous, of no added benefit and, for some people, may be dangerous. If you have been sedentary, however, you may have to work up to 60 percent gradually. Nor is it necessary to strive for 90 percent, unless you are very fit and you are benefiting from your efforts.

To be certain that your heart is beating within the target zone and you are getting the cardiovascular benefits of your efforts, you have to take your pulse as you exercise. Do a 10-second pulse check every 5 to 10 minutes and multiply the count by 6 to get your

TARGET ZONES

AGE	TARGET ZONE—60–90% (BEATS PER MINUTE)	AVERAGE MAXIMUM HEART RATE
20	120–180	200
30	114–171	190
40	108–162	180
50	102–153	170
60	96–144	160
70	90–135	150

heart rate. (Keep moving as you count; if you have to stop, record your heart rate immediately, since the heart rate drops very quickly when exercise ceases.) If your pulse is below the target zone, work a little harder; if it is above, slow down.

After a while, you will be able to tell without counting whether you are exercising at the target rate. In fact, some experts recommend a method called the rating of perceived exertion (RPE), in which you rate on a scale of 6 to 19 how hard you think you are exerting yourself. For example, a rating of 6–8, which corresponds roughly to a pulse rate of 60 to 80 beats a minute, is very, very light; a rating of 13–14, or somewhat hard, corresponds to a target heart rate of about 70 percent of maximum; and a rating of 19 is very, very hard. Others suggest that you exercise at a level at which you can still carry on a conversation. You should feel that you are pushing yourself; but if you work so hard that you are too winded to talk, this is too much exertion.

As you become fitter from regular exercise, your heart will beat more slowly. (It is not uncommon for your exercise heart rate to drop by 10 to 20 beats per minute during regular exercise training.) If you do not increase the intensity of the exercise, your pulse will not reach the target zone. So, every 6 to 10 weeks, you may find that you must step up your exercise program.

Cardiovascular conditioning is the main focus of the aerobic component of a balanced exercise program. However, aerobic exercise has other important benefits. Because it increases the body's metabolic rate (the rate at which it burns fuel), it is a key factor in weight loss and maintenance: The more you exercise, the more calories you burn. And exercise strengthens and improves the long muscles and the bones to which they are attached.

Best examples—brisk walking, running, jogging, swimming, cycling, aerobic dancing, jumping rope, stair climbing, cross-country skiing, rowing

RESISTANCE (WEIGHT) TRAINING A fit body is a strong body. Women need muscle strength for all the lifting and carrying and pushing and pulling that they do, and also to bear the effort of most aerobic exercise.

Muscles grow stronger, firmer, and somewhat larger when they work against resistance—lifting weights, for example, or pulling against an opposing force, or working against body weight in push-ups and chin-ups. Tendons and ligaments, which connect muscle to bone, also become stronger when they work against resistance. In addition, muscle action during exercise contributes to the building of strong bones by increasing their calcium uptake.

Regular resistance training builds and strengthens muscles, increases endurance, tones and trims the body, and helps prevent musculoskeletal injuries and back problems. Contrary to popular belief, moderate resistance training does not produce a bulky, body-builder look.

The role of resistance training in building strong bones is particularly important for women. With their thinner bones, women are at high risk for developing osteoporosis as they grow older. Many experts believe that resistance training can build up a protective reserve of bone mass sufficient to prevent this crippling disease.

A balanced weight routine designed to strengthen all the major muscle groups—legs, hips, chest, arms, shoulders, back, and abdomen—involves eight to ten exercises and takes 20 to 30 minutes to perform. The American College of Sports Medicine recommends a light to moderate routine two to three times a week, with a day off between sessions to allow muscles to recover.

Best examples—weight machines, such as Universal or Nautilus; hand-held or free weights, such as dumbbells and wrist/ankle weights; cross-country ski machines and rowing machines; push-ups and similar calisthenics. (Free weights may cause injury if used improperly. It is suggested that novices begin with weight-training machines and move on to free weights when they are stronger and more skilled.)

FLEXIBILITY Flexibility is the ability of a joint to move freely through its full range of motion—for example, arms and legs that can flex freely and extend,

EXERCISE AND CALORIES

How many calories you use when exercising depends on several factors:

• *How much you weigh.* The more you weigh, the more calories your body must use in moving around.

• *How long you exercise.* Exercising harder and faster only slightly increases the calories expended. The better way to burn more calories is to exercise for a longer time and increase the distance you cover.

• *Air (and water) temperature.* Exercising in cold air, especially when lightly dressed, uses extra calories because your body must keep warm. In cool water, the added metabolic stress is even greater because water conducts heat away from the body at a significantly faster rate than does air at the same temperature.

The following table shows the approximate calories used, per minute, in various activities, by a person weighing 127–137 pounds.

ACTIVITY	CALORIES
Aerobic dancing	6.58
Bicycling, 5.5 mph	3.58
10 mph	6.16
stationary, 10 mph	6.25
Calisthenics	4.50
Gardening, weeding and digging	5.75
Golf, hand cart	3.75
Hiking, 20-lb pack, 2 mph	4.50
Jogging, 5.5 mph	9.75
8 mph	11.90
Rope jumping, 55 per min	7.58
95 per min	9.75
Rowing machine, easy	4.50
vigorous	9.75
Sawing wood by hand	5.83
Skiing, downhill	8.83
cross-country, 5 mph	10.41
cross-country, 9 mph	14.83
Snow shoveling, light	9.08
heavy	15.66
Stair climbing, normal	6.70
rapid	14.80
Walking, 2 mph	2.80
4 mph	5.20

or a spine that can bend with ease. A flexible body bends and reaches without putting strain on the muscles. Flexibility is developed slowly, day by day, just as strength is.

Exercises for flexibility—stretches—are an essential part of any fitness program. Done correctly and regularly, stretching increases the joints' range of motion, improves athletic performance, and helps to prevent strains and injuries.

Flexibility may help prevent back problems, which affect approximately four out of five people in their lifetime. Experts agree that one of the best ways to prevent back distress involves keeping the hamstring (back of thigh), stomach, and hip muscles—all of which help support the spine—strong, well stretched, and flexible.

Flexibility also promotes good posture. In turn, the ability to carry oneself with seemingly effortless grace promotes self-confidence.

Most experts agree that 10 minutes or more of daily, light stretching is beneficial. Stretches should be done slowly, without bouncing, almost to the point of hurting. The idea is not to increase repetitions, as with weight training, but to hold the stretch and gradually increase its duration. You can begin by holding each stretch for at least 10 seconds and work up to 30 seconds.

The best time to stretch is not before exercising but afterward, when the muscles have warmed up and are less likely to be injured. (Do not confuse this with warming up the cardiovascular system before engaging in aerobic exercise. This warm-up is important, and it can consist simply of starting the exercise slowly—walking before you run, swinging your arms before aerobic dancing, and so forth.)

Best examples—calisthenics, Hatha yoga, t'ai chi, and movement-awareness approaches, such as the Feldenkrais Method and the Alexander Technique.

THE MINIWORKOUT

Experts usually advise that you work out 30 minutes or more, three times a week. However, a recent study at the Stanford University School of Medicine suggests that three daily 10-minute sessions may have the same benefits as the traditional 30-minute workout, when they are performed at the same intensity. These miniworkouts seem to increase metabolic rate and blood flow and improve oxygen intake just as much as the longer sessions.

If you cannot set aside a regular workout time, try to accumulate 45 minutes of physical activity every day by making small changes in your daily routines: climb the stairs rather than take the elevator, park the car at a distance, get off the bus or subway a few stops early, and so on. This approach is most useful for the sedentary, as it tends to provide the health benefits of exercise rather than the purely fitness benefits.

BEFORE YOU START

Before you embark on a vigorous new program, or significantly increase your present amount of exercise, it is a good idea to consult your doctor. A preexercise checkup is strongly advised for people over 40 who have not been exercising regularly and for anyone with a known medical problem. The American Heart Association recommends that you see your doctor first if you have uncontrolled high blood pressure; frequently experience pain or pressure in the chest, neck, shoulder, or arm after exercising; are extremely breathless after mild exertion; have bone or joint problems; often feel faint or have spells of severe dizziness; or if you have a medical condition requiring special attention, such as insulin-dependent diabetes.

If you are seriously overweight or are otherwise at risk of heart disease, your doctor may advise that you take an exercise-tolerance (stress) test to assess your cardiovascular fitness. In this test you pedal a stationary bicycle or walk on a treadmill at ever-increasing speed while an electrocardiogram is taken and the blood pressure and pulse rate (and possibly also oxygen consumption) are measured. Because there is some risk associated with a stress test, it should be done only by a health professional and only in a facility equipped to deal with any emergency that might arise.

THE EXERCISE ROUTINE

Creating a balanced exercise routine is highly personal: You need to find an activity you truly enjoy—and the time in which to do it. At first, fitting workout sessions into a busy week may require a bit of juggling. Yet once you experience its positive health benefits, the workout should become a natural and pleasurable part of your daily routine.

There is no one way to get fit. Your own personal likes and dislikes are the best guides to developing a program you can stick to. If you like disco music and have a good sense of rhythm, aerobic dancing would be a good choice. If you want companionship, you could take cycling, skating, or exercise classes at the local Y. If you prefer to go it alone, there is walking, jogging, or jumping rope. If you enjoy competition, tennis or racquetball might fit the bill. Other considerations: whether the exercise is an indoor or an outdoor activity as well as what it will cost in equipment, fees, and club memberships.

Cross training—alternating and combining several different activities—is one of the best ways to achieve a balanced workout. It is also one of the best ways to beat boredom, which is the main reason people give up exercise programs. Different activities develop different components of fitness. For example, bicycling is good for endurance and for strengthening your leg muscles, but it does not increase overall flexibility or exercise your arms; yoga is fine for flexibility, but it does not promote either strength or endurance. Cross training allows you to work your whole body, lessens the chances of injury from overdevelopment or overuse of the same set of muscles, and provides a sense of accomplishment and control. A mix of activities also makes it easier to combine exercise with socializing, which for many women is an important part of an exercise program.

The weekly schedule of a cross-training enthusiast might include a low-impact aerobic-dance class at the Y or exercise studio, swimming, a yoga class, and two resistance-training sessions. Or daily 30-minute aerobic walks might be supplemented by a twice-weekly stretch-and-tone video and a tennis date on the weekend.

Once you have found an exercise program you enjoy, you must fit it into your schedule. What time of day you work out is a matter of personal preference: There is no "right" time. Some people find that exercising early in the morning gets them going for the day; others like the change of pace that a midday exercise break provides; still others prefer an evening session that allows them to wind down after a busy day. Some women plan their workouts at the beginning of each week, just as they would schedule meetings and appointments. Others schedule a session each day, knowing that some will be forgone, in order to end up with at least three workouts a week.

STAYING INJURY-FREE

If you have not been exercising regularly, starting slow is imperative for protecting both your cardiovascular and your musculoskeletal systems. Warm up for at least 5 to 10 minutes to let your heart and

EXERCISING SAFELY

- Warm up before exercising by doing a slow and gentle version of the chosen exercise.

- Cool down after exercise, slowing down your activity and allowing your pulse to return to normal.

- If you have chest pains (which may be accompanied by pain in the arm, neck, shoulders, and jaw), stop exercising immediately and seek medical help.

- If you feel dizzy or nauseated or extremely breathless, stop exercising. Check with your doctor.

- If you experience pain in a joint or muscle, do not try to work through the pain. Switch to an exercise that does not hurt. If the problem persists, see your doctor.

- If exercising leaves you markedly fatigued, check with your doctor before working out again.

- Do not exercise when the temperature is above 90°F or the humidity is 80 percent or more. Humidity slows the evaporation of sweat, which allows the body temperature to rise, placing extra strain on the heart.

- Do not exercise when the wind-chill factor is −20°F. In very cold weather, protect your face and hands against frostbite and wrap a loose-knit scarf across your mouth to warm the air you breathe.

- Drink plenty of cool (not iced) liquids before, during, and after exercise, especially when the weather is hot and/or humid.

- Wait 4 hours or more after drinking alcohol before you exercise, and at least 2 hours after eating a heavy meal.

- Do not tackle too much too soon. Increase the intensity and duration of your exercise gradually.

- If you find you don't have enough breath to talk or sing during exercise, slow down. You are pushing yourself too hard.

muscles adjust. The easiest warm-up is simply to start your chosen exercise at a slower pace: If you plan to run, start by walking a few blocks, or take some slow practice swings before you start your tennis game.

Stretching is important, but you risk injury if you try to stretch cold muscles. You can stretch after your initial warm-up, but many experts advise stretching during your cooldown. To let your heart rate gradually return to normal, cool down for at least 5 minutes, longer if you stretch then.

Learn to recognize warning signs that you may be overdoing it (see box, "Exercising Safely"). Although it is manifested in different ways, pushing too hard can cause problems for amateurs and experienced athletes alike (see box, "Young Female Athletes: A Warning").

WORKING OUT AT HOME: EQUIPMENT

There are many advantages to working out indoors at home. There is no need for a gym bag, nor do you have to fit your workout into someone else's schedule. You do not have to contend with traffic or dogs or polluted air, or rainstorms and extremes of heat and cold.

Fitness equipment for use at home can run the gamut from a jump rope for a few dollars to a complete home-gym unit costing several thousands of dollars. The choice you make will depend on your exercise goals, the amount of money you have to spend, and the space you have available. For aerobic conditioning, you might consider getting a rowing machine, a stationary bicycle, an adjustable step, or a jump rope. For muscle building, there are home gyms with bars, weights, and steppers; free weights such as dumbbells and ankle weights; and jump ropes with weighted handles. An exercise mat is basic equipment for stretching and flexibility exercises. Be sure to try out any equipment before you buy it, at a friend's house, at a health club (as a guest or on a 1-day pass), or at the store. Many hotels now offer health facilities free or at a small daily rate to their guests, another good way to try out equipment, *if* the facility is supervised by knowledgeable staff. Some manufacturers allow you to purchase equipment on a 30-day trial basis.

YOUNG FEMALE ATHLETES: A WARNING

Both men and women are afflicted by athletic injuries, but young women athletes who engage in long-distance or endurance sports are especially vulnerable to knee problems, shin splints, ankle sprains, and stress fractures. This was confirmed in a 1993 report of a 13-year study of 60,000 young athletes in the Seattle area, in which female cross-country runners topped an injury list that ranked eighteen activities, even including damage-prone sports like football and wrestling. Female gymnasts and ballet dancers are also vulnerable to such injuries.

Biological factors predispose women athletes to certain injuries. For example, women have wider hips than males, and a sharper angulation of their thigh bones, meaning that the muscles on the insides of the knees are weaker than in men. This sets the stage for chronic knee problems at an early age among women runners.

Biological and hormonal factors also increase a woman's vulnerability to premature osteoporosis. Many of today's star athletes—especially Olympic long-distance runners, gymnasts, and skaters—start training at a very early age, usually before puberty. These young athletes have low levels of estrogen, and their intensive athletic training keeps them excessively thin. Consequently, many experience delayed puberty, and some never achieve their full growth potential because they do not undergo the normal adolescent growth spurt. Their continued low estrogen levels prevent them from developing maximum bone density, which normally occurs at about age 30. Some may even be losing bone mass at a time when they should be building it, leading to stress fractures and early osteoporosis.

Exercise physiologists generally recommend that young women should not run more than 30 to 40 miles a week, and for many, even that may be too much. Any woman who trains to the point where she stops menstruating should seriously reevaluate her priorities in light of the long-term consequences for her health.

WORKING OUT IN COMPANY

Many women have found that joining a health club is an important part of keeping fit. The club offers the companionship of other exercisers; instructors to provide supervision, ensure that the equipment is used to best advantage, and prevent beginners from doing too much too quickly; and sophisticated machines that provide positive reinforcement by reporting the number of calories burned and miles covered. Health clubs can be expensive, but if investing in a membership keeps you participating regularly, your dollars will be well spent. Many Ys have upgraded their facilities to be competitive with health clubs at a more moderate cost.

Evaluate several facilities before you sign a contract. (See box, "Considering a Health Club?") Request guided tours and when you've narrowed down your choice, ask for a 1-day pass so you can try out the machines or take an exercise class.

You do not have to join a full-facility health club to have companionship as you exercise. Commercial exercise studios offer a variety of options. Aerobic dance and other classes are available at many YWCAs and YWHAs. New Age centers offer classes in yoga and t'ai chi. And many colleges and schools make their swimming pools available to the public.

WALKING: THE BEST BASIC WORKOUT

There are numerous reasons why 30 million American women walk for exercise. Walking needs no special equipment, just a pair of good shoes. It can be incorporated into everyday routines. It is virtually injury-free (walking subjects the joints to stress that is equivalent to only one and one half times the body weight, in contrast to three to five times in running). Because walking is less tiring, it can be sustained longer, especially in hot weather. Fitness professionals and doctors alike consider walking the best basic workout for anyone of any age and body weight.

Casual walking is an excellent way for a sedentary person to begin to exercise, priming the body for future fitness. (See box, "Tips on Walking.") If you have been sedentary, start out with a leisurely 20-minute stroll every other day. When this regimen becomes comfortable, add 10 minutes to the walk, or increase your speed, or include another strolling day in your routine. Strolling (at about 2 miles an hour) limbers up the body and is a pleasurable activity.

TIPS ON WALKING

- Warm up first with 5 minutes or more of slow strolling and gentle arm swinging.

- Cool down after your walk, slacking your pace for the final 5 minutes. Then stretch the muscles of the legs, arms, and shoulders.

- Walk on a flat surface that allows you to move without interruption (a track is ideal).

- Do not overdo it. Consider alternating fast-paced-walk days with leisurely strolls.

- After 6 weeks of flat-surface walking, challenge yourself with hilly terrain or a long hike.

- In cooler weather, wear layers of loose, comfortable clothing (preferably cotton) that you can remove easily as your body heats up; top off your outfit with a visored hat and a jacket made of material that can withstand wet weather.

- Invest in a pair of good comfortable shoes. Shoes for walking should have moderately stiff sides to provide stability, a beveled "crash pad" on the heel to absorb the shock of the stride, and a moderately cushioned flexible sole.

However, it confers little cardiovascular benefit unless your fitness level is quite low. For most people, brisk walking (at 3½ to 5 miles an hour) is beneficial. Walking at this speed is often called fitness walking.

The technique of fitness walking is only a slight exaggeration of the normal walking style. It is not the odd gait of race-walkers, with their abrupt, switching movements of hips and shoulders.

Posture is important. Your chin should be tucked in, shoulders relaxed, stomach pulled in, and buttocks tucked under so that the small of your back is flat. As you stride out, your heel strikes the ground first, at a 45-degree angle. As your body moves forward, your weight rolls along the outside edge of your foot to the toes, for the push-off into the next step.

In regular walking, your arms swing at your sides, with very little muscular exertion. In fitness walking, they are held bent at a 90-degree angle and are pumped vigorously. On the forward swing, your elbows come up to chest height, on the backward swing, they are level with your shoulder blades. Your fists, gently clenched, just brush the sides of your body. These vigorous arm movements greatly increase the aerobic benefits of the walk as well as strengthen the torso and the arms themselves.

CONSIDERING A HEALTH CLUB?

If you are thinking about joining an exercise facility, consider first how you would use it. If you just want to take an aerobics class, you won't need a full-fledged health club. If you want to cool off in the pool after class, or have a snack or use the sauna, then a full facility may be right for you. Get recommendations from friends and visit several facilities. Make a checklist for evaluating them. Consider the following:

The Staff

Are the instructors certified? Reputable certifications come from the American College of Sports Medicine, Aerobics and Fitness Association of America, International Dance Exercise Association, Institute for Aerobics Research, and National Athletic Training Association. All of these groups require their instructors to be certified in CPR.

Are the instructors trained in the use of the equipment and in handling any medical emergency that might arise?

Does the staff take a medical history and design an individualized workout program for each new member?

If you are interested in taking exercise classes, be sure to observe one. Does the instructor give individual attention to students, correct technique, and make sure no one overdoes it? Is the emphasis on safety and having fun, or on pushing everyone to the maximum?

If you are interested in using weight machines and other equipment, will an instructor show you how to use them safely and effectively? Is the weight room staffed or will you be on your own once you learn the basics?

The Facility

Is the location convenient to home or work? Does the club have adequate parking or is it near public transportation?

Be sure to visit at the time you would use the facility. Is it crowded after work or understaffed at midmorning?

If you are interested in weight training or aerobic exercise machines, is there a variety of machinery—weight machines, stair climbers, rowing machines, treadmills, bicycles—to give you a complete workout? Are there enough of them or are people waiting in line to use them? Are they all in working order? Can they be adjusted to individual fitness levels?

Is the club—including locker rooms and showers—clean, well lit, and odor-free?

The Deal

Does the cost of membership include the use of all the facilities or must you pay extra for classes or court fees? If you do not intend to use the racquetball courts, for example, then a high court fee won't bother you, provided the basic membership is lower than at an all-inclusive club. However, if the options that interest you are not part of the standard membership, you may end up paying a lot more to use the facilities.

Is the membership flexible? If, for example, you become ill and cannot use the club for 3 months, is there a freeze policy that extends your membership?

Be very wary if you are being pushed to sign on the spot to get a better price, or if the club promises expansion in the future. Ask for a contract to take home and study.

When you are ready to sign up, ask for a trial membership or a guest pass. Take a class and speak to the instructor. Discuss any health problem or restrictions you might have and find out how willing the instructor is to adapt exercises to you.

Finally, talk to members. Are they satisfied with the level of service? Would they sign up again?

Managing Stress and Promoting Emotional Health

Defining stress would be the logical way to begin this chapter, but even the experts can't agree on a definition.

Dr. Hans Selye, who first researched stress and its health effects in the 1930s, defined it as the body's response to certain demands. Stress can be caused by monotony and boredom as well as change and excitement. Moreover, an event can be both stressful and pleasurable, and one person's stress may be another's pleasure.

The subjective nature of stress and its causes (stressors) has led to one theory that the major cause of stress is feeling a lack of control. Thus, when people feel they have no control over their relationships, their work, or their lives, they feel stressed. If that is true, then modern life is filled with stress.

Environmental circumstances, such as noise and odors, can be stressful, but here again, control is a significant factor. People can adjust to noise if they know they can control it, even if they decline to do so. In contrast, people who are exposed to a constant drone or a persistent odor that they cannot control may not be conscious of the irritant after time, but their bodies still may react to the low-level stressor. In some, this stress may lead to health problems; in others, it seems to have no ill effects.

Stress can also be caused by your perception of an event rather than the event itself, making it harder to recognize. For example, the stomach ache you develop while having dinner with friends may be written off as a stomach bug or a reaction to spicy food rather than as unrecognized conflicting feelings about someone at the gathering.

The seemingly arbitrary nature of stress and stressors makes it difficult to determine objectively how many of us are under stress, how stress affects health, and if women are affected more than men. Still, many people consider that they are under stress. Results from the 1985 National Health Interview Survey of 34,000 people found that 18 percent of men and 23 percent of women felt they had experienced "a lot" of stress in the 2 weeks prior to the survey. Moderate stress was reported by 31 percent of women and 32 percent of men. (See box, "Types of Stress.")

Stress seems to have a cumulative effect; the greater the intensity, frequency, and unpredictability of the stressors, the greater the chance that your health will suffer. Even so, not all stress is bad. In fact, without some stress, life would be dull and uneventful. Mild stress pushes us to achieve more and improve performance. Stress is also vital in times of real danger, producing sudden surges in strength, alertness, and reaction time to cope with unknown or dangerous situations. This response to stress accounts for superhuman feats in life-or-death situations, such as outrunning an attacker or singlehandedly lifting an impossibly heavy object to free a trapped child.

HOW THE BODY RESPONDS TO STRESS

Although the nature of stress varies considerably, the body's response to it is relatively constant. Faced with a perceived danger, the body channels all available energy into resisting or escaping it—the well-known "fight or flight" response. Instantaneously, the pituitary gland releases ACTH (adrenocorticotrophic hormone), which in turn spurs the adrenal glands, located atop the kidneys, to release several corticosteroid hormones, including noradrenaline and epinephrine (adrenaline).

These hormones act on different organ systems to halt temporarily unnecessary functions such as digestion and channel the body's resources to increasing the heartbeat, sharpening the senses, and raising the blood pressure. The liver quickly converts stored glycogen into blood sugar for instant energy. By increasing the amount of energy available to the brain, the muscles, and the heart, the body equips itself to "fight or flee."

While this response can be lifesaving in a dangerous situation, it can threaten your health when you are faced with chronic or frequent stress, especially in reaction to false alarms. For example, waiting in traffic or disagreeing with your boss can trigger the same metabolic responses as a narrowly avoided accident—your heart races, breathing gets shallow, blood flow to the muscles and the brain increases, muscles tense, and digestion slows down.

Without an outlet for the excess energy produced by this reaction, organs throughout the body may suffer. In fact, the American Academy of Family Physicians estimates that 50 to 60 percent of all illnesses are stress related. For example, frequent unresolved stress can lower resistance to disease by depressing the immune system. Increased blood pressure can damage the heart and blood vessels. Normal digestive and reproductive functions may also be hampered and the muscle tension caused by stress can lead to aches and pains.

Stress may be a factor in the development or outcome of a number of diseases, including peptic ulcers, ulcerative colitis, irritable bowel syndrome, and other intestinal disorders; heart disease, high blood pressure, asthma, rheumatoid arthritis, and allergies. People under stress often complain of anxiety, headaches, backaches, dizziness, palpitations, and fatigue. (See box, "Signs of Stress.") In women, stress may produce or worsen menstrual irregularity, premenstrual syndrome, and sexual dysfunction.

Stress may also contribute to substance abuse and addiction. For example, women under extreme stress often resort to alcohol or drugs to calm their nerves, promote sleep, or overcome fatigue. Food may also become a way to cope with stress: Overeating, bulimia, and anorexia nervosa have all been linked to stress.

Symptoms caused by stress, or illness exacerbated by it, is just as real as illness due to infection or injury, and should be regarded that way by physicians. In addition to (or instead of) conventional therapy, however, the doctor may recommend alternative therapies such as biofeedback training, dietary changes, meditation or other stress-management techniques.

TYPES OF STRESS

Stress can be classified into four types:

- ACUTE: a brief and intense reaction, such as to a narrowly avoided car accident

- SEQUENTIAL: when several stressors coincide, such as experiencing a near car accident, then arriving home to find the house has been burglarized

- CHRONIC BUT INTERMITTENT: such as a monthly doctor's appointment to monitor a disease in remission

- CHRONIC AND ONGOING: such as caring for an aging parent

SIGNS OF STRESS

Nervous habits: biting your nails, pacing, clenching or grinding your teeth

Physical symptoms: headaches, backaches, fatigue, digestive problems, and sexual or menstrual problems

Sleep problems: can't get out of bed in the morning

Lack of concentration: can't find your keys or remember what you were doing, or switch tasks every minute or so without following anything through

Skipping regular exercise routine

Guilt feelings about relaxation

Misusing food, alcohol, or drugs: Eating a pint of ice cream to cheer yourself up, having a drink to relax, or taking pills to help you sleep

STRESS, PERSONALITY, AND HEALTH

The so-called Type A personality, first described in the 1960s by Drs. Meyer Friedman and Ray Rosenman in their study of patients with heart disease and high blood pressure, has become a stereotype of the hard-driving, short-tempered executive barking orders while chain-smoking cigarettes.

While this may be extreme, many men do fit the definition: competitive, impatient, suspicious, hostile, and quick-tempered. (See box, "Signs of Type A Behavior.) Type A women, although they share the achievement orientation and "hurry sickness" suffered by Type A men, are seldom overtly antagonistic. In fact, they are apt to turn their anger inward while outwardly being cordial and considerate.

Type A men tend to focus their compulsions on work and perhaps sports. Many Type A women add marriage, parenting, and homemaking to that list. The pressures on these women can be enormous unless they can learn to modify some of their Type A traits or find appropriate outlets for relieving their stress.

A lack of these traits constitutes what Friedman and Rosenman called the Type B personality. However, labels can be somewhat misleading. Most of us do not fall neatly into either category. Some people may exhibit classic Type A behavior in one aspect of their lives and be very relaxed and noncompetitive (although no less successful) in most other situations. Other people may display some Type A qualities, such as achievement orientation and the need always to do two things at once, yet do not exhibit some of the more destructive traits, such as hostility or distrust.

Researchers have identified another stress-related personality trait—stress addiction, a tendency to find stress exciting and to actively seek out situations that test one's mettle and produce a surge of adrenaline. In fact, Dr. Paul J. Rosch, president of the American Institute of Stress, believes that stress addicts and Type A individuals may well be addicted to their own adrenaline. For example, business executives may be attracted to their particular job because of its fast pace and the constant source of stress it provides (and thus the steady stream of stress hormones).

Animal studies indicate that constant stress can eventually cause death. In people, results from the Boston Area Health Study, conducted by JoAnn E. Manson, M.D., show that Type A personalities may have an increased risk of heart attack because of lower levels of protective high-density lipoprotein (HDL) cholesterol. Dr. Manson's study found a 50 percent higher risk of heart attack in Type A personalities, presumably due to low HDL levels. (HDLs carry cholesterol away from body tissue, thereby reducing the buildup of fatty deposits in the arteries.)

SIGNS OF TYPE A BEHAVIOR

- Doing more than one thing at a time
- Irritability and impatience
- Interrupting others or finishing their sentences for them
- Competitiveness (even if it is not overt)
- Aggressiveness
- Suspiciousness and hostility
- Compulsiveness
- Chronic anger (in women, often suppressed)
- Perfectionism
- Excessive concern for approval from others
- Overscheduling and feeling constantly driven by time
- Feeling as if you were always in a hurry (also known as "hurry sickness")

Not everyone is affected by stress in the same way, however. In some situations, stress may actually have a protective effect. Researchers at the Minneapolis Veterans Administration Medical Center found that stress may induce the body to produce beta-interferons, which in turn produce lymphocytes, which help protect against disease. In a study conducted by the National Cancer Institute, it was shown that women with breast cancer who actively expressed anger and frustration with their disease had higher numbers of tumor-killing cells than women who were resigned to their condition. Perhaps in this case, the fight-or-flight response enables the body to fight the cancer.

THE CAUSES OF STRESS

By some definitions, just living causes stress. Anyone attempting to list the possible causes of stress might find a litany of opposites. (See box, "Some Causes of Stress.")

In the mid-1960s, two psychologists, Thomas H. Holmes and Richard H. Rahe, developed "The Social Readjustment Rating Scale," based on surveys of stressors men and women experience. They then ranked forty-two different life events according to stress level. The death of a spouse, for instance, was rated the most stressful, with a score of 100 points. A minor brush with the law (perhaps a traffic ticket) scored 11 points. The researchers concluded that a person whose life experiences produced a score greater than 300 points in one year had an 80 percent chance of becoming seriously ill.

More recently, Dr. Georgia Witkin, director of the stress program at Mount Sinai Medical Center in New York, found that many women could not identify with the Holmes-Rahe scale. Relationships, work, internal pressures, and having to juggle multiple roles all cause stress for them. To determine what stressors women would add to the list, Dr. Witkin polled 2,300 women in 20 states and also conducted 238 personal interviews. She found that they rated most stressors much higher than Holmes and Rahe. For example, in the 1960s survey, the death of a close friend was given 37 points; the 1990s survey gave that experience a score of 68. (See box, "Social Readjustment Rating Scale.")

The good news is that many stressors are also the best antidotes for stress. While marriage may be stressful, the companionship and partnership it offers can do much to relieve the pressures of a hectic work-

SOME CAUSES OF STRESS

This list illustrates how stress can be caused by myriad and seemingly opposite events and circumstances. This is just a partial list; feel free to add your own stressors.

RELATIONSHIPS

Marriage	Being single
Divorce	Making a relationship work
Raising children	Infertility
Proximity to family	Separation from family
Children growing older	Parents growing older
Demands of friendships	Lack of friendships
Obligations to the community	Feeling isolated and alone

WORK

Fear of failure	Fear of success
Tedious work	Demanding work
Too few resources	Not enough time
Lack of authority to make decisions	Too many decisions
Too much responsibility	Too little responsibility
Commuting	Setting up a home office
Working with others	Working alone
Lack of flexibility	Lack of routine

ENVIRONMENTAL AND OTHER SOURCES

Clutter	Housecleaning
Moving	Feeling financially trapped (by mortgage)
Job	Unemployment
Holidays	Everyday routine
Entertaining	Loneliness

day. And while work may be hectic and sometimes frustrating, a job well done offers a sense of achievement that can improve self-esteem, and work associates can become a supportive network in times of personal crisis.

WORK STRESS

Nearly 75 percent of all American women work outside the home, creating another major source of stress. The potential increases if the woman works in

SOCIAL READJUSTMENT RATING SCALE

LIFE EVENT	NEW POINT VALUE	OLD POINT VALUE
Death of spouse	99	100
Divorce	91	73
Marital separation	78	65
Jail term	72	63
Death of close family member	84	63
Personal injury or illness	68	53
Marriage	85	50
Fired at work	83	47
Marital reconciliation	57	45
Retirement	68	45
Change in health of family member	56	44
Pregnancy	78	40
Sex difficulties	53	39
Gain of new family member	51	39
Business readjustment	50	39
Change of financial state	61	38
Death of close friend	68	37
Change to different line of work	51	36
Change in number of arguments with spouse	46	35
Mortgage over $10,000	48	31
Foreclosure of mortgage or loan	55	30
Change in responsibilities at work	46	29
Son or daughter leaving home	41	29
Trouble with in-laws	43	29
Outstanding personal achievement	38	28
Spouse begins or stops work	58	26
Begin or end school	45	26
Change in living conditions	42	25
Change in residence	47	20
Change in school	36	20

Source: *The Female Stress Syndrome: How to Become Stress-Wise in the '90s*, Second ed., Georgia Witkin, Ph.D., Newmarket Press, N.Y., 1991. Used with permission.

a traditionally male-dominated field or if she constantly feels challenged to prove her worth.

Women who are successful in their careers may fear that this makes them less attractive to men. On the other hand, women who fear failure may be reluctant to take the necessary risks to succeed in the work world. Self-employed women (more than half of self-employed people are women) or those who run their own businesses may worry where the next check or client will come from.

Even though women have made inroads in the business world, they are more likely to hold positions of less authority. Women whose jobs involve very little autonomy—such as assembly-line workers or clerk-typists—have very high stress levels. Women who reenter the work force after spending several years rearing their children or following a divorce take on the additional stresses of adjusting to an office environment. Add to that the fact that women still earn about 70 cents for each dollar made by men—yet another source of frustration and stress.

However, staying home may not be the answer. Full-time homemakers certainly are not immune to stress. A job—even one with little autonomy and inadequate pay—can be an important step toward independence, self-esteem, and taking control of your life.

INTERNAL STRESSORS

Striving for unrealistic perfection may subject some women to excessive and unnecessary stress. They may worry unduly about their appearance or their health, and try every fad diet that comes along. Women often harbor negative thoughts—"I can't get that job," "I'm too fat," "I can't seem to make time for exercise," "I'll never get this work done on time"—instead of positive feelings: "It's worth a try," "I feel good at this weight," "I'm going to take the time to exercise," and "I know I'll do my best with this project."

Many women also seek approval from others rather than validating themselves. The very ability that allows women to be sensitive and considerate of others sometimes blocks their ability to trust their own feelings. Seeking self-confidence or self-esteem through the approval of others means relinquishing control. Trusting our own positive opinions about ourselves puts the control back in our hands.

MULTIPLE-ROLE STRESS

While going to work can be a relief from pressures at home, and sitting down to dinner with the family provide the best antidote to a bad day at the job, both situations can result in high levels of stress. This stress of multiple roles seems to be unique to women.

In a study of managerial employees at Volvo in Sweden, researchers found that while men's stress levels (measured by blood pressure and epinephrine levels) decreased markedly when they arrived home after work, the women employees' stress levels remained high. Having to prepare meals and do other household chores kept the women on edge, while the men took the opportunity to relax.

Sometimes the problem arises from unrealistic expectations about how roles should be fulfilled. Women who grew up in traditional households often expect to prepare a full dinner, keep the house spotless, and give the children undivided attention—just as their mothers did. Only, more likely than not, their mothers had all day to accomplish these tasks, instead of a few hours sandwiched into a workday. Women who take on multiple roles often need to let go of some of their high expectations and perfectionism in order to juggle their responsibilities more successfully.

Many men, too, have been brought up with an outdated role model—that of the father who sits down to read the paper or watch TV after work while his wife prepares dinner and tends to the house and children. Even though studies show that most men believe that working spouses should share household tasks equally, women still end up doing most of the chores.

Ironically, while taking on several roles can increase women's stress level, adding even more may reduce it. The nature of their responsibilities can have a great influence on mental and physical health, too. For example, sociologists at Indiana University have found that women who combine marriage, work, and parenting may experience more stress than women who take on one or two additional roles, such as part-time student or community volunteer. These roles may reduce stress by providing an outlet and a break from other responsibilities.

Another study, this one at the University of Pennsylvania, found that women who take on multiple roles actually were in better health than women who concentrated on performing just one function. This might be due to the increased social contacts and self-esteem that come from having many interests and activities.

RELATIONSHIPS

According to many women, relationships are the most frequent causes of stress. In fact, of the stressors most often added to Holmes and Rahe's original list (see section on "The Causes of Stress"), more than two thirds concerned interpersonal relationships.

Whether the cause is nature, nurture, or both, women tend to place greater importance on connectedness than men. Although relationships are very important to men, sociologists say, men focus more on independence and personal achievement than on intimacy and interdependency. While males see themselves in a hierarchical structure in which self-worth is measured by how far up the ladder they are, females view their friends and/or co-workers as peers with whom they gain favor by being connected.

Because women place greater importance on relationships, they often wind up taking on more responsibility for maintaining them. Connections to the larger communities of family, friends, and acquaintances figure prominently in the way they perceive themselves. They may regard failure to maintain a relationship as a personal failure. Depression in women has often been linked to changes in personal relationships. Still, these relationships are also an important source of joy and fulfillment and significantly reduce the detrimental effects of stress.

REDUCING STRESS

Considering where stress comes from is the first step toward reducing it; the next step is to develop ways to lighten the load. Managing time effectively, setting realistic goals and priorities, delegating responsibility, consciously letting go (as opposed to giving up), are all important ways to regain control over your life. You will be better able to manage the stress that you can't avoid if you get proper nutrition and sufficient exercise, and practice relaxation techniques. By making time for the basics, you acknowledge that your own emotional and physical well-being are important. That affirmation of the self may be the best medicine of all for stress.

GETTING ORGANIZED AND MANAGING TIME One of the most common sources of stress is having too many tasks and too little time to perform them. There are a number of good books that can help you make more efficient and effective use of your time and organize your life, your home, and your office. Most recommend that you establish goals, set priorities, and then arrange your life so that you will be able to manage them. Thinking about where you want to be 5 years from now can be daunting, however, when you are not sure how you will get through tomorrow. Ultimately, establishing short- and long-term goals is an excellent way of getting control of your life, but you may want to start with a few less "global" techniques.

Many women find that making lists can release pressure almost immediately. Just committing to paper all the must-do's can make you feel less anxious. Most list keepers describe a great feeling of satisfaction each time they cross a completed task off the list (and some even admit adding already completed tasks just so they can cross them off!).

Daily and weekly to-do lists are just the beginning. Think about developing a master shopping list, a list of gift ideas for family and friends (you would be surprised how many hints you can pick up in conversation during the year that will make birthday or holiday shopping less frantic), and a master house-maintenance list (so you'll know when to have the furnace serviced, for example). The more routines you develop, the less time you have to dwell on mundane things. Don't think of it as giving up spontaneity, think of it as stealing time to be spontaneous about the things that really count.

GETTING HELP, DELEGATING, AND LETTING GO Allow other people to help you. At home, children, spouses, or roommates can work together on chores such as cooking and cleaning. It's important to work together as a family to develop a household plan so that each member can have a say in the new system. Even young children can assist in the kitchen by setting the table (if you don't mind how they arrange the flatware!) or getting a pot out of the cupboard.

Families that can afford to hire someone to clean or cook often find it's more than worth it. Other chores that someone besides you can do are personal bookkeeping, laundry, grocery shopping, and gardening. Today, there are many creative businesses that will do your gift shopping, organize your wardrobe, or plan your child's birthday party, for example, so if possible, take advantage of their ingenuity.

Once you can accept help from others, you can start delegating authority. At home or work, try to farm out tasks that require the least amount of instruction to be done right. You can also assign several tasks at once and prioritize them to avoid constant interruptions.

After you have become accustomed to delegating tasks, you can begin to delegate authority. If you consciously decide to surrender control of a project, you are not giving up anything, but choosing instead to concentrate on things that are worth your time and energy.

Letting go can be very difficult for many women. They feel responsible for so many problems and conflicts over which they have no control. Women often think there must be a way to fix every problem, even those not theirs to fix.

When you delegate authority, you must learn to accept that other people will do things differently—and that is not necessarily bad. When the kids do the cooking, they may make a great mess; or your assistant may plan a meeting differently than you might have. Try to accept these differences. Remember that you are giving someone else the opportunity to grow. You may gain a new perspective or even discover a better way of accomplishing a task.

The final phase of letting go is coming to terms with not doing everything you once thought you should. What would happen if you skipped a meeting to take some time to be by yourself or with family and friends? Ask yourself what attending a particular event will mean to you in a few months or years. Then ask the same question about the necessity for meticulous housekeeping, gourmet meals every night, saying yes to everyone who asks your help.

PROPER NUTRITION Diet is often the first thing to suffer in times of stress. When your body does not get the nourishment it needs to function effectively, nutrient stores are depleted. You become fatigued and more susceptible to disease. Sugary snacks, caffeine, and alcohol may give temporary boosts, but all are self-defeating stopgaps. (See Chapter 9, "Healthful Eating for a Lifetime.")

EXERCISE Regular aerobic exercise helps fight stress and fatigue by strengthening heart tissue, lowering blood pressure, enhancing blood circulation, increasing muscle strength, and improving lung capacity. A physical workout can energize and relax the body at the same time.

Our stressful society provides ample opportunity to rev up our engines in anticipation of challenges.

However, societal restraints rarely allow appropriate outlets for this physiological preparation for "battle." Exercise is an ideal release for the pent-up tension and excess energy. Strenuous exercise may also increase the production of endorphins—body chemicals that enhance well-being—thereby countering stress. (See Chapter 10, "Keeping Fit.")

RELAXATION TECHNIQUES By consciously resting the body and clearing the mind of disturbing thoughts, relaxation techniques stop the brain from sending out messages of danger. The mind must send positive, rather than stressful, messages to the muscles. The real benefit of relaxation is to learn to turn off negative thoughts and give the body a break from the constant onslaught of stress.

Total relaxation is different from sleep. Relaxation is also different from inertia. It takes concentration and effort to relax because your mind remains awake, receptive, and alert while your muscles slacken and become limp. Very few people can relax on demand. In fact, the simple words "just relax" can often heighten tension.

There are various ways to relax, from something as simple as sipping a hot cup of herbal tea and reading a favorite novel to painting, gardening, listening to music, or walking. Spending time with close friends or family can also be relaxing. A recent study at the University of Miami found that people's blood pressure levels were highest in the presence of strangers and lowest when they were with their families.

While some people find it easy to relax once they have the time, others need more help. Many people learn more formal relaxation techniques from a book, therapist, or class. For instance, yoga and t'ai chi include specific movements to release tension from the muscles progressively, while meditation involves remaining still and focusing the mind on releasing tension.

You must find the technique that is appropriate to your needs and vary it to suit the circumstances. For example, you can use progressive relaxation to relax specific muscles during the day, while a half hour of meditation or yoga may be more appropriate after work.

PROMOTING EMOTIONAL HEALTH

Psychiatrists have long contended that women are more susceptible to emotional problems than men. Sigmund Freud, the founder of psychoanalysis, explained female psychology in terms of "penis envy,"

Progressive relaxation, developed in the 1930s by Dr. Edmund Jacobson, acknowledges the importance of relaxation and how difficult it is for many people. By practicing this technique regularly, Dr. Jacobson and his patients found that they could learn to relax almost instantly. Over the years, people have relieved headaches and backaches and managed stress by practicing relaxation techniques.

Progressive relaxation is based on the idea that by consciously tensing and relaxing a muscle, you can let go of residual tension in that muscle. To illustrate, shrug your shoulders up as high as you can. Hold them there for a few seconds, then breathe out and release the shoulder muscles. Feel the tension go out of your shoulders. This also helps identify tight muscles by pointing out the difference between tension and relaxation in a particular part of the body.

There are several different ways to practice progressive relaxation. Many people record the steps (see below) on tape and play them back, others have someone else read the steps aloud to them. And commercially made tapes are available that take listeners through the steps.

Most people start out sitting in a comfortable chair in a quiet, dimly lit room. If you find that you fall asleep, try changing the time of your practice session (wait at least 1 hour after eating) or hold something loosely in your hand. If you fall asleep, the item falling to the floor will wake you up.

For best results, practice progressive relaxation twice a day at the same times each day. It will take at least a week of regular practice to master the technique. Then you should be able to relax certain muscle groups almost instantly.

1. Sit with both feet on the ground and your arms at each side. Use a pillow to prop up your head. Close your eyes. Alternatively, this exercise can be done lying down (see Figure 11.1).

2. Start by relaxing the muscles in the face: Breathe in and squeeze your eyes tight shut. Hold your breath for 5 seconds, then breathe out and release. As you do this, say to yourself, "Relax and let go" or simply "Relax" or "Release."

Fig. 11.1 *By tightening each group of muscles in turn for 5 seconds and then relaxing them, you can learn to release tension and relieve stress.*

PROGRESSIVE RELAXATION

3. Push your tongue against the roof of your mouth. Hold for 5 seconds. Release.

4. Clench your teeth. Hold for 5 seconds. Release.

5. Frown as hard as you can. Hold for 5 seconds. Release.

6. Bring your chin to your chest. Hold for 5 seconds. Release.

7. Push your head into the pillow. Hold for 5 seconds. Release.

8. Shrug your shoulders. Hold for 5 seconds. Release.

9. Push your shoulders back. Hold for 5 seconds. Release.

10. Extend your arms in front of you and clench your fists. Hold for 5 seconds. Release.

11. Bend your arms and bring your elbows together in front of you. Hold for 5 seconds. Release.

12. Expand your chest. Hold for 5 seconds. Release.

13. Tighten your stomach muscles. Hold for 5 seconds. Release.

14. Tighten your buttocks. Hold for 5 seconds. Release.

15. Stretch out your legs in front of you and raise them a few inches off the ground. Hold for 5 seconds. Release.

16. With your feet on the ground, try to raise your toes off the ground. Hold for 5 seconds. Release.

17. Spend a few moments concentrating on breathing slowly. As you breathe in, scan your body for residual tension. As you breathe out, imagine pushing the tension out of that area.

18. Remain sitting quietly for 5 minutes. Imagine being in a relaxing place, such as a quiet beach or a deep forest.

19. Open your eyes. Continue to sit quietly until you are ready to resume your activities.

Variations:

1. If you find that you cannot release all the tension in your muscles on the first try, add one more release to each step. This time, relax completely for 15 to 20 seconds before going on to the next step.

2. The steps can be done in virtually any order that works well for you.

3. If some parts of your body are holding tension more than others, invent your own stretching and releasing exercises for those areas.

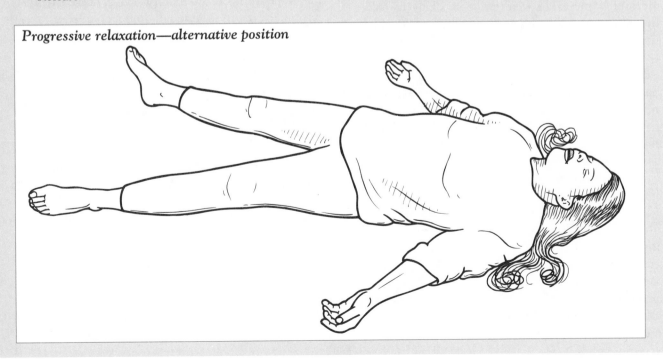

Progressive relaxation—alternative position

holding that male personality traits were the norm, and when a woman recognized that she could not be a man, she "retreated" into what he termed normal feminine personality traits, becoming childish, submissive, masochistic. According to this view, a woman forms dependent attachments to men as a substitute for her missing penis.

Fortunately, this nineteenth-century view of womanhood has changed, with the change in the roles of women in the home, workplace, and society. Some of the mental disorders, such as hysterical neuroses, that incapacitated so many nineteenth-century women have all but disappeared. Still, recent studies show that women today seek professional help for depression, panic attacks associated with agoraphobia (fear of being alone in crowds or open spaces), anorexia, bulimia, and other psychological problems more often than men do. (For specific disorders, see the Encyclopedia and Chapter 13, "Rethinking Body Image.") It is unclear whether women have more mental illness than men or whether they are simply more willing to seek help.

There are suggestions that a woman's social and economic status is an important factor in her mental health. A number of surveys show that women with depression outnumber men about two to one. However, when researchers at Rush-Presbyterian St. Luke's Medical Center in Chicago studied the incidence of depression among divorced and separated men and women, they found an equal distribution between the sexes, with one major exception. Women who had followed the traditional roles of wife and homemaker were twice as likely to suffer clinical depression as men or as women who worked outside the home and who held less traditional views of their role as women.

Even though the role of women in society has changed, there is no denying that women have certain inherent personality traits that differ from those of men. Male and female brains develop somewhat differently from before birth, and behaviorists believe these differences explain why males tend to be more aggressive than females. Gender-related hormonal differences also play a role in personality traits.

Perhaps more important, however, are undeniable cultural biases and traditions. From birth onward, girls are treated differently than boys, and this is reflected in emotional strengths and weaknesses. In almost every culture, little girls are groomed to be nurturing, a characteristic that can have two faces. It makes women more adept at forming friendships and emotional attachments than men, and many believe this explains why women generally fare better emotionally after the death of a spouse. By contrast, women who place overriding importance on being a wife and mother may be overly vulnerable to emotional problems if they are unable to fulfill these roles.

Stress and anger take a psychological toll on both women and men, but in general men cope with these emotions better than women. Typically, women tend to suppress anger and stress, a habit that can lower their self-esteem as well as create physical symptoms. Fortunately, there are a number of effective ways to deal with these problems, and seeking help from a mental health professional no longer has the stigma it once did.

GETTING HELP Help in dealing with mental and emotional problems generally takes three forms: drug therapy, talk therapy (psychotherapy), and self-help. Often, these approaches are used most effectively in combination. Following are brief descriptions of common types of psychotherapy and the mental health professionals that offer them.

TYPES OF THERAPY Psychotherapy of all types is based on verbal and nonverbal communication between the therapist and the patient. All have as their goals the relief of symptoms, which often take the form of painful emotions; changes in behavior and, sometimes, destructive personality traits; and ultimately, self-awareness and understanding. The role the therapist plays in the process, how information is sought, and the predominant goal of the therapy vary depending on the therapy. All of these therapies can take place in individual, group, couple, or family settings, although individual therapy is the most common.

There are basically four major types of therapy, as well as a number of new approaches, sometimes called experimental therapies, many of which help patients fulfill their human potential or achieve self-actualization.

• **Supportive Therapy.** Treatment in supportive therapy focuses on relieving symptoms and restoring coping mechanisms. The most common form of individual therapy, it concentrates on the manifestations of the symptoms rather than attempting to understand their root causes, although this understanding may come as a result. Instead of seeking to make major changes, the therapist guides the counseling process, gives advice and encouragement, and helps bolster the patient's defense mechanisms and coping strategies. Supportive therapy can be used for long-term treatment of psychiatric illness or personality disorders in patients for whom psychoanalysis is inappropriate, but it is more often used in short-term situations for individuals who are otherwise reasonably healthy but unable to cope with current emotional difficulties or a specific life crisis, such as loss of a job or a loved one.

• **Psychodynamic Psychotherapies.** Each of the three therapies in this category, which are based primarily on the work of Freud, have in common the belief that psychological distress and maladaptive behaviors result from unconscious conflicts that often date back to childhood. Rather than focusing on a specific behavior or thought process, psychodynamic psychotherapists help individuals gain insight into their past and the workings of their subconscious mind in order to resolve conflicts and change behavior.

In classic Freudian *psychoanalysis* the analyst plays a neutral role, sitting behind the patient, who lies on a couch and speaks freely. The patient, who may see the analyst 3 to 5 times a week for 3 to 5 years or longer, talks about whatever comes to mind in the process of trying to gain understanding. Freudian psychoanalysis may not be appropriate for a patient in a crisis situation or someone who would have trouble with intense self-analysis.

Psychoanalytic psychotherapy provides more support and intervention from the therapist than does psychoanalysis, is less intense (1 to 3 times a week), and generally shorter (2 to 5 years). Unlike psychoanalysts, who must undergo psychoanalysis themselves as part of their training, psychoanalytic psychotherapists have not necessarily done so.

As its name implies, *brief dynamic psychotherapy* is shorter and more directed than either of the other two preceding therapies. It generally lasts 3 to 6 months and concentrates on a specific problem.

• **Behavioral Therapy.** A type of short-term psychotherapeutic treatment that focuses on changing specific behaviors, this is also known as *behavior modification*. It assumes that behavior and feelings are habitual responses to past associations. It does not attempt to understand the underlying conflicts that may have produced the problem responses or behavior but, rather, concentrates on replacing them with more productive, less stressful actions. Behavioral therapy is particularly effective in treating such problems as anxiety disorders and phobias, eating disorders, and stress disorders.

• **Cognitive Therapy.** Like behavioral therapy, cognitive therapy is short-term, but rather than attempting to change behavior directly, it concentrates on changing distorted ways of thinking that contribute to problems. Its goal is to replace poor and counterproductive coping skills with more productive ones. The therapist helps the individual identify faulty thought processes, and proposes solutions, often assigning "homework" so that the patient can try out new behaviors or ways of thinking.

SELF-HELP So-called twelve-step programs, modeled on Alcoholics Anonymous, that offer a prescribed way to recover from addiction are available for various types of abuse or addiction, from drugs to gambling to overeating. There are also support groups for people who are divorced or widowed, have a chronic or terminal illness, have survived trauma or disaster, or are going through difficult situations. Groups for family members of people in these situations are also available.

Self-help groups offer a useful adjunct to professional therapy. In some cases, where therapy is not available or not affordable, they may provide the only support to an individual. However, many community mental health facilities offer free or low-cost services, and some private therapists have a sliding fee scale.

DRUG THERAPY Some people may resist taking drugs for mental and emotional problems because they fear becoming addicted or suffering serious side effects, or because they feel that drugs will cover up problems without treating them. These fears are for the most part unfounded or outmoded. Several new classes of drugs work extremely well without strong side effects, many of the more addictive drugs are no longer used, and physicians are now more attuned to the possibility of dependence.

Drugs can be particularly effective in helping patients get symptoms under control so that they can function in daily life while they work on understanding the causes of their feelings or behavior. Antidepressants and antianxiety drugs are key components in the treatment of depression, anxiety disorders, phobias, and schizophrenia.

MENTAL HEALTH PROFESSIONALS

• **Psychiatrists.** These are medical doctors (either M.D.s or D.O.s—doctors of osteopathy) who have completed at least 4 years of residency training beyond medical school, 3 of which focus on mental disorders. In addition, some psychiatrists study at a psychotherapy training institute, and the majority choose to become certified by the American Board of Psychiatry and Neurology. Most belong to the American Psychiatric Association.

Psychiatrists are unique among therapists in their ability to diagnose underlying physical illness that may cause or contribute to a mental problem, to prescribe drugs, and to arrange for hospitalization.

Although many psychiatrists act as primary therapists in private practice, others work in institutional settings in collaboration with other health professionals. In these cases, they may supervise medication or see patients referred to them by other therapists for medical evaluation.

• **Clinical Psychologists.** These therapists hold doctoral degrees, which generally require 5 years of course work in various therapeutic techniques as well as supervised clinical practice. In addition, they must pass a licensing exam. They offer a variety of therapeutic services and may work independently or in collaboration with a psychiatrist. Clinical psychologists may specialize in psychological testing and personality assessment or employ a range of psychotherapeutic techniques. Most belong to the American Psychological Association, and some have passed a competency examination given by the American Board of Professional Psychology.

• **Clinical Social Workers.** Social workers represent the largest category of mental health professionals. Also called psychiatric social workers, they hold a master's degree in social work and have completed 2 years of supervised postgraduate work. Some have additional training in psychotherapy. They may practice independently or in collaboration with a psychiatrist and are qualified to treat a full range of mental and emotional problems.

Social workers are licensed or certified in all states, but the accrediting bodies vary. The two major ones are the National Association of Social Workers and the American Board of Examiners in Clinical Social Work.

• **Certified Clinical Mental Health Counselors.** These therapists hold a master's degree in mental health counseling and have been certified by the National Academy of Certified Clinical Mental Health Counselors after completing supervised practice and a qualifying exam. About half the states require licensing for these professionals, but many do not even regulate the use of the title counselor, so it is wise to check credentials.

• **Psychiatric Clinical Nurse Specialists.** Most psychiatric nurses have training or experience beyond general nursing, and work in hospitals, but some who have special training provide psychotherapy to private patients. Psychiatric clinical nurse specialists certified by the American Nurses Association hold a master's degree, have completed supervised practice, have had 2 years of independent practice, and have passed a qualifying exam.

• **Certified Pastoral Counselors.** Although most members of the clergy do some counseling in the course of their work, some complete a training program at a psychotherapy institute or pursue a graduate degree that includes clinical training in crisis intervention. Most states do not require licensure, but the American Association of Pastoral Counselors offers a rigorous certification process for pastoral counselors who have received advanced training, and many of them become full-time therapists.

• **Marriage and Family Therapists.** This is not a specific category of professional therapist, but rather a specialization that may be offered by clinical psychologists, social workers, nurse specialists, or psychiatrists. These specialists treat couples (married or unmarried, heterosexual or homosexual) or families. Within this framework, they may employ various modes of therapy and see patients individually, together, or (with families) in various combinations. The focus is on fostering healthy relationships by improving communication among family members and changing destructive patterns of interaction. Although a few states license or regulate family therapists, in most states, anyone can use the title marriage counselor. In addition to licensing or certification in their professional category, marriage and family therapists may belong to the American Association of Marriage and Family Therapists or the American Family Therapy Association, but neither group certifies individuals.

• **Sex Therapists.** As with family therapists, sex therapists do not belong to a specific category, but some have attended medical-center or institute training programs and are certified by the American Association of Sex Educators, Counselors, and Therapists. (For more information, see Chapter 2, "Sexual Health.")

THERAPY IN PRACTICE Although the therapies described in the preceding section represent the major types, there are more than 450 kinds of therapy. There are also individual and various group settings.

Moreover, many counselors are experienced in more than one type of therapy and may use a hybrid approach or a combination of approaches, depending on what seems appropriate for the particular patient at a specific point in the process. If all this seems mind-boggling, the key factor to focus on is not the correct form of therapy or the right type of professional, but finding the best relationship for you. What makes therapy successful is developing rapport with someone you feel you can trust, who seems to be on your side, who treats you with respect.

CHOOSING A MENTAL HEALTH PROFESSIONAL

There are two general approaches to the search for a mental health professional. You can gather recommendations for therapists, call them and narrow your choices after brief phone interviews, and then make appointments with one or two to determine whom you feel comfortable with. Sources of names include your personal physician, clergy, friends and colleagues, the psychiatry department of a teaching hospital, a local mental health clinic or psychotherapy training institute, and the state or local offices of the associations that certify various mental health professionals. (See Resources.) This approach works well if you have a good sense of your problem—for example, if you are seeking bereavement counseling.

If your problem is more complex or you are not sure how therapy can help you, another approach is to go for an evaluation first. Local hospitals or mental health clinics and psychotherapy institutes often offer this service. You will usually have a single 40- to 50-minute session or possibly a second session if the evaluator feels that psychological testing would be valuable. The evaluator will want to know about your symptoms, your relationships with important people in your life, both past and present, and any other information that may help define your problem. He or she may also want to speak to your spouse or other family member. In the end, the counselor should be able to give you a preliminary diagnosis or explanation of your problem, a recommendation of the most appropriate kind of therapy, a general outline of what that therapy should entail, an estimation of the time it may require, and recommendations of two or more appropriate professionals (some evaluators may offer their own services). The value of this approach is that it focuses your search and may help you find an appropriate therapist sooner.

In either approach, you can expect your initial session with a potential counselor to be a time for questions—yours and the therapist's. Although you may feel uncomfortable revealing personal information to a virtual stranger, you should try to be honest and remember that therapists are accustomed to hearing intimate details about people's problems. When it is your turn, you should ask about the therapist's training and experience, what type of therapy he or she uses, how sessions will be conducted, how long the therapy can be expected to last, and what the fee will be.

If you do not feel comfortable with the first therapist you visit, see a second or even a third one. At that point, if you still haven't found someone you feel you can trust, it may be the idea of therapy itself, and not the therapist, that is causing your discomfort. In that case, you should start with the therapist that you find the least objectionable, with the understanding that you will benefit in the long run. Remember that there may be times in the best of relationships when the therapist will challenge your views or probe areas that you find painful to confront. If you have developed an underlying trust of the therapist, you should be able to weather these difficulties.

CHAPTER 12

Quitting Smoking

(and Other Harmful Habits)

Millions of people around the world consistently indulge in substances that alter their moods, energy levels, and emotional and physical rhythms. Along with the perception of pleasure, most of these substances produce adverse effects, some temporary, others permanent.

A woman who smokes a few cigarettes a month will probably not experience health problems. One who drinks a glass of wine each night may actually be healthier than a teetotaler. At the other end of the spectrum, however, are women whose health, relationships with family and friends, and careers have been severely disrupted or destroyed by substance dependence. For these women, quitting, recovering, and rehabilitating means choosing life after years of heading toward death. If a bad habit takes hold, there is a variety of helpful sources for people who want to quit. With a strong desire to stop and a supportive network in place, most people are able to release themselves from their addictive prisons.

SMOKING

Despite increased awareness of the health consequences of smoking, about 46 million people in the United States continue to smoke, and each year there are more than 400,000 smoking-related deaths. Currently, female smokers in the United States are quitting at a slower rate than male smokers. If the trend continues, the number of female smokers is expected to equal the number of male smokers within the next decade.

More than 22 million American women smoke—23 percent of the female population. Young people, especially girls, are taking up the habit at an earlier age. Each day, about 1,500 teenage girls set themselves up for long-term cigarette addiction and all the health risks associated with it.

WHY WOMEN SHOULD QUIT There are plenty of reasons why both men and women should quit smoking: In the United States, smoking is the leading preventable cause of sickness and death. The American Cancer Society, American Heart Association, and American Lung Association, as well as the U.S. Surgeon General, have done a masterful job of explaining the specific health risks that smoking holds for the general population. But the unique risks to women who smoke have not gotten as much attention. Here are some of the conditions that these women face:

• **Heart Disease.** According to the long-running Framingham Heart Study, smoking is a more serious heart-attack risk factor for women than for men. Smoking as few as four cigarettes a day doubles a woman's risk; fifteen to twenty-five cigarettes a day triples it.

A 1992 study at the St. Louis University School of Medicine showed a strong link between cigarette smoking and coronary artery spasm in women. In this disorder, the heart's blood vessels become dangerously constricted as a result of the contraction of the smooth muscle that surrounds the inside of the blood vessels. In addition to causing chest pain, dizziness, and fainting, a sustained coronary artery spasm can result in a heart attack or sudden death.

Women who smoke and take birth control pills are at higher risk of developing heart attack and stroke than women who do neither, although preliminary studies show that the risk associated with low-dose estrogen pills is less than that of the older, higher-dose formulations.

• **Lung Cancer.** Since the 1950s, lung cancer in women has increased by 400 percent, and it now kills more women each year than breast cancer. According to the 1989 Surgeon General's Report on Smoking and Health, women smokers are twelve times as likely to get lung cancer as women who have never smoked. Quitting decreases the risk considerably. In fact, for ex-smokers who quit 10 or 15 years ago, the risk is nearly as low as it would have been if they had never smoked.

• **Cervical Cancer.** The risk of cervical cancer doubles in women who smoke, according to the American Cancer Society.

• **Early Menopause.** Women who smoke experience menopause an average of 2 years earlier than non-smokers, which in turn increases the risk of heart disease and osteoporosis.

• **Fertility.** According to the National Institute of Environmental Health Sciences, women who smoke less than a pack a day are 25 percent less fertile than nonsmokers; if they smoke more than a pack a day, they are 43 percent less fertile.

• **Pregnancy.** A woman who smokes during pregnancy passes carbon monoxide and other noxious substances on to her unborn child, decreasing the fetus's supply of oxygen while accelerating its heartbeat. She also runs the risk of having a miscarriage or stillbirth.

Infants of smokers are usually underweight at birth; may have decreased resistance to disease; are slower to develop physically, intellectually, and behaviorally; and are at increased risk of sudden infant death syndrome (SIDS).

• **Breast-feeding.** The breast milk of mothers who smoke may be contaminated with nicotine, which can cause health problems in newborns. A 1989 study showed that these babies are more likely to be colicky. Nicotine can also suppress levels of prolactin, a hormone necessary for the production of breast milk, so smokers may have to stop breast-feeding earlier because of insufficient milk supplies.

• **The Skin.** People who smoke age more quickly. Smoking impairs blood circulation, so the body does not get as much oxygen or other nutrients that are necessary for repairing the wear and tear of living.

Cigarette smoke may also activate enzymes in the skin that help break down the fibrous proteins, called elastin and collagen, that provide support to the skin. Crow's-feet, or wrinkles around the eyes, may be more common in smokers because they squint to keep smoke out of their eyes. In a recent study, heavy smokers were nearly five times as likely to experience premature aging of the skin and excessive wrinkling as nonsmokers. Overexposure to the sun multiplies the wrinkling effect. Heavy smoking combined with an hour of sun exposure a day can increase the chances of premature wrinkling twelvefold.

• **Effects on Medications.** Smoking may interfere with the metabolism of certain prescription drugs, such as tranquilizers and antidepressants (which are mostly prescribed for women). According to the American Pharmaceutical Association, the drugs can be less effective because they may be eliminated more quickly from the body of a smoker. Thus, larger doses may be necessary.

SMOKING AND THE NONSMOKER Women who smoke compromise the health of those close to them. Nonsmokers who are exposed to the tobacco smoke of others are at increased risk for heart disease and lung cancer. In the United States, about 53,000 deaths each year are attributed to environmental tobacco smoke. The sidestream smoke that comes off the lighted end of a cigarette is not filtered and contains substantially higher levels of toxic and carcinogenic compounds, including nitrosamines and ammonia, than are found in mainstream smoke. "Passive" smoking can also aggravate many medical conditions, including asthma and blood circulation disorders.

Partners of smokers are at increased risk of coronary heart disease, or of more chest pain or a second heart attack if they already have heart disease. A 3-year study of nonsmoking women in five metropolitan areas found that their risk of lung cancer increased by 30 percent if their husbands smoked. The study, reported in 1991, also found a similarly higher risk for women who were exposed frequently to smokers on the job and in social settings.

Children exposed to secondhand smoke are more likely to suffer from upper respiratory problems, ear infections, and impaired lung function. Researchers at the University of Arizona College of Medicine in Tucson tracked asthma in children over a 7-year period. They estimated that passive smoking causes up to 100,000 new cases of childhood asthma in the United States each year.

A 1991 report by the National Center for Health Statistics showed that 4.1 percent of children who lived with smokers were in fair to poor health; only 2.4 percent of children who were never exposed to tobacco smoke at home fit into that category. The children of smokers also require a longer period of recovery from illness and they are much more likely to take up the habit than those of nonsmokers.

OTHER INCENTIVES The incentives to quit smoking encompass more than health considerations. In many social circles, smoking is no longer acceptable, and legislation restricting smoking in public places has made it more difficult to light up. In many companies, employees have been forced by nonsmoking policies to go outdoors to smoke, which can eat into productivity. Smokers may resent being treated like lepers, but for anyone who does not smoke, especially the ex-smoker, the restrictions are much appreciated.

Once they have quit, ex-smokers (and their families and colleagues) can count on a fresher breath, a sharpened sense of taste, clothing and furnishings that no longer smell of smoke, and the freedom that comes from being released from the cigarette ball and

chain. They can enjoy places where smoking is prohibited, rather than counting the minutes until they can light up again. They do not have to isolate themselves from nonsmoking friends at social functions. Ex-smokers express feeling a sense of relief when they walk down the street, go to the doctor or dentist, or eat out because they no longer have to worry about getting dirty looks or stern lectures.

The overwhelming evidence is that women who quit smoking live longer than those who continue to smoke, and their health benefits begin almost immediately. It is never too late to stop. A 5-year study of people over age 65, reported in 1991 in *The New England Journal of Medicine*, showed that even smokers who quit in their seventies can enjoy a longer life.

WHY NOT QUIT? Someone who has never smoked might wonder: Considering all the benefits of quitting, why don't more people join the ranks of ex-smokers? Anyone who has ever had a smoking habit understands all too well. They are addicted to nicotine, a chemical that causes a pharmacological and behavioral addiction stronger than that associated with heroin and cocaine. Some smokers believe that cigarettes calm their nerves. Actually, they have the opposite effect: Cigarettes raise the heart rate and blood pressure and can produce irritability and anxiety as the nicotine begins to wear off.

Most smokers admit that their habit is extremely harmful to their health, and studies show that four out of five smokers wish they could quit, but kicking the habit usually takes four to ten tries. (See box, "Common Rationalizations for Not Quitting Smoking.") The effort that succeeds is often sparked by a new attitude or incentive. Some people quit after seeing other smokers who look "old" before their time. Others realize that they are essentially slaves to tobacco and cannot enjoy even a movie or a good night's sleep without smoking. Some people respond to self-rewards: a health-club membership or a new car (one that will keep its "new" smell longer).

Women often find it harder to quit than men. Only 40 percent of women succeed in doing so, compared with 49 percent of men. Experts believe this disparity is caused by women's fear of weight gain, the lack of social support, and more severe withdrawal symptoms. Women may also use cigarettes to manage stress and depression. So many women juggle family and work responsibilities that smoking can be tempting, even though they know it is potentially deadly. Women may have a harder time finding substitute coping behavior that is effective.

Women's fear of gaining weight has been encouraged for years by cigarette companies, starting with a 1920s campaign that told women to "Reach for a Lucky Instead of a Sweet." These Lucky Strike ads are one of advertising's biggest success stories. In truth, some people do gain weight after quitting—5 to 8 pounds on average. One explanation for the weight gain is that smoking speeds up metabolism, so smokers burn calories faster. Other theories are that people who smoke often do so instead of eating, or that smoking reduces the appetite.

PREPARING TO QUIT More than 90 percent of Americans who have quit smoking have done it on their own. The majority have stopped "cold turkey" by throwing away their cigarettes and resolving not to buy any more. Others have cut down gradually by limiting the number of cigarettes they smoke each day. Some smokers try to quit by switching to a brand that is distasteful or contains less tar and nicotine. This method is generally ineffective; moreover, most people who smoke "light" cigarettes tend to smoke more of them or to inhale more deeply.

Cutting down can be done in a variety of ways. First, stop buying cigarettes by the carton. It may help to smoke only half of each cigarette, postpone lighting up for progressively longer intervals, or do things that are incompatible with smoking. For example, many people find that smoking cigarettes and drinking milk do not go well together. Exercising also discourages smoking.

Monitoring every cigarette during the preparation period helps increase your awareness of the habitual side of smoking. Be conscious of each cigarette by hiding the pack or giving it to a friend or spouse who will know about each cigarette you smoke. Keep from emptying ashtrays, so you will have a vivid reminder of how many cigarettes you have smoked. (For additional suggestions, see box, "Tips for Preparing to Quit Smoking.")

QUITTING DAY Setting a target date is the best way to make a commitment to quit. Sharing that goal with others makes it more difficult to ignore the date. When the day comes, throw away all cigarettes and remove ashtrays and lighters. Freshen the environment by washing the smoke smell out of clothes and furniture and by airing out rooms or buying flowers.

During the days that follow, plan to stay busy with nonsmoking activities. Many ex-smokers (and you should start thinking of yourself as one of them) find that they enjoy spending time at museums, libraries, department stores, and other places where smoking

RATIONALIZATION	RESPONSE
I'm under a lot of stress, and smoking relaxes me.	Your body's used to nicotine, so you naturally feel more relaxed when you give it a substance it's come to depend on. But nicotine really is a stimulant—it raises your heart rate, blood pressure, and adrenaline level. Most ex-smokers feel much less nervous just a few weeks after quitting.
Smoking makes me more effective in my work.	Trouble concentrating can be a short-term symptom of quitting, but smoking actually deprives your brain of oxygen.
I've already cut down to a safe level.	Cutting down is a good first step, but there's a big difference in the benefits to you between smoking a little and not smoking at all. Besides, smokers who cut back often inhale more often and more deeply—negating many of the benefits of cutting back. After you've cut back to about seven cigarettes a day, it's time to set a quit date.
I smoke only safe, low-tar/low-nicotine cigarettes.	These cigarettes still contain harmful substances, and many smokers who use them inhale more often and more deeply to maintain their nicotine intake. Also, carbon monoxide intake often increases with a switch to low-tar cigarettes, which decreases the amount of oxygen available in the blood.

COMMON RATIONALIZATIONS
FOR NOT QUITTING SMOKING

RATIONALIZATION	RESPONSE	RATIONALIZATION	RESPONSE
It's too hard to quit. I don't have the will-power.	Quitting and staying away from cigarettes is hard, but it's not impossible. More than 3 million Americans quit every year. It's important for you to remember that many people have had to try more than once, and try more than one method, before they become ex-smokers, but they *have* done it, and so can you.	Sometimes I have an almost irresistible urge to have a cigarette.	This is a common feeling, especially within the first 1 to 3 weeks. The longer you're off cigarettes, the more your urges probably will come at times when you smoked before, such as when you're drinking coffee or alcohol or are at a cocktail party where other people are smoking. These are high-risk situations, and you can help yourself by avoiding them whenever possible. If you can't avoid them, you can try to visualize in advance how you'll handle the desire for a cigarette if it arises.
I'm worried about gaining weight.	Most smokers who gain more than 5 to 10 pounds are eating more. Gaining weight isn't inevitable—there are certain things you can do to help keep your weight stable. (See box, "How to Keep Your Weight Down When You Quit.")	I blew it. I smoked a cigarette.	Smoking one, or even a few, cigarettes doesn't mean you've "blown it." It does mean that you have to strengthen your determination to quit and try again—harder. Don't forget that you got through several days, perhaps even weeks or months, without a cigarette. This shows that you don't need cigarettes and that you *can* be a successful quitter.
I don't know what to do with my hands.	That's a common complaint among ex-smokers. You can keep your hands busy in other ways—it's just a matter of getting used to the change, of not holding a cigarette. Try holding something else, such as a pencil, paper clip, or marble. Practice simply keeping your hands clasped together. If you're at home, think of all the things you wish you had time to do, make a list, and consult the list for alternatives to smoking whenever your hands feel restless.		

Adapted by the U.S. Department of Health and Human Serrvices from *Clinical Opportunities for Smoking Intervention—A Guide for the Busy Physician*, National Heart, Lung, and Blood Institute, NIH Publication No. 86–2178, August 1986.

TIPS FOR PREPARING
TO QUIT SMOKING

• Decide positively that you want to quit. Try to avoid negative thoughts about how difficult it might be.

• List all the reasons you want to quit. Every night before going to bed, repeat one of the reasons 10 times.

• Develop strong personal reasons in addition to your health and obligations to others. For example, think of all the time you waste taking cigarette breaks, rushing out to buy a pack, hunting for a light, etc.

• Begin to condition yourself physically: Start a modest exercise program, drink more fluids, get plenty of rest, and avoid fatigue.

• Set a target date for quitting—perhaps a special day such as your birthday, your anniversary, or the Great American Smokeout. If you smoke heavily at work, quit during your vacation so that you're already committed to quitting when you return. Make the date sacred, and don't let anything change it. This will make it easy for you to keep track of the day you became a nonsmoker and to celebrate that date every year.

• Bet a friend you can quit on your target date. Put your cigarette money aside for every day, and forfeit it if you smoke. (But if you do smoke, simply strengthen your resolve and try again.)

• Ask your spouse or a friend to quit with you.

• Tell your family and friends that you're quitting and when. They can be an important source of support, both before and after you quit.

• Have realistic expectations—quitting isn't easy but it's not impossible either. More than 3 million Americans quit every year.

• Understand that psychological withdrawal symptoms are temporary. They usually only last 1 to 3 weeks.

• Know that most relapses occur in the first week after quitting, when withdrawal symptoms are strongest and your body is still dependent on nicotine. Be aware that this will be your hardest time, and use all your personal resources—willpower, family, friends, and tips—to get you through this critical period successfully.

• Know that most other relapses occur in the first 3 months after quitting, when situational triggers—such as a particularly stressful event—occur unexpectedly. These are the times when people reach for cigarettes automatically, because they associate smoking with relaxing.

• Realize that most successful ex-smokers quit for good only after several attempts. You may be one of those who can quit your first try. But if you're not, don't give up. Try again.

Source: "Clearing the Air," U.S. Department of Health and Human Services, Public Health Service, National Institutes of Health, NIH Publication No. 92-1647. Revised April 1988. Reprinted December 1991.

is not allowed. Whenever possible, avoid cocktail parties or routines, such as driving, that you automatically associate with smoking. Socialize and carpool with nonsmokers. Whenever the urge to smoke hits you, engage in activities that are difficult or impossible to do with a cigarette in your hand: Write a letter, do needlework, get a manicure, play the piano, or swim.

Paying attention to personal hygiene can be therapeutic. After meals, for instance, a toothbrushing can substitute for your usual cigarette. Taking a warm bath or shower when the urge hits can be relaxing and distracting. In fact, a bath and a glass of fresh juice can serve as a bedtime treat that is far more

soothing than smoking a cigarette. Establish new routines to reinforce the benefits of quitting smoking.

A pat on the back for quitting is worth pursuing. Because most people are nonsmokers or ex-smokers, it should be easy to find support, especially among your family and close friends. Health care professionals, such as the family physician and the dentist, are usually happy to grant kudos. Chances are they will also provide helpful tips and advice to encourage you to stick to your goal.

WHAT ABOUT WEIGHT GAIN? The weight gain that so many people fear usually amounts to 5 to 8 pounds over a 5-year period. One in ten ex-smokers may gain 30 pounds or more. In terms of health, the extra pounds are a minor risk factor compared to smoking, so there is no excuse to continue the more harmful habit. Weight gain is not inevitable. Part of the solution is to keep low-calorie snacks such as carrot sticks, dietetic candies, sugarless gum, or air-popped popcorn within easy reach. Cutting down on alcohol consumption can not only help keep weight down, but may also help curb the urge for a cigarette for those women who always smoke when they drink. (For additional tips, see box, "How to Keep Your Weight Down When You Quit.")

Perhaps the most successful way to control your weight is to establish a regular exercise regimen. (See Chapter 10, "Keeping Fit.") Most smokers who get out of breath during exercise find that their lung capacity increases dramatically when they quit smoking. Exercise also breaks up old routines, combats the restlessness that cigarette withdrawal may provoke, and burns calories. Most of all, exercise makes you feel better, both mentally and physically.

PROGRAMS FOR WOMEN Most stop-smoking programs are based on principles that help men and may not be as effective for women. According to Sue Delaney, an ex-smoker and author of *Women Smokers Can Quit: A Different Approach*, the needs of women who want to quit smoking differ from those of men. For example, men and women are taught to deal with problems differently: Men are expected to solve problems independently, while women learn to solve problems by sharing feelings and bonding with others. Also, some studies have suggested that women tend to use cigarettes as a way of coping with stress and negative emotions.

For these reasons, Delaney recommends a multi-faceted program that includes a physician's advice and counseling, nicotine replacement therapy, behavior-modification techniques, and an ongoing program of self-help and long-term support to help prevent relapses. Women are more likely to succeed with a program that provides group support and encouragement and helps them deal with the emotional issues that arise once stress-management support is removed. Nutritional counseling and other techniques can help women maintain their weight or cope with the anxiety provoked by gaining a few additional pounds. Women who find that they remain depressed after they quit smoking should consider seeking professional help.

EXTRA HELP Stop-smoking aids have received a lot of attention since the nicotine skin patch was de-

vised. Because the patch delivers nicotine to the bloodstream through the skin, it allows smokers to deal with the psychological aspects of quitting before having to cope with physical withdrawal problems such as restlessness, anxiety, frustration, irritability, and increased appetite.

Another option is a gum that also releases nicotine but, unlike the more passive skin patch, requires active use. (See box, "Stop-Smoking Aids.") Both the patch and the gum need a prescription, and are designed to fit into a regimen that includes smoking-cessation counseling to help with psychological symptoms of withdrawal. Other techniques that may be helpful include hypnosis, acupuncture, and relaxation exercises.

Although less than 10 percent of all smokers who quit do so through smoking-cessation programs, these programs are often the best recourse for highly addicted smokers who have tried to stop many times before and are at the greatest risk of developing health problems. The support of a group of people going through the same thing is the key for some people; investing money in the quitting effort is what cinches the commitment for others. Smokenders, a

---

HOW TO KEEP YOUR WEIGHT DOWN WHEN YOU QUIT

• Make sure you have a well-balanced diet, with the proper amounts of protein, carbohydrates, and fat.

• Don't set a target date for a holiday, when the temptation of high-calorie food and drinks may be too hard to resist.

• Weigh yourself weekly.

• Chew sugarless gum when you want sweet foods.

• Plan menus carefully, and count calories. Don't try to lose weight—just try to maintain your pre-quitting weight.

• Have low-calorie foods on hand for nibbling. Some good choices are fresh fruits and vegetables, fruit and vegetable juices, low-fat cottage cheese, and air-popped popcorn without butter.

• Take time for daily exercise, or join an organized exercise group.

Source: "Clearing the Air," U.S. Department of Health and Human Services, Public Health Service, National Institutes of Health, NIH Pub. No. 92-1647. Revised April 1988. Reprinted December 1991.

STOP-SMOKING AIDS

In the struggle to stop smoking, badges of commitment have become a common sight. These badges are round transdermal nicotine patches, about 2 inches in diameter, that are worn on the skin. Marketed under such names as Habitrol, Nicoderm, and ProStep, they each deliver a steady dose of nicotine through the skin into the bloodstream, allowing a smoker to deal with psychological withdrawal symptoms before having to cope with troublesome physical symptoms.

Some patches, such as ProStep, deliver nicotine over a 24-hour period, an amount equivalent to fifteen cigarettes. Others are used in a 10- to 12-week regimen in which the nicotine dose diminishes with time. A 6- to 12-week supply of the patches costs about $200 to $300.

Although preliminary studies show that the patches can be successful for some people, they were approved by the Food and Drug Administration only in late 1991, and long-term follow-up studies are not yet available.

Another prescription stop-smoking aid, on the market since 1984, is nicotine chewing gum. Marketed under the brand name Nicorette, it releases nicotine that reaches the bloodstream through the lining of the mouth. An estimated 1 to 2 percent of all people who rely on the gum to stop smoking transfer their addiction to the gum, so it should not be used for more than 6 months at a time. The nicotine gum is less expensive than the patch. It costs about $20 to $30 for a box of ninety-six, and most people use four to eight boxes. Many people do not like the taste of the gum, however, and prefer the more passive patch.

Nicotine replacement may help suppress the minor weight gain that usually accompanies quitting smoking. In a study reported in 1992 in the *Archives of Family Medicine*, women who used nicotine gum gained less weight (about 0.7 pound) than those who used a placebo (about 3.7 pounds). The men in the study gained about the same amount whether they used the gum or not. Further studies will try to determine why the gender difference occurred and whether the effects would be the same with the nicotine patch.

The side effects of these products are usually minor. The gum can cause hiccups, a sore throat, jaw pain from chewing, nausea, and heartburn. The patch may produce minor skin irritation. A patch that delivers nicotine overnight can cause insomnia or other sleep disturbances. There is one extremely important requirement for people on nicotine-patch therapy: They must not smoke. Smoking and using the patch can lead to a nicotine overdose that may even lead to a heart attack. Other unpleasant side effects may include abdominal pain, mental confusion, nausea, and vomiting.

Studies show that smokers who use the skin patch are twice as likely to quit—at least temporarily—as those who are given placebos. Researchers stress, however, that the most successful patch users also enroll in a formal smoking-cessation program with behavior-modification techniques taught by a professional.

---

private company based in Irvine, California, is one of the oldest and most successful programs. In 20 years, it has treated more than 600,000 people, who pay about $300 for six weekly seminars. For a more modest fee, the American Cancer Society has a smoking-cessation program called FreshStart, in addition to self-help literature about quitting.

Some highly addicted smokers benefit only from residential programs that treat smoking as an addiction akin to alcohol or narcotics dependence. These inpatient programs can be very expensive. For example, a 12-day program at Glenbeigh Hospital in Hialeah, Florida, costs about $3,500. During their stay, patients cannot smoke or take in caffeine or sugar. Health care professionals—including therapists, cardiologists, nutritionists, and pulmonologists—help them get through the withdrawal period and learn a new life-style that includes a better diet and exercise. For hard-core smokers, this drastic approach may be a last chance, and if it works, it is well worth the cost.

THE AFTERMATH Within 12 hours after the last puff, your body begins to heal itself. The levels of carbon monoxide and nicotine rapidly decline, and the heart and lungs begin to repair any damage from smoking. Within a few days, the senses of taste and smell become sharper, breathing is easier, and the smoker's cough almost disappears. These positive signs may be temporarily offset by physical withdrawal symptoms (such as dry mouth, hunger, fatigue, and sleep problems as the body gets rid of nicotine), but this part of the recovery process rarely lasts more than 2 to 3 days.

For most ex-smokers, staying away from cigarettes becomes easier as the weeks go by. If you have been used to taking cigarette breaks at work, even if you are allowed to smoke at your desk or workstation, you will find yourself becoming a lot more productive. The most difficult times are stressful situations that involve relationships, working under pressure, or experiencing unfamiliar situations that create anxiety and nervousness. Learn to anticipate and quickly recognize these instances, and use the coping skills of quitting to overcome the urge to start smoking again.

One cigarette or even one pack does not make an ex-smoker a smoker. Be aware, however, that the first 14 days may be the most critical. A study published in early 1994 in the *Journal of the American Medical Association* showed that smokers who were able to abstain completely during the first 2 weeks of a quit attempt had the best chance of success in the long run.

If you slip up, do not be too self-critical. Analyze the circumstances that caused the backsliding and be aware of the potential next time. Do not hesitate to seek informal group or professional support if backsliding seems imminent.

Ex-smokers should reward themselves generously and frequently for their efforts. One way to do this is to celebrate the monthly anniversary of the quitting date. Or save each day the money you would have spent on smoking and buy something really indulgent at the end of 6 months.

ALCOHOL

One in twenty American women has a drinking problem, according to the National Institute on Alcohol Abuse and Alcoholism. In fact, women make up one third of the alcoholics in the United States. Drinking problems are on the rise among young women. Half of the women in alcohol treatment programs, are under age 35. A female alcoholic can be of any race, ethnic background, religion, marital status, sexual preference, or social class, although the perception of the problem may differ among these groups.

WHAT CONSTITUTES ALCOHOLISM? Alcohol is a powerful drug that changes both mood and perception. Ethanol, the main ingredient in all alcoholic beverages, acts as a depressant on the central nervous system. In low doses, it can have a disinhibiting effect—making people feel more outgoing. In higher doses, its action is similar to that of a sleeping pill and in very high doses, an anesthetic.

Excessive drinking is usually thought to be the cornerstone of an alcoholism diagnosis, but for women this is a weak criterion. In fact, a woman need not drink much to qualify as an alcoholic. If drinking interferes with her control over her own life and is destructive either physically or psychologically, she has a drinking problem. Specific instances of lack of control may include family conflicts, job difficulties, emotional disturbances, driving while intoxicated (DWI) citations, financial pitfalls, and health problems. If she continues to drink anyway, there is a good chance she is an alcoholic. (See box, "Are You an Alcoholic?") If she tries to stop at this point, she may experience withdrawal symptoms such as tremors, nausea, dry mouth, sweating, weakness, and depression. These symptoms make it difficult to quit without the aid of a structured treatment program that provides counseling support and, if necessary, temporary use of antianxiety drugs.

Alcoholism appears to have both biochemical and psychological components and, in many cases, it is probably inherited. A number of common "genetic markers" have been found in alcoholics and may explain the biological reason for developing a dependence on alcohol. Most research on heredity factors in alcoholism, however, has been done on men. One study reported in 1992 in the *Journal of the American Medical Association* indicates that from 50 to 61 percent of all alcoholism in women has a genetic component. There is no "cure" for alcoholism. An alcoholic who abstains from drinking, however, can recover and live a normal life.

ADVERSE EFFECTS ON WOMEN A given dose of alcohol is clearly more damaging to women than to men. First of all, the amount of water in a woman's body is lower than that of a man of comparable size, so even if they drink the same amount, the concentration of alcohol in her blood will be higher than in his. During menstruation this concentration may be even higher.

Women also appear to produce less of an enzyme called alcohol dehydrogenase that breaks down alcohol in the stomach before it enters the bloodstream. Even when a man and woman of the same size drink equivalent amounts, the alcohol is 30 percent more toxic to the woman because her body does not metabolize it as efficiently. In fact, years of excessive alcohol use decrease the production of alcohol dehydrogenase even more. In alcoholic women, the enzyme may be absent altogether. If this is the case, alcohol is absorbed directly, much as if it were injected into the bloodstream.

Increased toxicity of alcohol takes its toll in women. Since it takes less alcohol to produce liver damage, women alcoholics are more likely to experience liver disease. The disease also progresses more rapidly and is more likely to cause death in women than in men. Alcohol use in women has been linked to increased suicide rates, severe depression, breast cancer, and osteoporosis. A female alcoholic has an average life expectancy of 63, about 15 years less than the norm for women.

We see the most tragic results of alcoholism in pregnant women. Alcohol use is the leading preventable cause of mental retardation in newborns. Fetal alcohol syndrome (FAS) causes dysfunction of the central nervous system, slows down pre- and postnatal growth, and may produce facial malformations. The syndrome strikes 1 to 3 of every 1,000 newborns—about 3,600 to 10,000 babies per year.

BARRIERS TO TREATMENT For a variety of reasons, women alcoholics often are reluctant to come forward for treatment. Society persists in viewing alco-

ARE YOU AN ALCOHOLIC?

1. Do you end up having an argument with your spouse every time you drink?

2. Do you try very hard not to drink before a certain hour every day?

3. Do you ever drink because you are nervous about going to see a doctor? Going to the dentist? Starting a new job? Going to a funeral?

4. Do you ever drink because you are afraid of doing something and think a few drinks will make it easier and will relax you?

5. When you drink, do you make an effort to drink slowly so that people won't notice you?

6. Do you sometimes miss going to work on Monday morning (after a weekend of drinking)?

7. Do you sometimes keep a bottle in your car just so it's handy if you want it?

8. Have you ever had trouble finding your car when you've been drinking?

9. Do you ever feel uncomfortable about getting rid of empty bottles?

10. Do you ever try to find different places to get rid of your liquor bottles?

11. Do you ever have trouble stopping drinking once you get started?

12. Have you ever had trouble remembering things that happened while you were drinking?

13. Have you discovered that you get less flak from family members if you sneak a few drinks and don't do all your drinking in front of them?

14. Do you ever want to take a drink the next morning after drinking the night before . . . to recover faster?

15. Do you believe that you have a serious drinking problem but are afraid to mention it to anyone?

16. Have you ever told yourself that you really ought to give up drinking?

17. Do you find that drinking makes you feel less insecure and less vulnerable?

18. Have you found that it helps to have a drink or two before going to a party and that it makes you feel less nervous?

19. Have you ever bought your liquor at several different stores because you didn't want to go back to the same one?

20. Have you ever noticed any changes in your drinking habits (such as significant increases in intake)?

A social drinker, a person without an alcohol problem would have answered no to all twenty questions. Did you?

Source: *Goodbye Hangovers, Hello Life*; Jean Kirkpatrick, Ph.D., Ballantine Books, New York, 1986, pp. 29–30.

holism as a moral failing rather than as a physical disorder. In one study, male and female college students were shown videotapes and written descriptions of dating scenes. Their reactions showed a general acceptance that a woman who orders an alcoholic beverage is more likely to exhibit sexual behavior than one who orders a soft drink. The irony is that although alcohol causes disinhibition and may increase impulsive behavior, it actually diminishes sexual response in most women, and the majority of female alcoholics experience some type of sexual dysfunction.

Many celebrities have publicly confessed their drinking problems to try to dispel some of the myths surrounding alcoholism. Betty Ford, Elizabeth Taylor, Kitty Dukakis, Liza Minnelli, and others have become stars of rehabilitation. In spite of those efforts, most women do not identify with these high-profile role models. They are viewed as having had "better" excuses for depending on alcohol: the pressures of political life and show business.

Other barriers to treatment include the lack of financial resources, lack of child care, and fear of being identified as an alcoholic. Some women fear that they will be ostracized at work, face loss of respect at home, and even run the risk of losing their children through court action. In addition, women tend to drink more in the house, so family members may be the only ones who recognize the problem. Though they may try to help by such measures as removing alcohol from the home, family members may be reluctant to encourage a woman to seek treatment because of their own attitudes about alcoholism.

Often, women are just expected to solve their drinking problems alone. Rarely, however, are alcoholics able to just kick the habit without treatment. Despite their best intentions, they are almost always overwhelmed by the desire to obtain, conceal, and drink alcohol. They may enter treatment in response to pressure from loved ones or work colleagues. This lack of self-motivation, however, is not necessarily a barrier to successful treatment. One of the goals of treatment is to motivate the alcoholic to want a healthy existence badly enough to go through the necessary steps to achieve it.

TYPES OF TREATMENT Alcoholism is treated in essentially three ways: by individual counseling, inpatient and outpatient treatment programs, or self-help, which is usually combined with individual counseling. The type and length of a treatment course varies according to the effect drinking has had on an indi-

vidual. Some people are able to stop drinking by attending meetings of organizations like Alcoholics Anonymous (AA). Others require individual counseling at the same time.

When additional guidance is necessary, a brief stay at a residential treatment center may be in order, and in cases of extreme dependence, detoxification in a hospital and intensive inpatient rehabilitation may be the only ways of stopping the abuse. Tranquilizers that help ease the symptoms of withdrawal may be employed in this type of treatment, but care must be taken that drug addiction does not replace the alcohol dependence.

A variety of helpful sources exist. (See Resources.) AA, Women for Sobriety, and Rational Recovery are organizations that hold meetings where people talk anonymously about their problems with alcohol. In addition, local affiliates of the National Council on Alcoholism and Drug Abuse provide information and a wide range of professional services. Some large companies and unions sponsor treatment programs for employees and members. A family doctor or cleric may be able to locate other local resources, such as hospitals, mental health agencies, county and state medical societies, and university-affiliated agencies.

Inpatient treatment is not an option for some women. If they have children, they may not be able to secure child care services while they are in treatment. They also may have difficulty with the cost of treatment. For example, at the Hazelden Institute, a nonprofit treatment center in Minnesota, a typical 28-day stay runs about $8,000. The cost can soar to $25,000 or more for private clinics. These programs may or may not be covered by insurance.

THE GENDER DIFFERENCE Male alcoholics outnumber women two to one, and treatment programs are often quite male dominated. Women may feel intimidated by this. Many women alcoholics have been sexually abused, but may find it difficult to talk about sexual issues in groups that include men. Woman-specific treatment programs, though usually not as accessible, offer a special sensitivity to the problems associated with the female alcoholic: lack of self-esteem, possible drug dependence, anxiety disorders, depression, and the stigma of female alcoholism.

Alcoholics Anonymous (AA) has achieved its success rate by instructing alcoholics to turn their problems over to a higher power, admit their moral defects, and seek humility, but the woman alcoholic may already be struggling with feelings of powerlessness, humiliation, guilt, and low self-esteem. Women for Sobriety, an organization started by Jean Kirkpatrick, herself an alcoholic for 20 years, provides a program developed specifically for women. It emphasizes confidence-building, positive attitudes, and love of oneself—all desperately needed by most female alcoholics—and provides a forum where women can speak to and meet other women in treatment.

Rational Recovery was developed by a man who objected to AA's spiritually based guidelines. The program's principles revolve around the attitude that the alcoholic does have power over his or her addiction and that the dependence can be broken in a finite period of time.

Whether a woman chooses one of the alternative organizations (which are not as widely available) or a more traditional program, the important thing is that she find support. In the aftermath of alcoholism recovery, support is paramount in maintaining sobriety.

DRUG DEPENDENCE

Human beings have been searching throughout history for mood-altering drugs that do not have harmful side effects and an addictive potential. In the United States, 10 million people abuse tranquilizers, painkillers, and other prescription drugs, while 5.5 million are estimated to abuse such illegal substances as marijuana, cocaine, and heroin. Fortunately, these numbers seem to be declining.

LEGAL SUBSTANCES In the past 30 years or so, a number of excellent prescription drugs have emerged to help people get through temporary periods of anxiety and insomnia, alleviate pain, or allow those who have serious, long-term problems such as depressive illness to lead more normal lives. Unfortunately, some individuals take these drugs solely for their mood-altering effects or start off taking them for legitimate reasons and ultimately become addicted. Although more men than women take illegal drugs, women constitute the overwhelming majority of prescription drug abusers. Among the drugs that are commonly prescribed, and prone to misuse and abuse, are benzodiazepines, barbiturates, and pain-killers.

•**Benzodiazepines.** Americans annually consume about 3.7 billion benzodiazepine pills, (Valium, Xanax, and Ativan) to treat what is usually temporary anxiety and insomnia. One well-known benzo-diazepine-related sleeping pill is Halcion. Withdrawal reactions from regular use of benzodiazepines can occur within a few weeks and may consist of depressed mood, insomnia, convulsions, tremors, cramps, vomiting, and sweating. For that reason, most doctors monitor patients using these drugs frequently and decrease their use gradually if they have been taken for any extended period. Most physicians discontinue prescribing the medication under these circumstances, or require that the patient go for counseling, but some women simply go to another doctor for a new prescription rather than stop taking the drug or admit dependence.

•**Barbiturates.** Rarely prescribed nowadays, barbiturates are mostly sleeping pills such as sodium pentobarbital (Nembutal). These drugs are not only stronger than benzodiazepines, but they also have more troublesome side effects and are more likely to be habit-forming.

•**Analgesics.** Pain-killers that contain opium-derived narcotics also have a strong potential for abuse, although for acute short-term pain, such as that following surgery, they are appropriate and should not be refused for fear of addiction. Drugs such as meperidine hydrochloride (Demerol) and morphine are extremely effective at relieving severe pain and are usually prescribed regularly only for people with a debilitating or terminal illness, where dependence may not be a concern. Analgesics have strict prescribing guidelines that help guard against addiction.

•**Amphetamines.** Another group of drugs prone to abuse are amphetamines—stimulants originally prescribed for appetite regulation. They have been banned by the Food and Drug Administration for use as a weight-loss aid. Amphetamines are now prescribed only occasionally for depression and for a few uncommon medical conditions, but they are still available on the street. Sometimes amphetamines are abused by students or others who wish to stay awake for long periods of time. Chronic use of these stimulants can bring on restlessness, sleeplessness, overexcitability, psychiatric disturbances, hand tremors, and profuse perspiration, and it can place undue stress on the heart.

ILLEGAL SUBSTANCES Males who use illegal substances still outnumber females, but illegal drug use is on the rise in younger women. Although there are a few medical indications for prescribing these substances (marijuana can help control nausea during chemotherapy, and cocaine is a component of some local anesthetics), the following drugs are used for their mood-altering effects.

• **Marijuana.** Used primarily to attain a feeling of relaxation, marijuana is now known to do more damage to the body than was once thought. The drug can cause extreme, though temporary, anxiety and palpitations, especially among inexperienced users. Because it affects perception and memory, smoking marijuana can seriously affect motor activities such as driving. One study in Boston found that 16 percent of drivers responsible for fatal auto accidents were under the influence of marijuana.

Because it is so deeply inhaled, marijuana also has adverse effects on the lungs, damaging the cells that normally protect them from infection and causing changes that may be precancerous. Moreover, the marijuana available now is much more potent than that sold 20 years ago, and data on the effects of its long-term use are not yet available.

Although marijuana is not physically addictive, it sometimes creates a psychological dependence characterized by concern with maintaining a constant supply, an inability to cut down, and a resistance to recognizing the dependence. Quitting can cause mild withdrawal symptoms, for example, anxiety and irritability.

• **Cocaine.** Also known as "coke" or "snow," cocaine is sold as a white powder that is usually snorted through the nostrils. It also comes in injectable and smokable forms.

Cocaine quickly enters the bloodstream and produces a feeling of euphoria and increased energy that is relatively short-lived, about 30 minutes or so for the average high. Its addiction potential is strong because of the extreme high, which is followed by an extreme low as soon as the effects wear off, causing the user to desire another high as soon as possible. Occasionally, there is permanent heart muscle damage or erratic heart rhythms that in rare instances can cause premature death. Prolonged snorting can cause ulcers or bleeding in the nose. Other effects include convulsions and, if the cocaine is injected, skin abscesses. And those who share needles when they inject cocaine are at high risk of contracting AIDS.

About one third of all Americans who are addicted to cocaine are women, and it is estimated that more than half of those in treatment are under age 30. They suffer from increasingly lowered self-esteem, depression, anxiety, paranoia, psychotic reactions, fatigue, nervousness, inability to concentrate, and insomnia. Despite cocaine's reputation as a "love" drug, it eventually causes sexual dysfunction in both men and women. If used during pregnancy, cocaine can disrupt the oxygen supply to the fetus, which results in premature birth, low birth weight, irritability or tremors and, in severe cases, death.

• **Crack.** A smokable form of cocaine, crack is the quickest, cheapest, most addictive way to attain cocaine's characteristic euphoric high. Addiction to crack develops faster than addiction to any other drug except for nicotine.

• **Heroin.** Heroin was once legal and widely prescribed in the nineteenth century for all sorts of minor ailments and severe pain. Heroin can be snorted or injected, and its effects come on quickly and usually last for 3 to 4 hours. Chronic use can cause brain dysfunction, liver disease, and lung abscesses. These problems are not caused by the heroin itself, but by contaminants in the substances that are mixed with the drug and by infectious agents that enter the bloodstream during injection. Users who share needles with others are also at risk of AIDS infection.

Withdrawal from heroin is an extremely unpleasant experience, with symptoms that may include nausea, vomiting, tremors, insomnia, hot and cold flashes, extreme anxiety, and an overwhelming desire for the drug. However unpleasant, withdrawing from heroin is actually less dangerous than withdrawing from alcohol and many antianxiety drugs. Sometimes methadone, a synthetic opiate, is given to an addict to make the transition to nondependence.

• **Hallucinogens.** Substances that produce hallucinations and other mind-altering effects are found in a variety of plants, including peyote cactus and about one hundred species of mushrooms, and in synthetic drugs. LSD is perhaps the most notorious of these hallucinogens; PCP ("angel dust") and MDMA ("ecstasy") are others. Most people who use these drugs tend to do so experimentally, and long-term, frequent use is rare. The drugs are not necessarily addicting, although a small percentage of people do abuse them, but they can cause problems such as flashbacks.

TYPES OF TREATMENT A person who becomes addicted to a drug is seeking to alter mood and perception. The desire to escape or just "hide out" from reality fuels the dependence. (See box, "Signs of Substance Dependence.") In women, that desire to escape may arise in response to low self-esteem, lack of self-confidence, or an "empty" feeling. The perceived embarrassment of admitting addiction, especially if it involves an illegal substance, probably only heightens those feelings.

The first and most important step to recovery is talking to someone who cares and will not be judgmental—a friend, doctor, or members of a recovery group. Organizations such as Narcotics Anonymous (see Resources) have been successful in part because they give addicted people a chance to be with others who are in the same boat. These meetings, however, cannot offer complete treatment for drug addiction. With some drugs, withdrawal can produce symptoms that require medical supervision. For instance, withdrawal from barbiturates can cause life-threatening medical problems in some people who try to quit "cold turkey."

As with alcoholism, treatment for drug dependence may require hospitalization or short sessions in special treatment centers. In the course of treatment, a team of health professionals, including psychiatrists, psychologists, nurses, and social workers, use medication and talk therapy to help the individual relieve withdrawal symptoms and to work toward permanent rehabilitation. Eventually, a self-help group composed of other ex-addicts becomes a cornerstone of support. The individual is expected to help others who seek recovery, which can serve as a poignant reminder of what he or she has already overcome. Whether through self-help groups or individual or group therapy, an ex-addict must try to discover the value of life, and learn that even satisfying lives are riddled with stress and adversity from time to time. Attempts to escape from those difficult moments by turning to mood-altering substances can keep that person from really "living."

WOMEN IN RECOVERY Treatment for drug dependence poses several problems for women. If they have children, they may fear losing custody if they admit to the problem, and if they do seek treatment, they may be unable to secure or afford the required child care. Some self-help groups provide anonymity along with assistance and suggestions. However, some of these groups focus on the concept that individuals are powerless over their problems and must seek humility, which may not be appropriate for someone who has felt powerless and humble all her life. Nevertheless, all available sources of support should be investigated until the most suitable program can be found. In smaller communities, it may be necessary to take whatever is offered, even if it is not perfect, and try to get the most out of it. Any support is better than no support.

STAYING DRUG-FREE A crucial turning point comes when ending dependence becomes more compelling than continuing it. Preventing a relapse is an ongoing struggle, but the commitment to rehabilitation is strengthened by family support, community involvement, improved health, and increased job success. It may be extremely difficult to avoid temptation because it means staying away from anyone who uses drugs, whether friends, family, colleagues, or even a spouse. Women who radically change their lives, breaking old patterns and forming new associations, report the most successful rehabilitation. Changing jobs, making friends with non-drug users, moving to a new community, or becoming more involved in the present community all help to shake things up and create a new drug-free life.

SIGNS OF SUBSTANCE DEPENDENCE

A diagnosis of "psychoactive substance dependence" may be made if at least three of the following statements are true:

• The substance is taken in larger amounts or over a longer period than the person intended.

• There is a persistent desire or unsuccessful effort to stop.

• The person spends a great deal of time trying to get the substance (e.g., robberies to raise the money), taking it or recovering from its effects.

• Using the substance disrupts important social obligations or work activities.

• The person continues to use the substance despite knowing that it is causing problems (e.g., drinking even though it makes an ulcer worse).

• There is a marked tolerance: The person needs markedly increased amounts of the substance to become intoxicated or has a marked reduction of the desired effect if using the same amount.

• There are withdrawal symptoms.

• The substance is taken to avoid the withdrawal symptoms.

Adapted from *Diagnostic and Statistical Manual of Mental Disorders,* 4th ed., American Psychiatric Association, Washington, D.C., 1994.

Rethinking Body Image

The image of the "perfect woman" is everywhere, from billboards to magazine covers and fashion runways. What society considers perfect changes from generation to generation. (See Figure 13.1.) The boyishly thin "Twiggy" look, after a brief resurgence, is definitely out, but it has been replaced by an even more unattainable standard: the Barbie doll body—lean and sculpted, yet voluptuous, with large, even surgically enhanced, breasts. Professional models, who in 1967 weighed about 8 percent less than the typical American woman, now weigh 23 percent less. Only a fraction of women look like this. But the ideal continues to wreak havoc on both the minds and bodies of American women of all ages.

Despite the progress they have made in the workplace, many women believe that society continues to judge them more heavily by their appearance than by their accomplishments. Often, that is also how they judge themselves. A majority are unhappy with their appearance, particularly their weight. For example, in a study sponsored by the Melpomene Institute for Women's Health Research in St. Paul, women were asked to evaluate 5 female silhouettes that ranged from 10 to 20 percent underweight through normal weight to 20 percent overweight. When asked to choose which figure they would like to resemble, more than 80 percent of the respondents chose either the 10 percent or the 20 percent underweight figure. When asked to choose which silhouette looked most like theirs, almost 40 percent chose either the 10 percent or 20 percent overweight figure. In fact, 60 percent who thought they were overweight were in the normal weight range for their heights.

For some women, unhappiness with their bodies translates into serious problems. Adolescent girls are especially prone to this concern. Many become slaves to the mirror and the bathroom scale, which undercuts their self-esteem and saps energy from more important pursuits. In some cases, it may lead to eating disorders.

For the sake of their mental and physical health, women must learn to accept their bodies as they are, not as society dictates they should be. This chapter examines distorted body image, assesses its costs, and suggests ways to adopt more healthy, self-affirming attitudes.

WEIGHT LOSS: RISKS VS. BENEFITS

There is no question that obesity (usually defined as 30 percent above ideal weight for a particular height and age) poses serious, and growing, health risks. Americans, especially women, are heavier now than they were a generation ago, despite the emphasis on being slim.

Just how overweight does someone need to be before his or her health is jeopardized? No one knows for sure. Some experts contend that being even slightly overweight significantly increases the risk of women developing coronary heart disease, perhaps even more so than it does for men. The Nurses' Health Study has shown, for example, that a woman who is 5 feet 4½ inches tall and weighs between 137 and 145 pounds has a 30 percent greater risk of having a heart attack than a woman of the same height who weighs 125 pounds.

Other experts counsel against dieting, even for people who are clearly overweight. In fact, larger, long-term studies have associated a slight weight gain with advancing age to longevity. One caveat: Some of the studies that link being thin or underweight to shorter life expectancies fail to take other factors, such as smoking and illness, into account.

Fig. 13.1 *Our society's idea of the ideal female shape has changed dramatically over the years, earlier favoring a full-figured woman, then an hour-glass figure, a boyish look, and most recently, the athletic look.*

The ideal shape through the ages

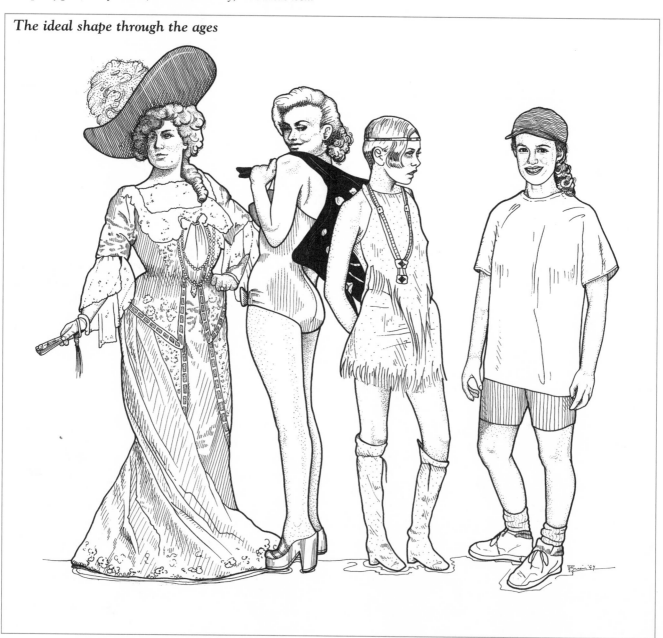

People with certain medical conditions, including high blood pressure, high blood cholesterol, heart disease, arthritis, and diabetes can obviously benefit from sensible weight reduction. And the more risk factors a person has, the more important weight control becomes. However, for moderately overweight people, the benefits of chronic weight-loss efforts may not outweigh the risks. Some studies have found that the greatest reduction in disease risk may come from losing just 5 to 10 pounds—but not the same 5 to 10 pounds over and over again. Yo-yo dieting, in which weight is repeatedly lost and regained can be especially harmful. (See Chapter 9, "Healthful Eating for a Lifetime.") It is not only bad for a dieter's morale, but it may make losing weight progressively more difficult and has even been associated with a lowered life expectancy. The biggest problems connected to weight loss, though, may stem from issues related to self-esteem.

How Much Should You Weigh? Defining the "desirable" or "ideal" weight isn't easy. For many years, the Metropolitan Life Height and Weight Tables provided the standard. The data were based on weights at which policyholders lived longest. Some of the tables took body frame size, a rather vague concept based on the width of elbows, wrists, and hips, into account, with lower recommended weights for smaller-framed people. The tables were revised in 1983 to reflect a more liberal range of acceptable weights.

Then, in 1990, the federal government published its *Dietary Guidelines for Americans*. These went a step further, promoting an even more lenient weight range that made it all right for people to weigh a little more as they aged (see box, Chapter 9, "Appropriate Weight in Youth and Middle Age"). Yet, even according to these guidelines, about 25 percent of Americans are overweight.

The government tables correspond closely to BMI, or body mass index, a weight-to-height ratio that can also be used to determine appropriate weight. (See box, "How to Determine Body Mass Index.")

How body fat is distributed is also a key factor. Fat that is located around the hips and thighs (the typically female "pear" shape) may pose less of a risk to cardiovascular health than central obesity, or the more typically male "beer belly." One way to assess body-fat distribution is by determining your waist-to-hip ratio: Measure your waist (without sucking in your stomach). Then measure your hips at their widest point. Divide your waist measurement by your hip

---

How to Determine Body Mass Index

Body mass index (BMI) is considered a more meaningful figure than weight alone, since it accounts for height. The BMI equals your weight divided by the square of your height, and it is usually expressed in metric measurement. To determine your BMI:

1. Convert your weight to kilograms by dividing your weight in pounds (without clothes) by 2.2: _____.

2. Convert your height to meters by dividing your height in inches (without shoes) by 39.4 (_____). Then square it (multiply it by itself): _____.

3. Divide (1) by (2). Body mass = _____.

If you are aged 19 to 34, a desirable BMI ranges from approximately 19 to 25; if you are 35 and older, it ranges from 21 to 27. In general, a BMI in the range of 25 to 30 means you are overweight, and a BMI of higher than 30 means you are obese.

---

measurement to get your waist-to-hip ratio. A figure of .80 or above for a woman (.95 to 1.0 for a man) may indicate increased cardiovascular risk. However, you should remember that body-fat distribution is only one of many risk factors for cardiovascular disease. In young women with no other risk factors, a few extra pounds around the middle are no serious cause for concern.

THE DAMAGE OF DISCONTENT

It is not unusual, and probably not very harmful, for you to be dissatisfied with your body, especially as you age, so long as you keep things in perspective. Many men and women find fault with some aspects of their bodies, but women are much more likely to have a negatively distorted body image. (In fact, some studies show that men are more likely to perceive their bodies in an overly positive light.) Women tend to rate their bodies as heavier than those they believe men find attractive and up to 95 percent think they are more overweight than they actually are. Women are also far more likely than men to weigh themselves daily or several times a week, to diet—up to at least one half of American women, compared with one quarter of men—and to develop eating disorders.

Teenage girls are particularly afraid of being overweight, regardless of what they actually weigh. Perhaps because they do not realize that a changing body shape is a normal part of growing up, many teenagers develop unhealthy eating habits. The statistics are appalling:

• One out of three American girls aged 11 to 18 is on a weight-reduction diet, according to researchers at the University of Michigan.

• A study of nearly 500 girls in San Francisco found that almost 50 percent of the 9-year-olds and 80 percent of the 10- and 11-year-olds were dieting to lose weight. While 58 percent of the girls in this study described themselves as being overweight, only 17 percent actually were.

• In a study of more than 300 upper-middle-class high school girls, almost 75 percent reported being on a diet. More than 50 percent weighed themselves at least every other week, and 4 percent weighed themselves more than once a day. Up to 51 percent of the *underweight* girls reported extreme anxiety about weighing too much. Not surprisingly, their normal-weight and overweight peers were even more concerned.

Surveys have shown that, unlike their male counterparts, girls experience a notable drop in self-confidence and self-satisfaction in adolescence, a time when parental support and guidance can be crucial (see box, "Giving Girls a Healthy Start"). An unhealthy preoccupation with weight loss at a time when young bodies are still developing can also result in nutritional deficiencies. However, the most serious fallout from teen dieting is the possibility of developing an eating disorder.

IDENTIFYING AND TREATING EATING DISORDERS

ANOREXIA NERVOSA Unfortunately, the recent spotlight on the eating disorder called anorexia nervosa, spurred in part by celebrities' confessions of their own battles with compulsive self-starvation, has done little to stem the tide of new cases among the most vulnerable group—young women. An estimated 1

GIVING GIRLS A HEALTHY START

Parents, especially mothers, and other adults play a key role in helping girls and young women develop self-esteem and good eating habits. Many girls who are anorectic inherit their preoccupation with weight loss from their mothers. The following suggestions can help you guide your daughter toward establishing healthy patterns for life:

• Be a responsible role model. Do not judge yourself by your weight or shape. Make healthy eating habits and regular exercise a part of family life, not an obsession.

• If your daughter seems to worry needlessly about her weight, ask other adults she respects, such as coaches, dance teachers, or the pediatrician, to help reassure her that her weight is appropriate, and that she is a worthwhile person at any weight.

• If your daughter is overweight, discuss sensible strategies for slimming down. That usually means sensible eating, not drastic calorie-cutting, combined with moderate exercise. Also discuss what *doesn't* work—fad diets and quick-weight-loss gimmicks.

• Ask your daughter how she feels about the images of women she sees on television and in magazines. Some questions to help spark conversation: Do most women look like this? What's important about a woman besides weight? What messages do these super-slim images send women? Do not preach; just raise the issues.

• Ask your daughter what fears and expectations she associates with weight loss or gain. Does she believe that being thin will guarantee her popularity or success?

• Praise your daughter's personal qualities and achievements, not just her appearance.

• Do not tease your daughter about overeating or about her "baby fat."

• Prepare balanced, varied meals. Do not fuss over what your daughter does or doesn't eat at any individual meal. Do get involved—in a non-critical, supportive way—if your daughter lacks appetite or sharply changes her normal eating patterns over several weeks.

• Encourage nutrition education in your children's school, including a discussion of appropriate weight and body image.

out of every 200 girls aged 12 to 18 suffers from the disorder. Dancers, athletes, and others whose success depends on remaining thin are especially affected.

Anorectics (as those who have the disorder are known) become convinced that they are overweight even when they aren't. (See Figure 13.2.) They subsist on an extremely low calorie intake, insisting that they are not hungry and that there is nothing abnormal about their behavior. To be diagnosed as anorectic, a woman must show all of the following symptoms:

• a refusal to maintain at least the minimum weight considered normal for her age and height

• an intense fear of gaining weight or becoming fat, even though she is underweight

• a distorted body image

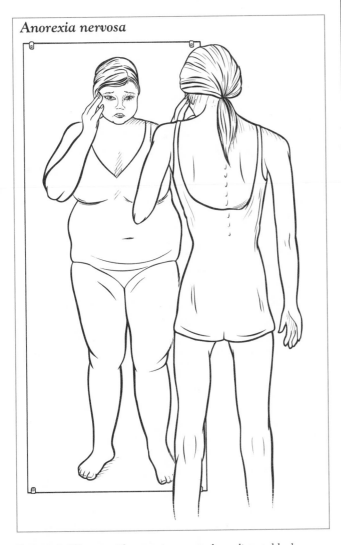

Anorexia nervosa

Fig. 13.2 *Women with anorexia nervosa have distorted body images, believing that they are fat when they are actually considerably underweight.*

• the loss of regular menstrual cycles—three consecutive missed periods not due to pregnancy

Anorectics may also exercise excessively, display obsessive eating habits (cutting food into tiny pieces, pushing it around on the plate, and refusing to eat with the family), and resort to binging or purging. (See section on "Bulimia.")

Anorexia most often begins in adolescence as an "innocent diet," but it can occur at any age, and it has been reported in children as young as 5.

Anorexia nervosa is more prevalent among white and middle- to upper-middle-class individuals. Anorectics are likely to be perfectionists and are prone to bouts of depression. They are often high achievers, eager to please their families and others, but lack self-esteem.

The condition may go away on its own, or it may grow steadily worse. In advanced cases, starvation causes the body to shut down vital metabolic processes. Blood pressure drops, breathing rate slows and menstruation ceases (or fails to begin). Other symptoms include hormonal imbalances, dry skin, brittle hair and nails, joint pain, and intolerance to cold. In up to 20 percent of these advanced cases, the condition is fatal.

Parents, teachers, and coaches should be alert to the warning signs of anorexia: severe weight loss, a preoccupation with being thin, a body image that is seriously out of kilter, and depression. (See box, "Signs of Trouble.") If you as a parent suspect a problem, let your daughter know that you are concerned and try talking to her about what may be causing her eating disorder. Arrange for a consultation with a professional specializing in these kinds of problems.

Once a person becomes anorectic, early treatment is vital. Commonsense advice, threats, and pleading are, in general, useless; most cases require professional help. The longer anorexia is allowed to go untreated, the more deeply entrenched the behavior becomes, and the more damage to the body results.

Convincing an anorectic to enter treatment isn't easy and it usually involves overcoming a great deal of denial. Recovery can be lengthy and difficult. Since anorexia is often a manifestation of emotional problems, such as deep insecurity and the need to control one's life, those issues must be addressed before real improvement can occur. Treatment may include psychotherapy, behavior modification, nutritional counseling, and self-help groups. Family support is essential. If symptoms are

SIGNS OF TROUBLE

For most adolescents, a few binges or food fads are normal. But be alert for these signs of unhealthy dieting in teens, especially girls:

• Refusing to eat with the family

• Large amounts of food missing (this may indicate binging)

• Leaving the table right after meals (this may denote purging)

• Evidence of using diet pills, emetics, or laxatives

• Exercising compulsively, and becoming very upset when the exercise routine is interrupted

---

severe or life-threatening, hospitalization may be required, at least initially.

BULIMIA An estimated half of anorectics also suffer from bulimia nervosa, or binging and purging. Other individuals suffer only from bulimia. Unlike anorectics, bulimics may be at normal or near-normal weight.

What constitutes bulimia? An occasional blowout with a box of cookies does not—even if you vomit afterward. Bulimics can eat anywhere from 1,000 to 55,000 calories of food in an hour, usually averaging about 5,000 calories. Then they induce vomiting or take large doses of laxatives to prevent digesting or retaining the food and thus gaining weight. The American Psychiatric Association (APA) characterizes this serious eating disorder as:

• recurrent episodes of binge eating (a minimum of two a week on average for at least 3 months)

• feelings of lack of control over eating behavior during the binges

• efforts to prevent weight gain by regular use of self-induced vomiting, laxatives, diuretics, strict dieting, fasting, vigorous exercise, or a combination of any of these

• persistent overconcern with body shape and weight

Bulimia is difficult to diagnose because, without drastic weight changes, bulimics can often hide their condition successfully for many years. A widely publicized 1981 study found that bulimia affects as many as 19 percent of female college students. However,

these subjects included a preponderance of dancers, who must remain thin and are at high risk for bulimia. More recent studies on broader samples, especially those using the APA's strict definition of bulimia, have found that only 1.3 to 3.8 percent of female college students (among males, it is 1 to 2 tenths of 1 percent) are bulimic.

The causes of bulimia are still not completely understood. Like anorexia, it may result from social pressure to be thin, coupled with a poor self-image and a tendency toward depression. The success (at least in the short term) of certain antidepressant medications in the treatment of bulimia suggests that the same problem with the brain's neurotransmitters, or chemical messengers, that is believed to cause depression may be to blame for bulimia as well.

Whatever the cause, bulimia wreaks havoc on health. Purging upsets the body's balance of electrolytes, such as sodium and potassium, which can result in irregular heartbeat, fainting, and fatigue. Nutritional deficiencies can develop, too. Regular vomiting can also damage the stomach and esophagus, and can cause erosion of tooth enamel, swollen glands, and liver damage. Overuse of laxatives can cause rectal bleeding and irritation of the large intestine.

Early intervention and long-term treatment, preferably by both mental health professionals and nutrition counselors, are keys to a successful recovery. Hospitalization may be necessary in advanced cases. While antidepressants may accompany treatment, they should not be the only form of therapy.

BINGE EATING In addition to anorexia and bulimia, researchers have identified what may be an even more common problem, "binge-eating disorder," frequent, uncontrolled eating binges, often driven by emotional distress. In fact, research suggests that the problem may be linked to anxiety or depression. These binges, unlike those associated with bulimia, are not followed by purging, and may account for many cases of persistent or recurrent obesity. Binging, which occurs at least twice a week on average, involves rapid eating to the point of uncomfortable fullness, followed by feelings of distress, guilt, and shame.

Controlling the condition requires treating the underlying depression and anxiety, identifying and avoiding situations that trigger binges, and establishing more normal eating patterns. Self-help groups, such as Overeaters Anonymous, can provide much-needed support to chronic binge eaters, but should be an adjunct to professional counseling.

EXERCISE ADDICTION

An obsession with exercise may be another sign of a distorted body image. Compulsively trying to burn off calories by exercising too long, too hard, or too often is common among those suffering from anorexia. Other people may become dependent on exercise, whether or not they are concerned with weight control. Some studies have shown that they suffer anxiety, guilt, tension, and irritability when they slow down or stop exercising (often because of injury). A popular theory holds that exercise stimulates the release of mood-altering chemicals called endorphins, which are responsible for the so-called runner's high, and may lead to exercise dependence. But this is only one of several theories, most of which postulate some brain-related changes produced by exercise.

Too much exercise can result not only in injuries and exhaustion, but it can also disrupt the body's normal processes. Amenorrhea, or lack of menstrual periods, for example, is common among very active women. Elite athletes and other women who get large amounts of exercise tend to have lower levels of body fat and thus a lower level of estrogen, which would normally be stored in this body fat. This may put them at risk for thinning bones and fractures.

Professional dancers and athletes, of course, must maintain extraordinary levels of physical exertion to remain competitive. These women have a particularly hard time recognizing when they are pushing themselves too hard. How can you tell if you are overdoing it? Signs include:

- exercising so much that you end up neglecting your family, job duties, or household responsibilities

BUILDING A BETTER BODY IMAGE

Getting into shape and staying that way are worthy goals. But learning to accept your physical limitations and imperfections is essential. Here are some steps you can take to improve your body image:

Analyze your feelings about your body

- Think about the messages your family gave you about your body while you were growing up. Were they complimentary or derogatory? Do they correspond to your current image of yourself?

- Ask yourself if you are unhappy with other aspects of your life. Is underlying unhappiness affecting your body image?

- If you are truly overweight, keep track of everything you eat for at least a week. Next to each item, write down your mood. Were you angry? feeling stressed? Think about what role food plays in dealing with your feelings.

- Make a list of goals or activities you have put off doing because of the way you look, and start doing them one at a time.

Put your image in perspective

- Study classic paintings and sculptures and note that most of the images we have come to see as beautiful are imperfect. Look for those depicting idealized female forms that are plumper than today's ideal. Thus, you will see that an "ideal" weight is relative and changes with the times.

- Look at favorite pictures of yourself. Do they jibe with your body image or have you been concentrating on the negative?

- Ask a good friend or partner to tell you what he or she finds attractive about you. Reevaluate your body image in light of what you hear.

Play up the positive

- Stand in front of a mirror and look at each part of your body. Write down all the parts that you like. Find something special. Is it your eyes? your smile? your hands? your hair? your ankles? Concentrate on how you feel about your best parts. How can you accentuate them?

- Consider which clothing styles make you look best, which outfits make you feel good, which ones bring you the most compliments. Wear these often.

- Wear colors that look good on you. If you're not sure which these are, consider having an analysis by a "color specialist." You may be surprised at the difference flattering colors can make in the way you look and *feel*.

Experience your body through your senses

- Take up an activity that is good for both your body and mind, such as walking, swimming, yoga, or regular stretching.

- Indulge yourself with scented body oils, bubble baths, massages, or herbal wraps.

- exercising to the point where the activity is no longer pleasurable, and you begin to dislike it

- ignoring injuries or exercising when you are in pain or against a doctor's advice

- a prolonged lack of menstrual periods (more than 3 months) not due to pregnancy or other medical causes

- setting unrealistic goals and being obsessed with attaining those goals, sometimes through the use of steroids

- an inability to vary your exercise schedule or skip a session without feeling guilty or distressed

If exercise is becoming a burden, physically or psychologically, it's time to reexamine your priorities. And if you cannot adopt a more reasonable program of physical activity, professional counseling may be in order.

COSMETIC SURGERY

Each year, about 150,000 American women receive surgical breast implants, more than 80 percent of them for cosmetic reasons alone. Another quarter of a million women undergo liposuction, a procedure that suctions out fat cells, reshaping fat-prone areas such as the thighs. Countless others are going under the knife for everything from nose jobs to tummy tucks in search of the perfect body. Although any surgery carries risk, some of these procedures are riskier than others. Breast implants, for example, can result in later complications and may make it more difficult to detect potentially cancerous breast lumps; liposuction may result in infection.

The question is whether the risk of breast augmentation or any other procedure to reshape the body outweighs the benefits to one's self-image. Ideally, a woman who chooses to undergo such a procedure should do so only for her own satisfaction or, in the case of breast reduction, physical comfort. And many women who are self-conscious about overly large breasts or a crooked nose find that corrective surgery changes their mental outlook. But some contemplate cosmetic surgery with pleasing men as their objective. Studies suggest that women overestimate male preferences in breast size and body weight, and some women who undergo cosmetic surgery may have unrealistic hopes pinned on the outcome. Before committing yourself, you should be clear about your expectations for the surgery, and consider whether it will really answer your needs. (For more information, see Chapters 14 and 15.)

TOWARD A BETTER SELF-IMAGE

Coming to terms with your body is a challenge you will meet at every stage of life. That means recognizing that physical attributes are just one part of yourself, and learning to judge your self-worth by measures other than the amount of weight lost or hours exercised.

In the long run, a tolerant and forgiving attitude toward your body can also make it easier to get into better shape. (See box, "Building a Better Body Image.") Women who see themselves as heavy or ugly are more likely to fail to take off weight and keep it off. How you feel about your body is very important to your overall well-being. Once you can accept yourself for who you are, attaining your "ideal" body weight won't matter as much.

CHAPTER 14

Breast Care

There is hardly another organ in your body that undergoes as many changes throughout your lifetime as your breasts. Breasts usually begin to grow shortly before puberty, and it takes several years before they reach their mature structure. (See Figures 14.1–14.6.) During pregnancy and after childbirth, they adapt to nursing. In every menstrual cycle, breast tissue responds to the ebbs and flows of female hormones. As you reach menopause, the breast structure alters again. These transformations can give rise to a variety of symptoms, including swelling, pain, tenderness, and lumps, and breast disorders are extremely common, although the vast majority are benign.

To provide the best care for your breasts, you must be attuned to any symptoms they may exhibit. By learning to recognize what is normal, you can spare yourself a great deal of anxiety and avoid unnecessary surgery and checkups, as well as quickly identifying any possibly abnormal symptoms.

SIZE AND SHAPE

Breast size is largely determined by genetic factors. It can also be affected by the amount of fat the breasts contain, and some women may find that their breasts shrink when they lose weight. Overweight women often, albeit not always, have large breasts because they contain a great deal of fatty tissue. Breasts have no muscle, and it is impossible to increase their size by exercise. (See Figure 14.7.) However, exercise can build up the underlying chest muscles, making the breasts protrude and appear larger. Good posture can also make the breasts look more prominent. Hormone therapy can increase breast size, and some women taking birth control pills notice that their breasts expand somewhat. But hormones should not be taken merely for this purpose.

Despite the claims of some manufacturers, there are no creams or other remedies that can enlarge the breasts or make them firmer. Firmness depends mainly on the amount of glandular tissue, the milk-producing part of the breast. The breasts of older women are usually softer than those of younger women because with age, glandular tissue shrinks and is gradually replaced by fat.

In view of the fashion to go braless, the question arises whether not wearing a brassiere will make the breasts sag. Women with small, light breasts do not need a bra, but if yours are heavy, you need good support to prevent the skin and supporting ligaments from stretching.

Many women are unhappy with the size or shape of their breasts. In particular, small-breasted women sometimes wish their breasts were bigger. However, this may be an unrealistic ideal. In one study conducted at the University of South Florida in Tampa, students were shown five drawings of women that differed only in the size of their breasts, and were asked to rate them in terms of attractiveness. Female students were also asked which figure they thought men would prefer. The researchers found that the size of breasts that male students preferred was a great

Breast development

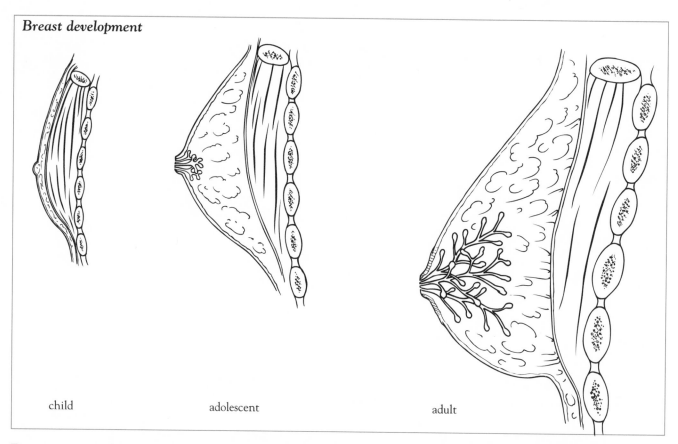

child   adolescent   adult

Fig. 14.1–14.6 *In children, breasts of boys and girls are indistinguishable. When a girl approaches puberty, her breasts begin to take on shape as first the nipples and areolae and then the breasts themselves begin to stand out from the chest wall. The lobes and alveoli of the milk-production system begin to grow inward from the nipple, and fat deposits accumulate until the breasts take on their adult shape. During pregnancy, glandular tissue expands, the areolae darken, and the Montgomery glands (which appear as bumps on the areolae) enlarge. The alveoli increase in number and size and, in the last trimester, colostrum—the forerunner of breast milk—is produced. During nursing, the breasts may be double or triple their usual size. With age, glandular tissue shrinks and is replaced by fat, making the breasts softer.*

Breast changes

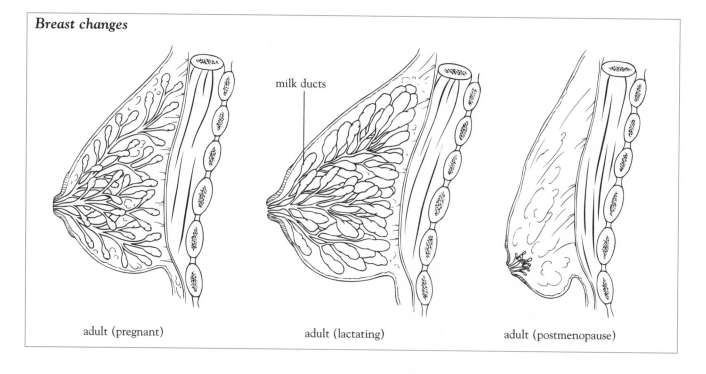

milk ducts

adult (pregnant)   adult (lactating)   adult (postmenopause)

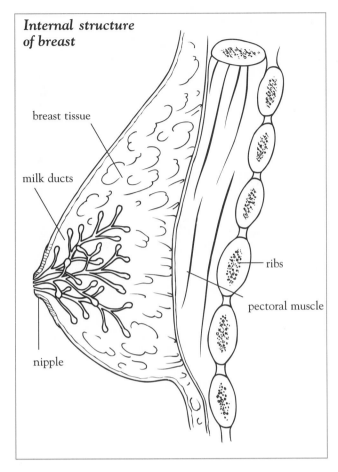

Internal structure of breast

breast tissue

milk ducts

nipple

ribs

pectoral muscle

Fig. 14.7 *The breasts have a complex structure of glands designed to sustain an infant. For many women, they are also a site of sexual stimulation.*

deal smaller than that which the women considered was the male ideal.

If you are truly dissatisfied with the size or firmness of your breasts, several cosmetic surgical procedures have proved successful in enlarging, reducing, or lifting them. (See section on "Cosmetic Breast Surgery.")

PREGNANCY AND BREAST-FEEDING

The most dramatic changes in the breasts take place during pregnancy. They become firmer and larger as the glandular tissue swells and expands. In some women, the breasts double or triple in size in preparation for breast-feeding. The areola—the dark ring around the nipple—grows darker or, in blondes, may become pinker. Sometimes, a second dark ring, called the secondary areola, may temporarily surround the areola. During the last 3 months of pregnancy, the

breasts become more engorged and the nipples often start secreting a discharge that is the forerunner of breast milk. (See box, "Caring for Your Breasts During Pregnancy.")

Immediately before and for a day or two after delivery, the breasts produce colostrum, a thick, milky fluid that precedes true milk. Afterward, whenever the baby suckles or the breast is stimulated manually, signals are sent to the mother's brain, triggering the release of the hormones prolactin and oxytocin. These hormones in turn stimulate the secretion of milk and its flow along the milk ducts to the nipple. (See Figure 14.9.) In response to the baby's suckling, the nipple and areola contract, which causes the ducts to squeeze and facilitates the flow.

Some women fear that breast-feeding will "ruin" their breasts, but in fact it will have no effect on their subsequent size and shape. Pregnancy itself, however, may change their appearance somewhat. Some women retain additional glandular tissue, which means their breasts will be larger than before pregnancy, while in others the glandular tissue may

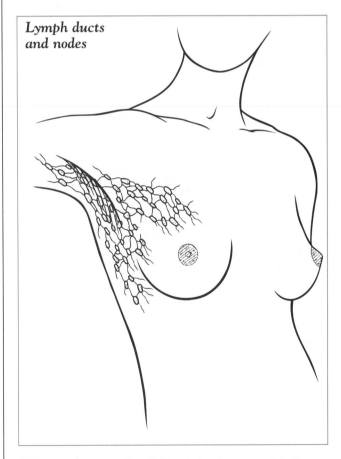

Lymph ducts and nodes

Fig. 14.8 *A system of lymph ducts and nodes surround the breasts, draining excess fluid and debris from the cells. Throughout the body the lymph system helps fight against disease and infection.*

CARING FOR YOUR BREASTS DURING PREGNANCY

• As your breasts become larger and heavier, wear a maternity bra that provides good support. It will keep your breasts from bouncing and may help reduce the tenderness that is particularly common in early pregnancy. Some women find it economical to purchase nursing bras (with cups that open) for use during the last few months of pregnancy as well as during breast-feeding.

• A good bra may also prevent the skin from stretching excessively under the weight of the breasts, helping them to return to their previous shape after pregnancy. Contrary to popular belief, skin lotions will not prevent stretch marks.

• You can rub your breasts with cocoa butter, lotions, or ointments if the skin is dry. Usually, the Montgomery glands—small bumps located throughout the areola—secrete sufficient fatty material to lubricate the areola and the nipple.

• Toward the end of pregnancy, as your breasts begin to leak a clear or milky substance called colostrum, you can wear pads, a folded handkerchief, or a soft tissue inside the bra. Do not, however, try to squeeze out the discharge, which is completely normal.

• In preparation for nursing, you can begin during pregnancy to toughen your nipples by rubbing them with a terry towel. You may also tug and roll your nipples between your thumb and fingers. These techniques can often prevent the sore, cracked nipples that often occur during breast-feeding for women with thin, fair skin.

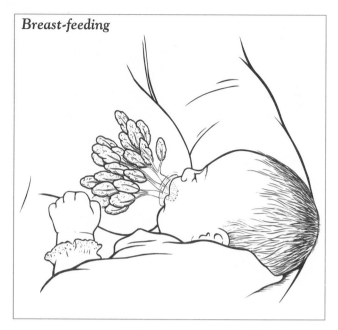

Breast-feeding

Fig. 14.9 *During breast-feeding, suckling triggers the release of the hormone oxytocin, which causes the cells lining the alveoli to contract, forcing milk into the ducts and reservoirs and then through 15 to 25 openings in each nipple into the baby's mouth. This process, known as the letdown reflex, can sometimes be triggered by seeing the baby or hearing its cry.*

CARING FOR YOUR BREASTS DURING BREAST-FEEDING

• If your breasts are sore, apply cold or warm compresses to alleviate the discomfort.

• Keep your breasts dry between nursing sessions to avoid skin irritation. To avoid chafing your skin by constant wiping, you can expose your breasts to the air, position them several inches from a lamp, or use a hair dryer to dry them.

• Do not wear bras with plastic nipple linings because they tend to collect moisture.

• If you have sore, crackled nipples, wash them with warm water without soap before and after nursing and apply lanolin or olive or peanut oil after feedings. You may give your baby expressed milk for a day or two to allow the crack to heal.

• Do not wear a bra that is too tight, as it may stop milk production—unless that is your intent.

• If pain and tenderness persist, especially if they are confined to one breast, call your doctor. It may be a symptom of mastitis, an infection that must be treated with antibiotics. (For more information, see the Encyclopedia.)

shrink, making them smaller or softer. Nursing does not make the breasts sag, although the inevitable stretching of the skin and supporting ligaments during pregnancy may alter the way they look. (See box, "Caring for Your Breasts During Breast-Feeding.")

BENIGN BREAST DISORDERS

Sometimes swelling and tenderness, called mastodynia, occurs in the breasts just before the onset of menstrual periods. This discomfort tends to disappear when the flow starts or reaches its height, only to recur the following month. (See Chapter 1, "The Female Body," and Chapter 4, "Menstruation," for more information.)

Along with the swelling, many women feel a lumpiness. This is a perfectly normal cyclical change. In preparation for pregnancy, the milk-secreting glands multiply during the first half of the menstrual cycle. After ovulation, other hormones continue the milk-readiness process. If there is no pregnancy, the fluid and tissue cells that have been produced are simply reabsorbed by the breasts.

With age, your milk-producing glands thicken and your body has more difficulty absorbing the excess fluid and tissue each month. The fluid may become trapped, forming cysts, which may persist for a month or two or become permanent. This disorder is known as fibrocystic breast disease. This and another benign breast disorder, fibroadenoma, are discussed in the Encyclopedia.

BREAST CANCER

Breast cancer, perhaps more because of the possibility of disfigurement than pain or death, is more frightening to women than any other form of cancer. Such statistics as one in nine women will develop breast cancer by age 85 cause many women to lose sight of the fact that breast cancer is treatable and often curable. Thousands of women treated for the disease survive 5 to 10 years or even longer. For example, the 5-year survival rate for women with localized cancer is 92 percent. The overall 5-year survival rate, even including women whose cancer has spread to distant sites, is 77 percent.

Breast cancer that is discovered before it has spread to the lymph nodes (see Figure 14.8) and generally before the primary tumor exceeds an inch in diameter means the chance of recovery is usually better than when it is discovered in a more advanced stage. Although in some cases, cancerous cells are thought to spread to distant parts of the body (metastasize) early in the course of the disease, physicians believe that, in general, the early removal of a cancerous tumor can prevent it from spreading. Moreover, small tumors can more often be treated with breast-sparing surgery than large ones.

There are certain risk factors for breast cancer, of which everyone should be aware, but half of all breast cancers develop in women who have no risk factors. There are some measures women can take to lower the risk, but the evidence for their efficacy is tenuous. Surgical treatment has been considerably refined in the last two decades. Radiation, chemotherapy, and the drug tamoxifen have been successful in treating breast cancer and in preventing its recurrence. But the best hope remains early detection, and scheduling regular physical and radiological examinations remains each woman's paramount responsibility.

BREAST CANCER PREVENTION

Most known risk factors for breast cancer are beyond control. One is increasing age, since breast cancer is largely a disease of older women. The risk begins to rise sharply after age 50. Heredity also plays a role, although it may not be as important as many women believe. Breast tumors are so common that two or more cases may occur in one family by chance. You are usually considered at increased risk if your mother or sister, or both, developed breast cancer before menopause. Women treated for cancer in one breast are increasingly likely to develop a malignancy in the other. Women who have had ovarian, uterine, or colon cancer, as well as cancer of the salivary glands, are at greater risk of developing breast cancer.

Another factor that increases the risk is early menstruation (before age 12), which means that your body will produce estrogen over a longer period of time. Estrogen, which plays many necessary, positive roles in the female body, also promotes the growth of some types of cancerous tumors. For the same reason, late menopause also increases the risk, as does having a first baby after age 30 or having no children at all. White women have a slightly greater risk than women of other races.

Markedly overweight women, particularly if they continue to be obese after menopause, are believed to be prone to developing several cancers, including those of the breast. While technically controllable, obesity is notoriously difficult to reverse.

One potential risk factor that can be controlled is alcohol intake. Many studies have linked drinking with an increased breast cancer risk, but others have found no such connection. It is possible that there is an association, but there is not yet enough evidence to state that women who drink moderately (no more than one drink a day) need give it up. More than two drinks a day, however, increases the risk for various diseases and may double that of getting breast cancer.

The most controversial risk factor for breast cancer is diet. Various studies have suggested that a high-calorie or high-fat diet increases the risk, while a diet high in fiber and vitamins A, C, and beta-carotene tends to lower it. Dietary fat spurs the development of cancer in the mammary glands of laboratory animals. In women, dietary fat may stimulate the ovaries to produce more estrogen, which is known to promote growth of malignant breast tumors. It may affect hormone levels in the body indirectly, by changing the amount and composition of body fat.

According to a recent theory, fat may also play a role that is unrelated to hormone production. In one small study, researchers found that the breast fat of women with breast cancer contained 50 to 60 percent more of certain contaminants, such as polychlorinated biphenyls (PCBs) and pesticides like DDT, than the breast fat of women without the cancer. Both chemicals have been banned for years, but they are still present in the environment and tend to collect in the fatty tissue of fish and animals.

Although the hypothesis linking fat to breast cancer is plausible, the evidence is inconclusive and there have been no controlled studies because of the difficulty of strictly monitoring what people eat. Much of the evidence comes from studying different cultures. In the United States, Canada, and industrialized European countries, where dietary fat makes up about 34 to 40 percent of calories, the rate of breast cancer deaths is almost four times higher than in some Asian countries where dietary fat is minimal. However, other life-style or environmental differences may affect a greater or lesser cancer risk. Some

HOW TO DO
BREAST SELF-EXAMINATION

While examining your breasts, make sure you examine all the breast tissue, which can extend to the armpit, the collarbone, and the breastbone. Breast self-examination is performed in several steps:

1. Stand before a mirror, arms by your sides, and see if you notice anything unusual about your breasts—a change in shape, discharge from the nipples, dimpling, puckering, or scaling of the skin.

2. Raise your arms, tighten them, and clasp them behind your head. This will tighten your chest muscles and thrust your breasts forward, helping you examine them in a different position. (See Figure 14.10.)

3. Put your hands firmly on the hips, bow slightly toward the mirror while pulling your shoulders and elbows forward, and closely look at the breasts again. (See Figure 14.11.)

4. Raise your left arm and, using the pads of three or four fingers—not the fingertips—of your right hand, carefully examine your left breast while applying sufficient pressure to feel the underlying tissue. You can start at the nipple and move in circles to the outer edge, or start at the outer circle and progress toward the nipple. You can also move the fingers in vertical or horizontal lines, from left to right or top to bottom. Alternatively, picture the breast as a wheel and examine every spoke, from center to the outer rim. Whatever method you choose, be sure to cover the entire breast. Then repeat the procedure on the second breast. Soaping your fingers will help them glide over the skin, making it easier to feel the texture underneath. Some women perform this part of the examination in the shower. (See Figure 14.12.)

5. Repeat step 4 lying on your back. This position flattens the breasts and makes them easier to examine. It often allows you to feel cartilage or bony structures of the rib cage that may at first be mistaken for lumps. Placing a pillow or folded towel under the shoulder helps shift the breast to the center of the chest. (See Figure 14.13.)

If you have large breasts, you may find it easier to examine them using both hands. Support your breast with one hand underneath while you use the other to examine the top surface. Change hands to examine the lower part of your breast. Repeat with the other breast. (See Figure 14.14.)

6. Report to your doctor any of the following signs:

• a lump or lumpiness

• dimpling or puckering of the skin anywhere on the breast

• any change in size, shape, or color of the nipple

• turning in or drawing back of the nipple

• discharge from the nipple

• rash on the nipple

• swelling of the upper arm or enlarged glands under the arm

Steps in breast self-examination

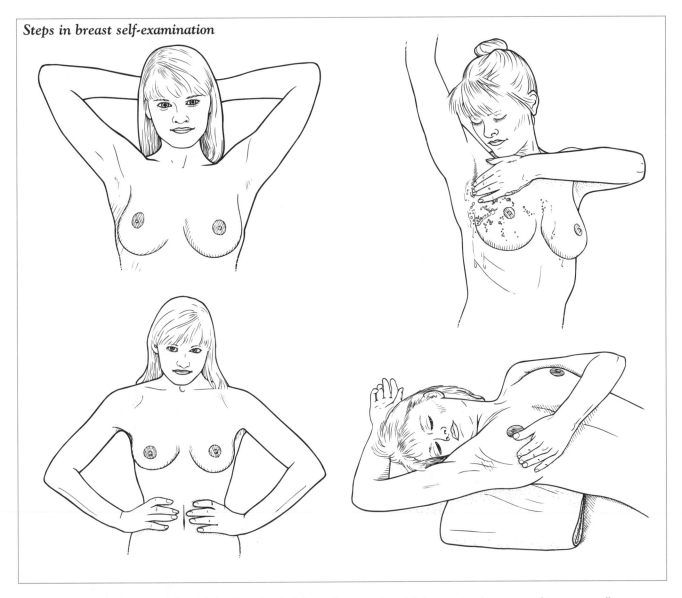

Fig. 14.10–14.13 *Clasping your hands behind your head while you flex your chest and then putting them on your hips as you pull your elbows forward allows you to see each breast entirely and in several positions. Although the manual breast exam can be done in front of a mirror, many women find that it is easier to do in the shower with soapy skin. The final part of the exam is performed by lying down.*

epidemiologic studies have failed to show a link between a high-fat diet and breast cancer. In 1992, the Nurses' Health Study, which has been following the diets and other health and life-style factors of more than 120,000 women since 1976, found no association between either fat or fiber intake and risk of breast cancer. However, it did find a clear positive correlation between total fat and animal fat intake and the risk of developing colon cancer. Some researchers point out that this study compared high-fat diets with medium-fat diets and postulate that the risk is lowered only with low-fat (20 percent of calories or less) diets.

There is some reason to believe that tamoxifen, a drug commonly used to treat breast cancer and prevent its recurrence, may prevent its development in healthy low-risk women. To test this hypothesis, the National Cancer Institute launched in 1992 a 5-year study of 16,000 women considered to be at high risk of breast cancer. Because the preventive value of tamoxifen is unclear, the drug may have serious adverse reactions. Its long-term effects are unknown and it should not be used by healthy women outside the study.

Hair dyes and reserpine, a drug used to treat high blood pressure, have been studied for a possible link

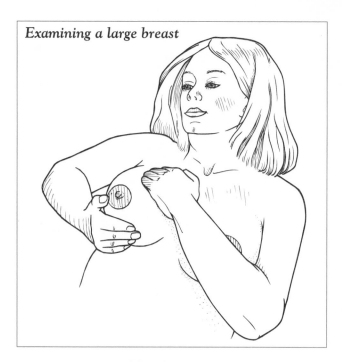

Examining a large breast

Fig. 14.14 *Women with large breasts may find it easier to firm and steady the breast with one hand underneath it while examining it with the fingers of the other hand.*

to breast cancer, but no connection has been found. Some studies have linked breast cancer with birth control pills or hormone replacement therapy given to women after menopause, but others have failed to establish a relationship. Contrary to popular belief, breast-feeding does not protect against breast cancer. (See box, "Reducing Your Risk of Breast Cancer.")

EARLY DETECTION OF BREAST CANCER

• **Breast Self-examination.** Many women are familiar with breast self-examination as a way to detect cancer, but its value in helping prevent unnecessary surgery is probably not as well known. A woman who examines her breasts regularly may be spared a biopsy should a doctor find a suspicious lump because she knows whether the lump is indeed new or has been there for years. To be beneficial, however, breast self-examination must be thorough and consistent. It should be performed once a month and takes about 10 minutes if done properly. If you are premenopausal, you should perform it between the 7th and 10th days of your cycle (7 to 10 days after your period starts), when your breasts are at their smallest. Women who examine their breasts properly can find lumps that are as small as ¼ inch in diameter. The majority of breast lumps are found by women themselves. (See box, "How to Do Breast Self-Examination," and Figures 14.10–14.14.)

• **Examination by a Physician.** The second important method of early cancer detection is to have a physician examine your breasts. Health and medical organizations are in agreement that this should be done annually. Examination by a doctor is especially important if you do not practice breast self-examination.

• **Mammography.** Mammography, or X-ray screening of the breast, can detect tumors that are very small and cannot be felt by the fingers. (See Figures 14.15 and 14.16.) It can significantly improve breast cancer survival for women over 50, reducing deaths

REDUCING YOUR RISK OF BREAST CANCER

The causes of breast cancer are not sufficiently understood to develop preventive measures, but you can take certain steps to reduce your risk of developing the malignancy. If you are considered to be at high risk of breast cancer, you should pay special attention to these recommendations:

• Avoid unnecessary X rays, particularly during puberty or pregnancy when the breast tissue undergoes rapid changes. Ionizing radiation is carcinogenic in large amounts, but it is best to avoid even small exposures to it unless medically justified. Your breasts should be covered with a breast shield during X rays for the lower back, and you should request a lead apron and collar when dental X rays are taken. Radiation levels to which breasts are exposed during mammography are believed to be too low to cause breast cancer.

• Maintain a normal body weight. Try to reduce if your weight is 40 percent or more above the level considered desirable for your height. (At that level, you are also at increased risk for cancer of the uterus, ovaries, gallbladder, and colon.)

• Although the role of dietary fat in the development of breast cancer is unclear, it may be prudent to decrease the amount of fat you eat. The American Cancer Society recommends keeping fat intake to no more than 30 percent of calories to reduce the risk of several cancers, including those of the breast and colon.

• While the role of alcohol in causing breast cancer is not conclusive, avoid heavy drinking, if for no other reason than it can cause liver problems, exacerbate cardiovascular disease, and increase the risk of developing several other cancers.

Mammography

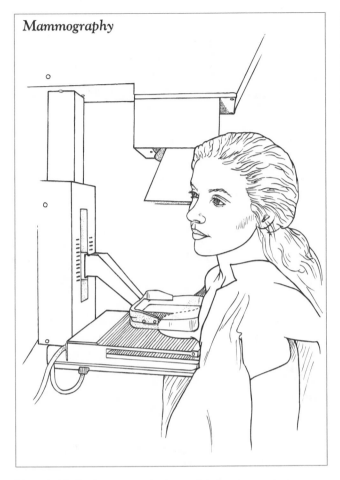

Fig. 14.15 *During mammography, each breast in turn is compressed between two plastic plates. The breasts are X-rayed in at least two positions, sometimes more if they are large. Compressing the breasts, which some women find uncomfortable, minimizes the amount of radiation necessary to get a clear image.*

Normal and abnormal mammogram

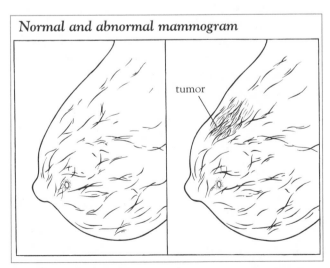

tumor

Fig. 14.16 *On a mammogram, a tumor appears as a white, denser area in the breast. Although mammography can help distinguish cysts and other benign conditions from tumors, a biopsy is necessary to confirm or rule out cancer. Eight out of ten breast lumps turn out to be benign.*

by about one third. (See box, "Where to Have a Mammogram.")

Mammography has its limitations, however. On the one hand, it does not detect approximately 10 to 15 percent of tumors. On the other hand, a mammogram reveals areas of the breast that are suspicious but not necessarily cancerous, and thus a benign lump can be mistaken for cancer.

• **Mammography in Younger Women.** Mammography is clearly justified in women under 50 who have a strong family history of the disease, have been treated for breast cancer in the past, or have been previously diagnosed with carcinoma *in situ*, which increases the risk of invasive breast cancer. For women under 40, in whom breast cancer is less common, mammography appears to be a less effective screening device. It is also less accurate in younger women because their breast tissues are more dense.

Experts disagree, however, about the value of mammography for women between the ages of 40 and 50 who are not at high risk. The American Cancer Society and the National Cancer Institute recommend that women start having regular mammograms in their forties, while the American College of Physicians, the American College of Surgeons, and the U.S. Preventive Services Task Force do not. Indeed, the United States is the only major country where mammography is still recommended for women under 50. The two major issues with respect to screening in this age group are whether or not mammography can cause cancer in younger women, and whether or not it can save lives in women under 50. (See box, "When to Have a Mammogram."

The answer to the first question appears to be no. Mammography equipment today uses very low levels of exposure that do not increase cancer risk. The answer to the second question may also be no. All major studies except one have shown that women under 50 derive no benefits from mammography in terms of breast cancer survival. However, the quality of the mammography performed in some of the studies has been questioned. Only the Health Insurance Plan Study of Greater New York, launched in 1963, showed that in women under 50, there were fewer breast cancer deaths among women who were screened with mammography compared with those who were not. In light of these conflicting recommendations, if you are under 50 you should consult your doctor before making a decision about mammography.

BREAST RECONSTRUCTION AFTER MASTECTOMY

Treating a small, early-stage tumor usually means performing a lumpectomy, removal of the tumor, leaving the rest of the breast intact. Treatment of larger tumors or cancers that have spread to the surrounding lymph nodes may involve some form of

WHEN TO HAVE A MAMMOGRAM

AGE	RECOMMENDATION	FREQUENCY
Under 40	Not recommended	
40 to 50	Possibly recommended—check with your doctor	Every 2 years
	Definitely recommended if you:	Annually
	have a strong family history of breast cancer	
	have been treated for breast cancer	
	have been diagnosed with carcinoma *in situ*	
50 to 75	Recommended	Annually
After 75	Not recommended	

WHERE TO HAVE A MAMMOGRAM

In 1987, the American College of Radiology (ACR) started an accreditation program that evaluates mammography facilities for the quality of screening they provide. For a list of accredited facilities in your area, you can call the ACR's toll-free number, 1-800-ACR-LINE. If you go to a facility that has not been accredited, the ACR recommends that you ask the following questions:

1. Is the radiologist certified by the American Board of Radiology or the American Osteopathic Board of Radiology?

2. If not certified, has the radiologist had at least 2 months of training in reading mammograms?

3. Are the technicians certified by the American Registry of Radiological Technologists or a state licensing board?

4. Is the X-ray equipment designed specifically for mammograms?

5. Is mammography a regular part of the facility's practice?

In addition, the Center for Medical Consumers, a public interest organization based in New York City, recommends that women inquire about radiation exposures at the facility. Limits for various types of mammograms set by the Quality Assurance Program of the New York State Department of Health can be used as a reference:

• 0.1 rads per view for film-screen systems without a grid

• 0.3 rads per view for film-screen systems with a grid

• 0.4 rads per view for xeromammography

The center also recommends that you keep the mammogram, or purchase a copy of the original, to make sure that it does not get lost or destroyed. You may need it in the future for comparison with other test results.

mastectomy. These treatment options, as well as radiation and drug therapy, are discussed in the Encyclopedia. This section describes your reconstruction options following mastectomy.

Breast cancer surgery need no longer be viewed as a permanently disfiguring procedure. Even if a diseased breast has to be removed, it can be reconstructed at the same time or, if preferred, at a later date. Most often, breast reconstruction is performed at the same time as mastectomy, which spares you the trauma of waking up without a breast. It may be done in two separate steps: reconstruction of the breast, followed about 3 months later by reconstruction of the nipple. If you face having a mastectomy, you should discuss reconstruction with your surgeon because the incisions for the mastectomy can be placed in ways that will facilitate certain reconstructive techniques.

Although breast reconstruction can greatly improve the quality of life, relatively few women undergoing mastectomies have their breasts reconstructed. Over the last decade, the number of reconstructions performed annually has more than doubled, but many women still hesitate to ask about the procedure because they are unaware of how successful the surgery can be, or perhaps they fear being perceived as vain or self-indulgent. Some may be concerned that reconstruction might increase the risk of the tumor recurring or make it more difficult to detect a malignancy should it develop. There is no evidence to support either of these fears. Indeed, besides its psychological advantages, reconstruction has numerous physical benefits, such as avoiding the sweating, skin irritation, neck and back pain, and posture problems associated with wearing a prosthesis.

Many health insurance policies cover breast reconstruction, and some states mandate its inclusion in policies that cover mastectomies. However, surgery on the opposite breast, which may be needed to create symmetry, may not be covered by insurance. Women who are evaluating various reconstruction options should find out exactly what their policy will cover.

TYPES OF RECONSTRUCTION When making a decision about what type of reconstruction is best for you, you should weigh the advantages of each method against the disadvantages. Sometimes surgery must also be performed on the healthy breast to create a match for the one that has been reconstructed. The nipple and areola are usually created several weeks after the initial reconstruction. An areola may be tattooed on the skin, or it may be created by a skin graft from another part of the body, such as the upper inner thigh. The nipple may be reconstructed by using a skin flap from local tissue on the breast mound, or by removing part of the healthy nipple if it is sufficiently large.

The major reconstruction techniques are:

• A breast implant—the same type as used in breast enlargement—can be inserted under the skin and muscle of the chest wall. If there is enough loose skin and muscle to cover the implant sufficiently, a permanent device is used. If the skin is too tight, a temporary implant with a filling valve is inserted first. This tissue expander is filled with saline (salt water) and enlarged gradually over a month or two to stretch the muscle or skin and create a pocket for the implant. Adjustment of the expander requires repeat visits to the surgeon but can improve the shape of the reconstructed breast, which might otherwise be too round and flat. This procedure may have the same complications associated with other breast implant techniques (see section on "Risks of Implants"), but it is the simplest of all reconstruction methods.

If there is not enough skin or muscle over the rib cage, tissue from another part of the body can be used to make a "flap." The three flap options are:

• Latissimus dorsi myocutaneous flap (LD flap). In a procedure used since the late 1970s, a wedge of a large muscle from the lower back is flipped over (through a tunnel under the skin) to the chest to create a breast. The muscle remains attached to the body by a thin bridge of tissue containing blood vessels and nerves. Although this technique leaves a scar on the back, it can be placed low enough to be hidden by a bathing suit. An implant is usually needed, but the flap can fill in the hollow left by extensive breast surgery. A variation on this technique, called the peg procedure, leaves a peg-shaped piece of skin attached to the muscle, which can be used to fill the hole left when the nipple is removed.

• Transverse rectus abdominus myocutaneous (TRAM, or RAM) flap. (See Figures 14.17–14.21.) First introduced in 1980, the TRAM flap involves reconstructing a breast by taking a portion of the lower abdomen that contains skin and fat, leaving it attached to the underlying muscle by a thin bridge of tissue, and rotating it up onto the chest wall. The result is a soft and natural-looking breast, usually without the need for an implant. In addition, the procedure creates a simultaneous tummy tuck.

For women who have abdominal scars, the TRAM flap is possible but must be modified. The procedure is not recommended for obese women or for smokers, whose small blood vessels may have been damaged by nicotine and cannot supply adequate blood (and thus oxygen) to the new tissue. Nor can it be performed on women who have no fat below the navel.

TRAM flap reconstruction has some drawbacks: It leaves a scar on the abdomen, can lead to wound-healing problems and occasional complications, and involves a longer recuperation period than with an implant. It usually requires a blood transfusion, preferably with your own blood donated in advance.

• Free flap. This procedure involves transferring a tissue wedge from the thigh or buttocks to the chest, where it is reconnected to the blood vessels. Such portions of tissue are referred to as "free flaps" because they come from areas located far from the breast and need to be detached from the body completely during the transfer. The procedure is long and complicated, and there is an approximately 5 percent risk that the flap will not heal. However, it eliminates the need for an implant and helps create a natural-looking breast.

TRAM *flap*

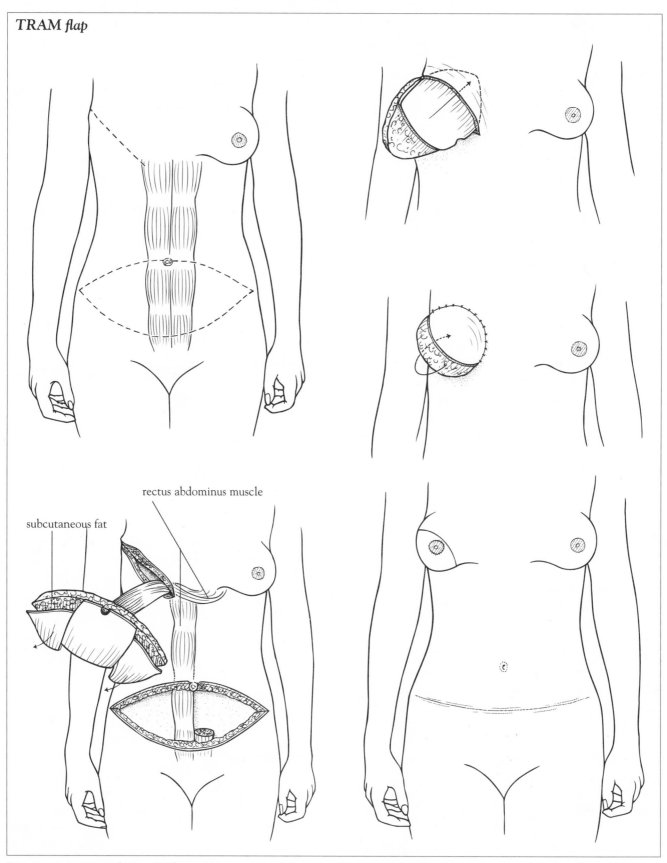

subcutaneous fat

rectus abdominus muscle

Fig. 14.17–14.21 *In the TRAM flap procedure, a portion of skin and fat is excised from the abdomen but left attached to a band of muscle. The tissue is threaded up through a tunnel below the fat of the abdominal wall and out through the incision left by the removal of the original breast. Then the excess skin is removed, the underlying fat fashioned into a breast, and the remaining skin attached to the chest. Later, a nipple may be fashioned, usually from the skin of the transplanted tissue.*

COSMETIC BREAST SURGERY

Surgical remodeling of breasts can improve your appearance, boost your self-confidence, and increase the variety of clothing styles you can wear. Although almost always elective surgery, some breast reduction procedures are performed for medical reasons.

As with any elective procedure, the decision to have cosmetic breast surgery should not be made lightly. Some women attach considerable symbolic significance to their breasts and can invest unrealistic hopes in having them reshaped, particularly if they are going through periods of emotional stress. Cosmetic surgery should not be expected to solve life's problems. (See box, "Choosing a Plastic Surgeon.")

BREAST ENLARGEMENT In breast enlargement, or breast augmentation, the surgeon makes an incision around the areola, under the breast or in the armpit, and inserts an implant—a soft, round envelope filled with saline. (See Figures 14.22 and 14.23.) The implants can be placed under the breast tissue or underneath the chest muscle. (See Figures 14.24 and 14.25.) Implants come in various sizes, but most women choose moderate enlargement, to a B or C cup size. If one breast is larger than the other, the asymmetry can be corrected by selecting implants of different sizes. The surgeon's fee for this procedure, which may or may not include the cost of the implant, ranges from $750 to $7,000, with the average being about $2,750. (All fees in this chapter are 1992 figures provided by the American Society of Plastic and Reconstructive Surgeons.)

Breast enlargement is relatively simple to perform but it is highly controversial because of ongoing concerns about the safety of breast implants. Critics say implants should be banned because they can cause serious problems. Advocates argue they must remain on the market, citing polls showing that the vast majority of women are satisfied with the devices. Underlying the debate is a deeper argument over stereotypes of beauty and women's right to take risks related to their own bodies. In a compromise decision, the Food and Drug Administration ruled in the spring of 1992 that silicone-gel breast implants would be available only through controlled clinical studies. Women who need such implants for breast reconstruction after cancer surgery are assured access to these studies, but not all women who simply wish to enlarge their breasts. Saline implants will remain available for cosmetic and reconstructive procedures.

Until restrictions were applied, more than 90 per-

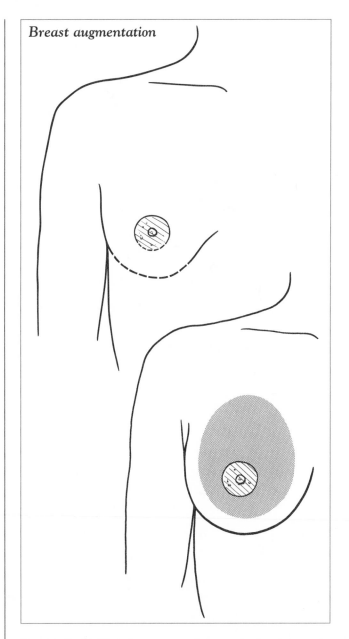

Breast augmentation

Fig. 14.22–14.23 *In breast augmentation, an implant is inserted through an incision at the margin of the areola, under the armpit, or in the crease under the breast. Once in place, the implant gives a natural appearance to the breast.*

cent of all implants were filled with silicone gel. Devices filled with saline were less popular because many surgeons felt they produced a less natural appearance of the breast. Also, when they leak, they deflate immediately. The third type, called a double-lumen implant, contains two envelopes, one filled with silicone gel encased inside another containing saline. The outer shell of all the implants is made of rubbery silicone, which may be glossy or textured. Injecting silicone directly into the breasts is dangerous and illegal.

Breast implant positions

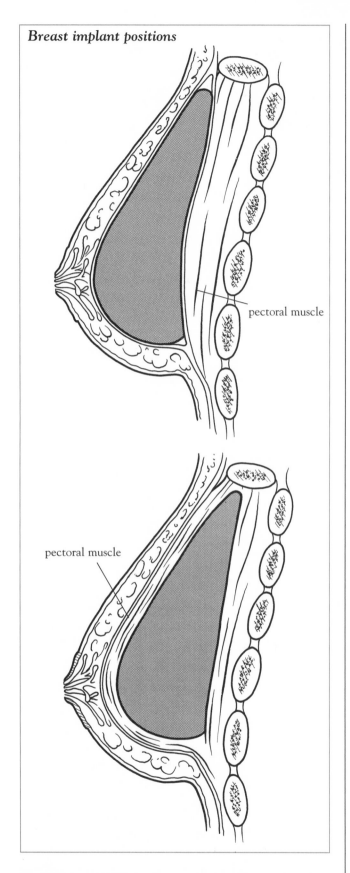

pectoral muscle

pectoral muscle

Fig. 14.24–14.25 *The implant may be placed between the breast and the underlying muscle (top), or placed beneath the muscle layer (bottom). In thin women with smaller breasts, the latter technique is commonly used.*

CHOOSING A PLASTIC SURGEON

• Although any medical doctor is allowed to perform cosmetic surgery, only a surgeon who is certified by the American Board of Plastic Surgery is likely to have the expertise. To find such a doctor in your area, contact the toll-free referral service of the American Society of Plastic and Reconstructive Surgeons: 1-800-635-0635.

• Find a plastic surgeon who specializes in breast surgery or at least performs a large number of cosmetic breast operations.

• Ask the surgeon if you can see photographs of women who had good, average, and poor results with the operation of your choice. If the physician shows you only the best results, you might have unrealistic expectations.

RISKS OF IMPLANTS Although breast implants have been used for some 30 years and inserted in over 1 million American women, they are not without problems. A number of research studies have examined the various complications of implants, but at this point they seem to be inconclusive.

One serious problem is breast hardening, known as capsular contracture. It occurs when a layer of scar tissue forms around the implant, squeezing it and causing it to feel hard. (The implant itself does not actually harden, but it feels that way because it has been compressed.) The breast becomes unnaturally firm and can appear deformed. It is not known how often this occurs, but in a 1990 survey, conducted by the American Society of Plastic and Reconstructive Surgeons, 18 percent of women with implants reported that they had "somewhat bothersome" breast hardening and 8 percent said that they had "very bothersome" firmness. The hardening is believed to be less common when the implant is placed underneath the chest muscle.

Capsular contracture can be relieved by removing the scar tissue in an operation called open capsulectomy, but hardening may recur. In the past, some surgeons disrupted the scar tissue by squeezing the breast, but this approach is not recommended because it can cause the implant to rupture.

The risk of rupture is a major problem with implants. It is unknown how long the devices can last, and there is a concern that a certain percentage of women may be unaware that the silicone gel from their implants has leaked. Manufacturers say that rupture without symptoms occurs in 0.2 to 1.1 percent of implants, but outside experts suggest that this figure may be as high as 4 to 6 percent. Even if the implant stays intact, microscopic droplets of silicone gel can seep through its shell; it is not known yet if this can cause disease. Some women with implants have developed immune disorders that theoretically can be triggered by reaction to a foreign material such as silicone. At present, no link has been established between the implants and disorders of the immune system. However, women who already have such a disorder, or a family history of immune problems, should probably not have breast implants.

There are two other major concerns: Can implants cause cancer and can they interfere with its early detection? At present, there is no evidence that silicone can cause cancer in humans. Implants covered with polyurethane foam were removed from the market after the coating was found to cause cancer in rats, but it is not recommended that women who already have such implants have them removed because the risk posed by the foam is believed to be too small. Women with implants should take special precautions in screening for breast cancer because the devices can obscure a tumor on a mammogram (see box, "Caring for Breasts with Implants"), and women who are at high risk of breast cancer should take this into consideration in weighing their decision to have implants.

Finally, in a small number of women (under 5 percent), breast implant surgery can reduce sensation in the nipples and interfere with breast-feeding, particularly if the implants are inserted through an incision made around the areola. If silicone enters the breast milk, the amounts are probably too small to hurt the baby, but this issue has not been sufficiently studied to make recommendations about breast-feeding after breast enlargement. To avoid serious complications, such as galactorrhea, or persistent milk formation, implants should never be inserted during pregnancy.

BREAST LIFT A breast lift, known technically as mastopexy, is an operation in which sagging breasts are reshaped and uplifted. Breasts may sag after a weight loss or childbirth. Sometimes they grow looser and more droopy during aging; the skin loses elasticity and the glandular tissue, which gives the breast its firmness, is gradually replaced by fat. More than half of the women who have their breasts lifted are over age 35. But even a young woman's breasts may sag if they are very large or if they grew too fast during puberty, irreversibly stretching the supporting ligaments.

During mastopexy, the surgeon moves the nipple and areola to a higher position, shifts the underlying breast tissue upward, and reshapes the breast by removing excess skin and tightening it up. (See Figures 14.26–14.27.) The volume of tissue within the resultant breast remains the same, although the breast may appear smaller because it sits high on the chest and no longer sags.

To enlarge the breasts, implants may be inserted. The incisions are usually made around the areola, vertically down from the areola and horizontally along the crease underneath the breast, to make the scars less conspicuous. Depending on the surgeon's preference and the appearance of the breast before surgery, an incision can be made only around the areola. This may tend to flatten the breast and create radial folds around the areola that may not completely disappear. In either case, the incision scars may fade with time, but they are permanent.

Women who expect to have perfect, youthful breasts after a breast lift are often disappointed to find

CARING FOR BREASTS WITH IMPLANTS

• For breast cancer screening, seek a mammography facility that has technicians who are experienced in examining breasts with implants. The technician must be skilled in preventing the implant from rupture and also in pushing the device to the side to obtain a good image. You will need four views of the breast instead of the usual two in order to be properly screened.

• Have your breasts examined twice a year by your plastic surgeon, gynecologist, or any other doctor familiar with breast disorders, and examine them yourself once a month.

• If you notice anything unusual about your breasts or feel unusual symptoms elsewhere in your body, report it to your physician immediately.

• Implants that rupture must be removed immediately and the spilled silicone gel must be scraped out. However, the prevailing medical opinion is that implants that produce no symptoms may be left in place.

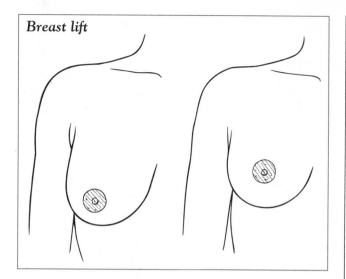

Breast lift

Fig. 14.26–14.27 *In breast lift surgery, a keyhole-shaped incision is made around the areola. In some cases additional incisions may extend vertically to the crease under the breast and may follow the crease under the breast. The nipple remains attached to the underlying tissue and nerves and is repositioned higher on the breast. The breast tissue remains intact, but a portion of the skin below the nipple is removed. The remaining skin is "cinched" together to make a firmer, higher breast. The final suture lines are shown at right.*

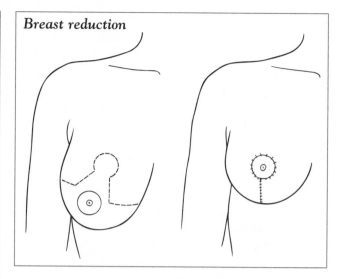

Breast reduction

Fig. 14.28–14.29 *In breast reduction surgery, skin and underlying breast tissue are excised (left). The nipple may remain attached to the underlying tissue to be repositioned on the breast or it may be moved as a free graft. The areola may be reduced in size to match the smaller breast.*

out that there will be scars. Another major problem with breast lifts is that the results may not last a lifetime. Under the pull of gravity, the skin will eventually stretch again, particularly if the breasts are large. (However, the nipple will not descend again.)

Moreover, as with any surgery, there may be postoperative complications, such as infection. These complications are rare, but since the goal of breast lift is purely cosmetic, they must be weighed against the operation's benefits. The surgeon's fee for this procedure ranges from $750 to 8,000, depending on its complexity, and averages about $3,000.

BREAST REDUCTION Some women with disproportionately large breasts are perfectly happy with their bustline, while others are self-conscious about it and feel that it interferes with athletic activity or poses other disturbing problems. (See box, "If You Plan a Breast Reduction.") Overly large breasts can create a host of medical difficulties, including back and shoulder pain, posture abnormalities, and skin rashes under the breasts.

Women who think their breasts are too big can have them reduced. This is called reduction mammaplasty. It is usually performed in a hospital under general anesthesia and lasts 3 to 4 hours. The surgeon removes part of the breast tissue; reshapes the remaining tissue; if necessary, reduces the areola to match the size of a smaller breast; and moves the

nipple and areola to a higher position. The resculptured breast is not only smaller but sits higher on the chest. (See Figures 14.28–14.29.)

After the operation, the breasts may take 3 to 12 weeks to assume their final shape. The nipples may be numb at first, but in 80 percent of cases, sensation returns to its former level almost immediately or within a few months; in the rest, sensation may be reduced or absent.

Breast reduction is a largely safe procedure, although it does carry a certain risk. Also, it inevitably leaves scars. Incisions are placed around the areola, down from the areola and along the crease underneath the breast, so that they do not show when you wear low-cut clothing. However, the scars are generally rather extensive because the operation involves a major remodeling of breast tissue. The width and appearance of the scars varies from one woman to another, but they are likely to be visible.

Despite these disadvantages, the operation, which may cost from $2,000 to $9,000, and averages about $4,500, brings a significant improvement in the quality of life to many women. It is usually performed after the age of 16, when the breasts are fully developed. Overweight women are advised to lose weight before the operation. Losing weight after surgery can cause the breasts to sag. Moreover, some breasts contain a great deal of fat and may decrease in size with weight loss, eliminating the need for a reduction.

IF YOU PLAN A
BREAST REDUCTION

1. Find out whether your insurance policy covers breast reduction. Many do. It is best to get a *written* approval from the insurance company before the operation is performed.

2. Let your surgeon know if you intend to breast-feed in the future. To preserve the milk ducts intact, the doctor may avoid detaching the nipple and areola from the breast. However, the ability to breast-feed cannot be guaranteed. If you plan to have children in the near future, you may wish to postpone the operation.

3. Let your surgeon know what size breasts you would like to have. Remember that it is easier to reduce breasts that are still too large after the operation than to enlarge breasts that are too small.

4. If you have a strong family history of breast cancer or if you are over 35, have a mammogram before the operation. Some 6 months after the breast reduction, get another mammogram done that you can use as a basis for comparison in future screenings for breast cancer. Otherwise, breast-reduction scars can be mistaken for tumors on subsequent mammograms.

5. Donate a unit or two of blood and ask the hospital to store it in case you require a transfusion during the operation.

6. Involve your partner in your decision to have breast reduction. He or she may play an important role in your adjustment to a new body image.

CHAPTER 15

Body Care: Preventive Maintenance

Whise good nutrition, regular exercise, and efforts to reduce stress can have profound effects on overall health, your individual body parts—skin, hair, eyes, teeth, nails, back, and feet—will profit from proper daily maintenance routines and preventive care. Developing good habits may not only stave off bothersome problems such as acne and eye strain, but also may prevent such debilitating conditions as gum disease and lower back pain and even help avert skin cancer.

SKIN

PREVENTING SKIN CANCER A deep, dark tan has long been considered a sign of health in this country, but skyrocketing skin cancer rates show that many women are paying a steep price for this dubious fashion. More than 700,000 new cases of basal-cell and squamous-cell carcinomas occur each year, making cancer of the skin the most common malignancy.

Fortunately, these two types are usually quite treatable and have an excellent cure rate.

More disturbing are the figures for malignant melanoma, a potentially deadly form of skin cancer, which are rising at a faster rate than any other cancer. In 1991, the lifetime risk of developing melanoma was 1 in 105; by the turn of the century, some researchers predict it will reach 1 in 75. According to the Skin Cancer Foundation, young women are the hardest hit. Melanoma is now the most frequent cancer in American women aged 25 to 29 and the second most frequent (after breast cancer) in women aged 30 to 34. Many environmental scientists cite the deterioration of the earth's ozone layer, which helps screen out ultraviolet radiation, as a major factor in this increase—all the more reason to rely on other forms of protection from sun exposure.

At highest risk for melanoma are people with fair skin, red or blond hair, and light eyes who have a history of blistering sunburn. The darker the skin, the lower the risk, although even very dark-skinned individuals occasionally develop melanoma, especially on the palms, soles of the feet, and nails. The risk increases with age; it rarely occurs before puberty. Other contributing factors include a family history of melanoma or dyplastic nevus syndrome, a proliferation of moles (often more than 100) that tend to be irregular in size and shape. Dark moles present from birth, especially large ones, also increase the risk.

• **Protection.** Since sun exposure is responsible for more than 90 percent of skin cancer, to protect yourself, follow these precautions:

• Stay indoors or in the shade between 10:00 A.M. and 2:00 P.M. (standard time) or from 11:00 A.M. to 3:00 P.M. (daylight savings time), when ultraviolet rays are strongest. This means total shade, not merely remaining under an umbrella at the beach, where the reflection off the sand can cause a burn.

• Use a sunscreen rated SPF 15 or higher. Many dermatologists recommend using the sunscreen daily, all year round, from the age of 6 months. Wear it alone or under makeup. Many manufacturers are now producing moisturizers, lip glosses, and lipsticks with built-in sunscreen. These products can be just as effective as sunscreen applied separately, as long as their labels specify SPF 15 or higher. These combination products may not be waterproof, however.

• Do not assume that sunscreen is sufficient protection. Wear sunglasses, broad-brimmed hats, and protective clothing whenever you are outdoors.

• Never deliberately seek a tan, whether from the sun or from artificial sources of ultraviolet light, such as tanning parlors.

• Remember that the sun's rays are stronger at higher altitudes and toward the equator and that ultraviolet rays can penetrate many materials. For example, 40 percent of the sun's rays penetrate water and up to 80 percent penetrate clouds. The intensity of UV rays can actually be magnified when they are reflected off snow (85 percent), sand (25 percent), and water (5 percent).

Until recently, only the ultraviolet B (UVB), the "burning" rays of the sun, were considered harmful. Evidence now indicates that ultraviolet A (UVA), the "tanning" rays, also inflict skin damage. And, unlike UVB, UVA does not diminish as dramatically during the winter months. There are several brands of sunscreen that are designed to protect against both UVA and UVB rays.

• **Early Detection.** Early detection and treatment of skin cancer can dramatically boost your chances for survival. The cure rate for malignant melanoma is 100 percent when it is confined to the epidermis, the outer layer of skin, but it declines as the melanoma grows deeper into the skin.

Some experts now advocate quarterly or even monthly self-exams for everyone and a yearly skin exam by a dermatologist for people in the high-risk category. A self-exam is quite simple and takes 10 minutes using two mirrors. (See Figure 15.1 and box, "Skin Cancer Self-Examination.") You may want to have a dermatologist help you do the first one, however, so that you can be reassured that freckles and existing moles are normal. Then you can look for new growths or changes in old ones. Here's what to look for:

• moles, growths, or spots that have grown larger and appear "pearly" with tiny capillaries running over

SKIN CANCER SELF-EXAMINATION

To check your body for suspicious-looking moles, the Skin Cancer Foundation recommends that you perform the following skin exam every 3 months:

• Examine your face, especially the nose, lips, mouth, and ears, front and back.

• Inspect your scalp, using a blow dryer and mirror to expose each section to view.

• Check your hands, palms and backs, between the fingers and under the fingernails.

• Standing in front of a full-length mirror, begin at your elbows and scan all sides of your upper arms.

• Next, focus on your neck, chest, and torso, lifting your breasts to view the undersides.

• With your back to the full-length mirror, use a hand mirror to inspect the back of your neck, shoulders, and upper back.

• Still using both mirrors, scan your lower back, buttocks, and backs of both legs.

• Sit down. Prop each leg in turn on a chair or stool. Use the hand mirror to examine your genitals. Check front and sides of both legs, from thighs to toes.

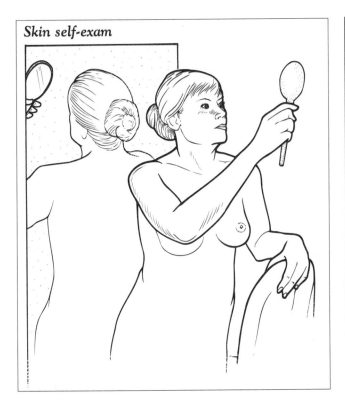

Skin self-exam

Fig. 15.1 *Skin cancer experts advise carefully examining your skin every three months, using a mirror when necessary to see all parts of your body.*

DETECTING MELANOMA EARLY

Melanomas usually look different from benign growths. Check for the following distinguishing features:

A—ASYMMETRY. While benign moles are often symmetrical, evenly shaped on all sides, melanomas tend to be asymmetrical—if a line were drawn through the middle of the growth, the two halves would not match.

B—BORDERS. The borders of benign moles are usually smooth and even, while the edges of early melanomas are more likely to be uneven or notched.

C—COLOR. While benign moles usually have a uniform color, the first sign of a melanoma is often mottling, or different shades of brown or black within one mole. Broken blood vessels may also be evident.

D—DIAMETER. Melanomas tend to grow larger than 6 millimeters in diameter, about the size of a pencil eraser. Any mole that rapidly increases in size should be examined by a doctor.

them, or are translucent, tan, brown, black, or multi-colored

- rough lesions that may be ulcerated and red

- moles with asymmetrical shapes or irregular borders

- any mole or spot that has increased in diameter or elevation, or changed color

Although most melanomas develop from existing moles, up to 10 percent occur on normal (clear) skin. (See Figure 15.2 and box, "Detecting Melanoma Early.") Any of the conditions noted above or any sore that persistently itches, bleeds, crusts, scabs, or hurts should be examined by a doctor. An open sore that does not heal within 3 weeks should also be reported.

BASIC SKIN CARE Many of the promises of the cosmetics industry are based on the premise that you can actually change the texture of your skin by slathering on various creams, oils, and emollients. The fact is, the skin cells to which you apply all this expensive goo are already dead. (See Figure 15.3.) What you actually want to do, then, is get rid of the cells, not plump them up or smooth them out. What you do with the skin left underneath is elementary: If it's too

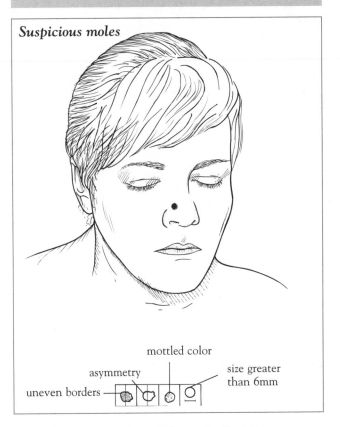

Suspicious moles

mottled color

asymmetry

uneven borders

size greater than 6mm

Fig. 15.2 *Most skin growths are benign, but distinctive characteristics of size, shape, and color can help distinguish those that are not.*

Cross-section of skin

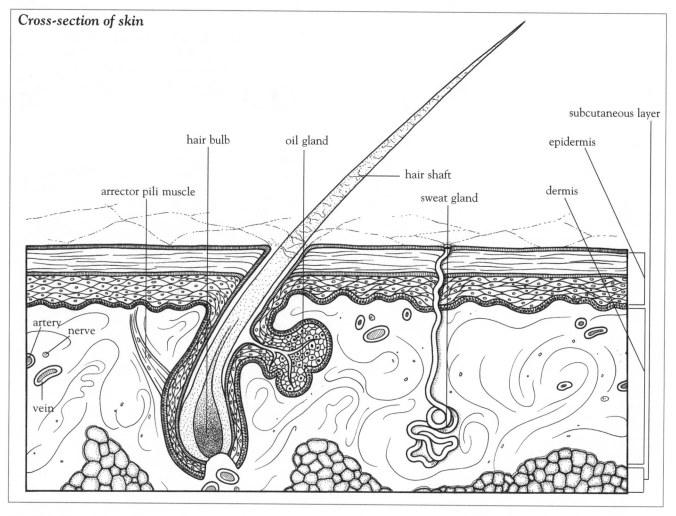

hair bulb   oil gland

arrector pili muscle

hair shaft

sweat gland

subcutaneous layer

epidermis

dermis

artery

nerve

vein

Fig. 15.3 *Most of the epidermis consists of waxy, lifeless cells that protect the underlying skin from injury and harmful substances while preserving its moisture. The rest manufacture the pigment melanin, which protects against ultraviolet light. The dermis layer has structures such as blood vessels and nerve fibers common to other organs but it also has hair follicles, sebaceous (oil) glands, and sweat glands.*

dry, try to conserve its natural moisture; if it's too oily, try not to add any more oil; and if it's normal, leave it alone.

If you remember those principles, your skin-care routine can be simple and effective. You should wash your face morning and night to remove dirt, dead cells, excess oil (if any), and makeup. If you have normal skin, use water and a mild, neutral soap, such as a transparent variety. For oily skin, which is primarily seen in younger women, you can use a stronger soap, one that is especially formulated for oily skin, or a rinsable cleanser for oily skin. If your skin is dry, which occurs as women age (see section on "Dry Skin"), do not use soap but a simple rinsable cleanser with no fancy additives. Avoid heavy creams that must be tissued off because they do not remove dirt and dead cells and may leave your skin dull-looking.

Remember to use sunscreen or a foundation containing sunscreen under makeup. Suit your makeup

according to your skin type. If you have normal skin, you can use just about any kind of makeup. For oily skin, put on a mild astringent first, then follow it with sunscreen and a water-based or oil-free makeup. For dry skin, always use moisturizer under cream- or oil-based makeup. Especially dry skin may require a heavier moisturizer, one containing urea or lactic acid, at night.

DRY SKIN What keeps your skin healthy is the constant shedding of individual skin cells, a process called exfoliation. Although the rate of shedding varies over the body, surface cells are replaced on average every 28 days—in young skin. As we age, the skin thins and flattens and the rate of cell replacement slows down. The dry, dead cells tend to stay on the surface longer, even when the moisture content of the underlying skin is unchanged, and often make you itch. Women's skin seems to be more prone to dryness than men's, although dermatologists do not know why.

Trying to restore normal balance to dry skin by applying oils and creams is pointless. The oil in your skin comes from within and cannot be replenished. However, you can make sure that you get adequate amounts of vitamins A and C (from fruits and vegetables) in your diet, because a deficiency in these vitamins can result in dry, rough skin. And you can conserve and restore the water or moisture in your skin. That's when moisturizers are useful. They do not soak into the skin, but they increase the skin's ability to retain moisture.

Here are some tips for treating very dry, itchy skin. You can modify them where appropriate:

• Avoid hot water and a lot of soap. Both remove the fats that normally form a barrier in the outer layer of skin and prevent evaporation of moisture from the cells. Use cool or warm water and a very mild, super-fatted soap only where necessary (underarms, genitals, feet). Use a rinsable cleanser on your face. Consider bathing only every other day and do not soak in the tub after washing.

• To help the skin retain water, pat on a moisturizer immediately after bathing while your skin is still wet. Use a moisturizer that contains 10 percent urea or lactic acid.

• Limit your exposure to cold, dry air, sun, and wind.

• Use a humidifier if the air in your home is dry.

WRINKLES, BAGS, AND SAGS Aging skin not only loses moisture, but also elasticity and resiliency, which ultimately causes sagging and wrinkles. Heredity plays a large part in determining how soon this will happen. Other factors include sun exposure, cigarette smoking, climate, hormonal balance, and overall health. Although you cannot influence heredity and not everyone wants to live in a humid climate, the message is clear: If you want to preserve your skin, stay out of the sun, do not smoke, and stay healthy. If you already have lines and leathery skin, there are a number of treatments available.

First, what doesn't work: cosmetics. Despite various claims, nonprescription cosmetic creams cannot reverse wrinkles or restore youthfulness. They may hide wrinkles (heavy pancake-type makeup does this but its two chief ingredients, soap and clay, are very drying). They can distract the eye (frosted cosmetics may give the skin a pearly glow, but actually contain minerals that soak up moisture). The best most of these products can offer is a temporary softening and plumping of the skin (cosmetic creams containing small amounts of estrogen and other hormones cause the skin to swell slightly, which can make fine lines appear less noticeable for a short time after treatment).

Scientific-sounding ads for products containing collagen are particularly deceptive. Since the protein collagen is a major component of skin cells, it sounds logical that adding it to a product would help restore the skin. In truth, collagen molecules are too large to pass through the epidermis to reach the deeper layers and be absorbed into the skin. All they can do is sit on the surface combating dryness like other, less expensive moisturizers.

•**Retinoic Acid.** One cream that does seem to work is retinoic acid, a vitamin A derivative, which is available by prescription as Retin-A. Dermatologists have been using Retin-A for years to treat acne successfully. They began to notice that their patients' skin started looking younger. The simple explanation is that, as a mild acid, Retin-A actually peels off the top layer of skin, leaving a smoother, pinker layer underneath. Because this layer has not been exposed to the sun, it has fewer lines and brown age spots. Actually the process is more complex: Retin-A appears to thicken the epidermis, which tends to thin with age; speed up exfoliation; stimulate blood circulation and produce new blood vessels, giving the skin its pinker tone; and stimulate collagen production in the dermis layer, which helps firm it up.

Retinoic acid must be used indefinitely. It takes at least 3 to 4 months to see any significant changes, and in the meantime the skin may appear red and irritated. Retin-A can also cause scaly patches and itching. Most women who stick with it find that this stage passes, but some cannot tolerate it. Retin-A also makes the skin more sensitive to sun damage, so that you *must* use a sunscreen scrupulously. One caution: Do not be fooled by over-the-counter creams that contain vitamin A or retinol. These do not have the same effect.

•**Alpha Hydroxy Acids.** A new group of cosmetic products offer a nonprescription alternative to retinoic acid. Alpha hydroxy acids (AHAs) are natural substances found in sugar cane (glycolic acid), citrus fruits (citric acid), soured milk (lactic acid), grapes (tartaric acid), and apples (malic acid). Despite manufacturers' claims to the contrary, and prices that vary from $4 to $125 an ounce, there is very little difference among them. They all act as exfoliants and, to some extent, humectants—substances that absorb moisture and hold it on the skin's surface. Higher concentrations are sometimes used by skin salons and dermatologists for facial peels to remove fine lines and help control acne by unclogging pores. The cosmetic products seem to be effective, resulting in somewhat smoother, pinker, more glowing skin. Un-

like Retin-A, however, they are not regulated by the Food and Drug Administration (FDA) and the long-term effects of their use are unknown.

The acid content of AHA products, not always listed on the label, ranges from under 2 percent to

Eyelift

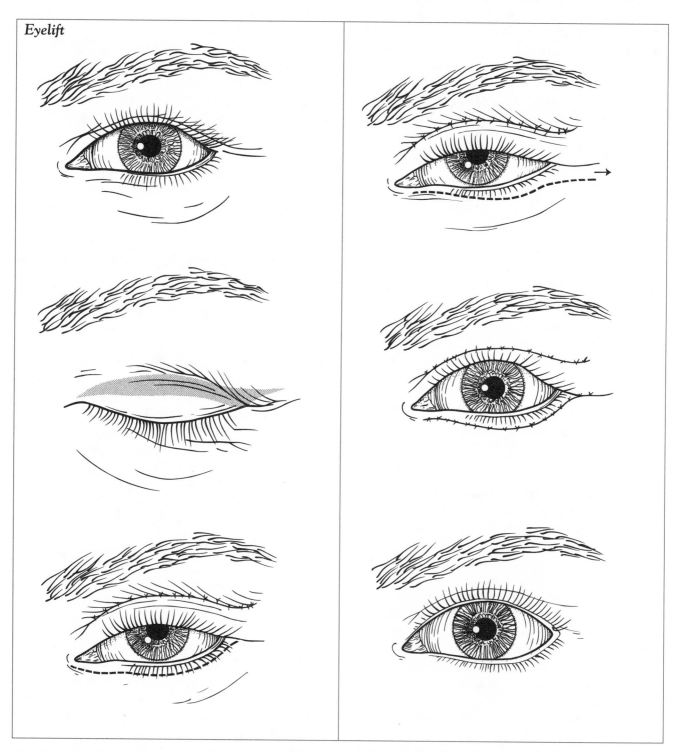

Fig. 15.4–15.9 *Eyelift surgery can remove the loose and sagging tissue, puffiness, and lines around the eye seen in the first picture. First the excess skin and fatty tissue between the natural horizontal creases in the upper lid (shaded area) are removed and the lid sutured. Then an incision is made in the lower lid and the skin pulled toward the outer corner of the eye to tighten sags and wrinkles. The scars left by the incisions are almost invisible.*

Facelift

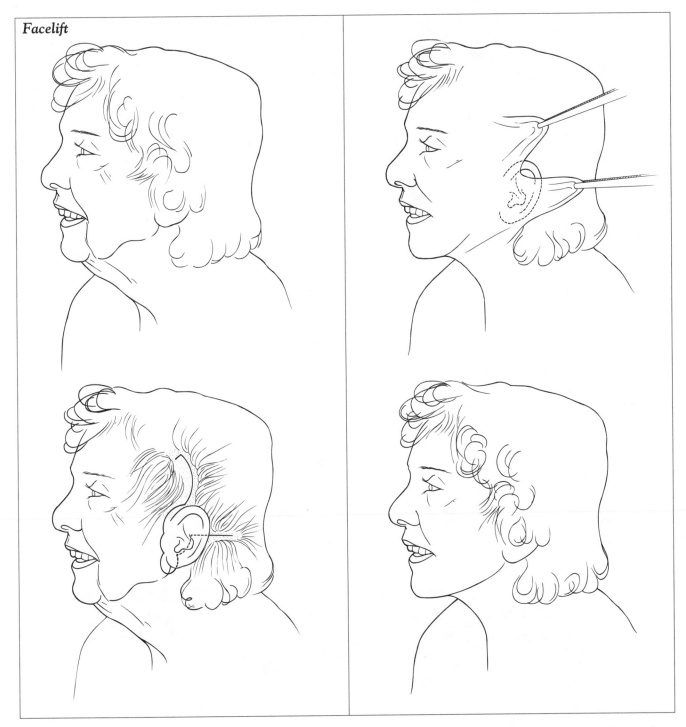

Fig. 15.10–15.13 *Sagging skin on the neck, jaw, and cheeks can be tightened via a rhytidectomy, or face lift. An incision is made around each ear and under the hairline at the temples. Then the skin is loosened and pulled upward and backward. Any excess skin is excised, and the remaining skin is sutured. The scar lines are nearly invisible and mostly covered by the hair.*

12 percent. You may want to start with a lower acid concentration and move up if necessary, or begin by using the cream or lotion only every other day.

•**Collagen Injections.** Unlike collagen creams, which sit on the surface, injected collagen works in the deeper layers of the skin. Bovine collagen is used to replace the body's natural collagen, a substance that cushions and supports the skin but is gradually worn away by the aging process. It pushes the skin up from underneath, filling in wrinkles and creases around the mouth, nose, and eyes, and on the forehead. The number of injections needed depends on how deep the lines are.

Collagen injections are generally quite safe, but can cause an allergic reaction in a small number of people, so dermatologists usually test it on the forearm first. The problem is, collagen is gradually absorbed by the body and thus must be repeated every 6 to 18 months. At about $300 per injection, the treatment can be quite expensive.

• **Silicone Injections.** Since the 1940s silicone injections have been used to smooth wrinkles, but have never been approved by the FDA except for experimental use. As problems with breast implants brought attention to the subject, the FDA reiterated its position that the use of silicone injections without specific authorization is illegal. Unfortunately, many doctors continue to use it routinely. In 1990, the American Academy of Cosmetic Surgery, which does not recommend them, found silicone injections were the ninth most popular procedure in cosmetic surgery.

• **Cosmetic Surgery.** More permanent solutions to wrinkles include face lifts and eye lifts. These procedures, illustrated here, can have dramatic results and provide a real ego boost, but they should not be undertaken lightly. They are expensive, and they are not without risk. The fees vary regionally and from surgeon to surgeon, but the surgery fee alone can be $600 to $7,500 for blepharoplasty (eyelid surgery), depending on whether lower lids, upper lids, or both are done (see Figures 15.4–15.9), and $1,800 to $8,000 for rhytidectomy (face lifts) (see Figures

15.10–15.13). Most important is finding a competent surgeon with whom you are comfortable and then discussing the procedure carefully to be sure that you have realistic expectations about results.

To find a surgeon, inquire of friends who have had similar procedures whose results you find pleasing, or call the American Society of Plastic and Reconstructive Surgeons or the American Society for Aesthetic Plastic Surgery (see Resources), for referrals to their members in your area. At an initial meeting with a potential surgeon, you should be sure that you understand exactly what the surgery will entail, the fees, the risks, and how long the hospitalization and recovery periods will be. Ask to see his or her before-and-after pictures of women with facial structures similar to yours to get an idea of the surgeon's skill and what the procedure can accomplish.

ADULT ACNE A skin problem universally associated with puberty, acne can persist throughout adulthood. In adults, however, it is usually has a different cause. In teens acne is almost always hormone related, due to normal surges in androgen that can quadruple in this period. Androgens promote male sexual maturation, but females normally have androgen as well. The side effect, in both sexes, is the stimulation of the oil-producing glands in the skin. The excess oil begins to clog the pores and the result is acne. (See Figure 15.14.) It can range from mild to serious; in either case, it usually clears up by age 20.

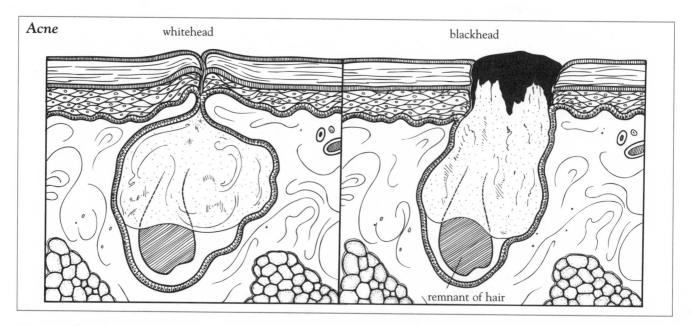

Fig. 15.14 *Acne is caused by a buildup of sebum, an oily substance produced by the sebaceous glands to keep the skin lubricated. A mixture of sebum and sloughed-off cells that clogs pores at the surface causes open comedones, or blackheads; a buildup below the skin surface creates closed comedones, or whiteheads.*

By the time you are in your late twenties or early thirties, the acne may return. Or you may experience your first serious eruptions. Other than premenstrual flareups, the cause may be an adrenal or ovarian disorder. However, this is rarely the case. More commonly, the culprits are oral contraceptives or other drugs (such as corticosteroids, Dilantin, and Danacrine, used to treat severe endometriosis), emotional factors, or climatic effects.

A major cause of first-time acne in adult women is makeup. In fact, dermatologists call this condition acne cosmetica. It may begin as a mild case that becomes worse when a woman tries to cover it up with heavy makeup. Or she may switch to a water-based or so-called oil-free makeup (some of which do, in fact, contain organic oils), but ends up putting more of it on because these products do not cover very well. Another scenario: Afraid of dry skin, she uses oily makeup, heavy moisturizers, and thick cleansing cream until her skin rebels.

Fortunately, some very good treatments are available, ranging from over-the-counter preparations for mild cases to systemic drugs for more serious ones. Besides easing up on cosmetics and adopting a sensible cleansing routine (see section on "Basic Skin Care"), acne sufferers can try nonprescription preparations containing benzoyl peroxide. For mild or occasional acne, these medications often do the trick, reducing inflammation and bacteria levels on the skin. Start with a 2.5 percent lotion, if you can find it (or have your pharmacist order it). It is also available in 5 and 10 percent solutions, if there is no improvement with the milder formulation.

More serious cases may require a visit to the dermatologist. A commonly used and very effective treatment is retinoic acid (see previous section). Resistant and severe cases may respond to antibiotics like tetracycline, which is generally safe but may produce annoying side effects such as mild gastrointestinal irritation or vaginal yeast infections. Accutane is usually the drug of last resort because it is potent and must be taken for several months. However, it can bring remarkable results, sending acne into long remission or curing it completely. Caution: Neither of these drugs should be taken during pregnancy. Tetracycline can cause problems with developing teeth, and Accutane can cause more serious birth defects. Some doctors will not prescribe either drug to women of childbearing age; others insist that birth control be strictly practiced.

HAIR

The hair shaft, like the top layer of the skin, is composed of dead cells. The cells of the outermost layer of the hair shaft, or cuticle, overlap to help prevent the evaporation of needed moisture. When the cuticle cells are properly aligned, and each shaft of hair lightly coated with natural oil, your hair has a smooth, even appearance (even if it is curly). When each strand of hair is smooth, light reflects evenly off your entire crowning glory, which is what gives your hair a shiny, healthy look.

The cuticle cells can be pulled out of alignment when your hair is stressed by excessive blow-drying, bleach, permanents, straightening, and other treatments. Light no longer bounces evenly off these misaligned cells and the result is dull-looking hair. Too little oil, too much oil, or residue from shampoo, mousse, and other hair-care products can also take the shine out of hair. While dull hair cannot actually be "nourished" by conditioners or body builders, these products coat the hair with oil and straighten out the cell structure of each shaft, so that its shine is restored. Basic hair care helps keep it that way.

BASIC HAIR CARE Hair needs to be brushed daily with a firm brush. Brushing helps get rid of surface dirt and dust and loose hair. It helps remove dead skin cells from the scalp and distributes oil from the scalp evenly over each hair shaft. Brush your hair for several minutes until your scalp feels warm. This helps stimulate circulation by massaging your scalp.

Be sure to wash your brush often, at least twice a week, to avoid redistributing the dirt and oil as you brush. To clean the brush, use a capful of shampoo, a few drops of ammonia, or both, in a sink full of water.

The variety of shampoos available is almost dizzying—there is a product for every type of hair problem, real or imagined. Finding the right one is often a matter of trial and error, since the same shampoo can behave differently on different people. There are basically two types—soap based and detergent based. In areas where the water is very hard (has a high mineral content), soap-based shampoos are less likely to leave a residue. Beyond this, there are formulations for normal, oily, or dry hair. Generally, the best shampoos are well balanced, but a slightly acidic shampoo (many contain lemon juice) may be best for oily hair.

It is not necessary to wash your hair every time you shower, although this will probably do no harm if you use a very mild shampoo. More regular shampooing can be helpful in controlling excess oil and dandruff (see next section).

DANDRUFF Dandruff is a condition that develops when the dead cells that are shed constantly from the surface of the scalp are trapped by the hair. It shows up as an embarrassing collection of white flakes on the hair and shoulders. Mild cases of dandruff in people who have normal hair can be treated simply by more regular and thorough brushing and shampooing to loosen and wash away the dead cells. A special dandruff shampoo is not necessary.

For people with oily hair, a dandruff shampoo containing coal tar may help slow down the rate at which dead cells are formed. These shampoos tend to irritate the scalp if used too frequently, so they should be alternated with regular shampoo.

Dandruff in people with dry hair may respond to dandruff shampoos containing zinc, which breaks up the clumps of dead cells so they can be washed away. As with shampoos containing coal tar, use these products only as long as necessary to control the condition.

HAIR DYES When the cells that give hair its color stop producing pigment, the hair gradually grays. No lotion or vitamin can halt or reverse the graying process. The only way to regain the original color is to replace it artificially with dye.

Generally, hair-dye products are safe and do not damage the hair unless they are used improperly. (In contrast, bleach can be damaging to the hair.) Permanent hair dyes, which penetrate the hair shaft so that the color change is long-lasting, contain p-phenylenediamine. This chemical can cause allergic reactions in some women ranging from rashes and redness to hair loss and scarring.

Experts advise doing a patch test on your skin and waiting 24 hours to see if irritation develops before treating your entire head with a dye. Wear rubber gloves and immediately wash off any dye that gets on the skin. The patch test must be repeated each time you use the dye because allergies, when they develop, only do so after repeated exposure, and the number of exposures needed to provoke an allergic response in someone predisposed to allergy varies from person to person.

For women allergic to p-phenylenediamine, there are semipermanent hair colors, temporary rinses, and henna. These coloring products work by coating only the outside of the hair shaft with pigment, so the results are often short-lived. Although they fade gradually over several weeks, they have the advantage of not producing an obvious color line as the roots grow out.

PERMANENTS AND HAIR STRAIGHTENERS Permanent wave solutions range from those that give a full head of curls (or relax already curly hair) to those that give hair increased body and produce only a slight wave. All contain an alkaline solution that breaks the chemical bonds that hold the protein molecules in the hair together in their normal fashion. After the solution is applied, the hair can be reshaped on rods or rollers to form tighter or looser curls. Then the solution is neutralized to stop its action.

Three basic types of permanent wave products are available in both home permanent kits and in salons, although the home-use kits tend to contain weaker chemicals. The chemicals in conventional wave solutions are generally safe and well tolerated. They range in concentration from gentle, which produces a body wave and is good for treated hair, to strong, which produces curls in even the most wiry hair. Acid wave solutions are less alkaline than the conventional type and better for treated hair, but are more prone to cause allergic reactions. Manufacturers advise doing a patch test behind the ear 24 hours before using the solution, to check for reddening that would indicate an allergic reaction. The third type of permanent is the soft wave, which lasts only a few months but is best for fragile or double-processed (bleached and then tinted) hair.

Conventional wave solutions can also be used by black women to relax their curls. Known as curly perms, they come in formulations specifically for black hair, which tends to be dry and much more fragile than most white women's hair. Although these perms are generally safe and less damaging to hair than other methods, they do not straighten hair completely. For that, many black women rely on hot combs or chemical relaxers. Hot combs, which are used in combination with hot oil, have been around for almost a century in salons and more recently for home use. They must be used extremely carefully, however. The oil can get very hot and if too much is used it can burn the scalp or run down and burn the face or neck. It is best to have it done in a salon, or if you are considering doing it at home, to get an experienced hairdresser to show you how.

Chemical relaxers are strong chemicals, much stronger and longer lasting than those used in curly perms. With some of them, pomade or oil must be spread over the scalp and surrounding area first to protect the skin. They must be used with extreme care; both a patch test and a strand test are strongly recommended. To patch-test, dab the solution behind your ear, wait 24 hours, and check for darkening or irritation that indicates an allergic reaction. If there is no reaction, the relaxer is safe to use, but only testing a strand according to package directions will tell you how long the relaxer must be left on to work without damaging the hair.

EXCESSIVE HAIR GROWTH Hirsutism, or excessive hair growth in women, is a condition marked by the abnormal growth of thick, pigmented hair on the face, chest, back, or extremities. (Normally, this type of hair, called terminal hair, is found only on the scalp, eyebrows, eyelashes, armpits, and groin.) Five to 10 percent of all women suffer from hirsutism, which ranges in severity from scattered patches of hair to a full beard. (See Figure 15.15.)

Often, hirsutism is simply a variation on normal hair-growth patterns and does not signal any abnormality. It may run in families, and it is more common among people from Latin and eastern Mediterranean countries.

In 95 percent of cases, hirsutism is associated with a rise in the blood level of the male hormone testosterone. It may occur, for example, when a woman gains a great deal of weight (because male hormones are manufactured from substances in body fat) or during menopause, when estrogen levels drop. In some cases, excess hair grows during times of emotional upheavals or extreme stress, which can trigger hormone imbalances.

In serious cases, excessive hair growth may signal a disturbance in ovarian function called polycystic ovary disease. Other symptoms of this condition include enlargement of the ovaries (which fill with cysts), irregular menstruation, and infertility.

In rare instances, the cause of the hair growth is an ovarian or adrenal gland tumor, which produces testosterone. This is usually accompanied by changes in the menstrual cycle as well as enlargement of the clitoris and deepening of the voice. Removing the tumor usually brings a return to normal ovulation and hair growth.

•Treating Excessive Hair Growth. If your hair growth appeared suddenly or worsened quickly, consult an endocrinologist. If the excessive hair stems from a hormonal problem, drugs may be recommended, depending on your age and general health. Oral contraceptives, which suppress testosterone production, may also be prescribed. Time is a factor: The longer the hair follicles have been exposed to testosterone, the less likely they are to return to normal.

In mild cases, the best treatment may be cosmetic therapy, such as shaving and tweezing. Waxing, performed at home or in a salon, can last up to 8 weeks because the entire hair is pulled out from the root, but it can sting, be messy, and lead to ingrown hairs. Chemical depilatories last slightly longer than shaving, but are not always effective on thick, coarse hair, and they can irritate the skin.

Electrolysis is the only permanent way to remove hair; however, the process is expensive and can be painful. You may need several treatments in the same area to achieve permanent results. Seek out a licensed practitioner to avoid scarring.

EXCESSIVE HAIR LOSS Hair loss can be due to age, heredity, various illnesses or disorders, or simple mismanagement (see box, "Minimizing Hair Loss.") Hair loss or thinning, especially at the crown and the hairline, is hereditary and often occurs after menopause. (See Figure 15.16.) Thinning hair can also plague women for up to 2 years after pregnancy. Hair loss, or alopecia, may occur in a small patch on the scalp or over the entire body. It can be caused by X rays, chemical agents such as permanents, emotional stress, thyroid disease, skin diseases, and certain drugs, especially those used in cancer treatments.

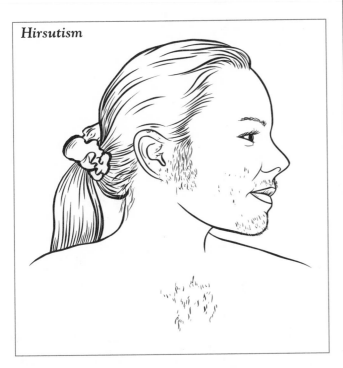
Hirsutism

Fig. 15.15 *An oversupply of testosterone, a male sex hormone found in small amounts in women, is the most common cause of excessive hair growth on the face, chest, and back.*

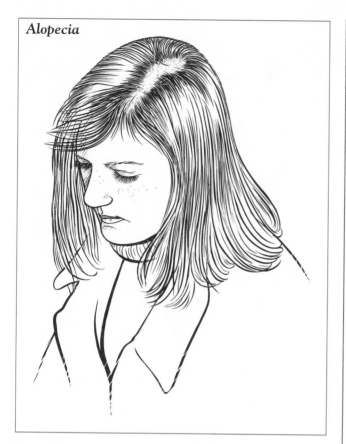

Alopecia

Fig. 15.16 *Excessive hair loss in women may be temporary (as happens after pregnancy) or progressive and be caused by many things, from stress to x-ray exposure to disease, but it is most often hereditary.*

MINIMIZING HAIR LOSS

• Do not pull your hair or massage your scalp too vigorously when shampooing. Towel-dry gently or let your hair air-dry.

• Comb or brush your hair gently and no longer than necessary. Use a conditioner to ease tangles.

• Avoid tight buns, ponytails, and other hairstyles that pull on the hair.

• Do not overheat your hair with hot rollers and curling irons. If you must use a dryer, set it on low. Wear a hat in the sun.

• Use a mild shampoo. If hair loss is excessive, avoid dyes, permanents, and other treatments that contain harsh chemicals. If you must use these products, stick to temporary or semipermanent dyes and soft-wave permanents.

• Wear a bathing cap in chlorinated pools and use shampoos that are specially formulated for chlorine-exposed hair.

• Eat a well-balanced diet. Proper nutrition is essential for hair growth.

Alopecia caused by an underlying condition, such as thyroid disease, is often reversible when the condition is diagnosed and treated. Unfortunately, most treatments for hair loss in patches, called alopecia areata, are not completely effective. Sometimes steroid therapy helps, but hair loss usually recurs when treatment is stopped. Because steroids can have serious side effects, they generally should not be used over a long period of time.

• **Treating Excessive Hair Loss.** Although proper nutrition is important for normal hair growth, there is no evidence that vitamins, food supplements, or other products taken orally prevent baldness or grow hair. In fact, the FDA has banned the sale of nonprescription creams and lotions promoted as hairgrowing agents. The only FDA-approved product to treat hair loss is minoxidil (Rogaine), available only by prescription.

Minoxidil works best when treatment is started during the early stages of hair loss. It must be massaged into the scalp twice a day for at least 4 months before it produces results, and it must be used indefinitely to keep new hairs intact. The treatment is expensive, and does not work for everyone. In one series of studies, 13 percent of women who used minoxidil experienced moderate improvement after 8 months, half saw minimal improvement, and a third experienced no improvement at all.

NAILS

Hair loss is often accompanied by lines and pitting on the nails. In fact, the nails mirror many physical and emotional disturbances. Severe infections, anxiety, or long-term insomnia, for example, may show up as lines and ridges. People with anemia may have nails with large depressions in them (called spooning), while someone with cirrhosis of the liver may have white marks on the nails. (See box, "What Your Nails Tell About Your Health.")

The nails are damaged by daily tasks as well. Detergents, frequent immersion in water, excessive use of nail polish remover, and using your nails as tools can all cause weakening, cracking, and splitting. Nails (especially the toenails) may also be plagued by fungal infections that form in the growing nail itself and cause thickening and lifting from the nail bed.

Sometimes even the treatments intended to beautify nails actually disfigure them. Sculptured or porcelain nail tips, which are added on to the ends of natural nails with a mixture of acrylic powder, solvent, and instant glue, can produce allergic reactions ranging from nail tenderness to loss of the nails.

The instant glue that is contained in press-on plastic nails can also produce allergic reactions. Some polishes, hardeners, and other products contain formaldehyde and toluene, chemicals that can irritate the skin. Many cuticle-removing solutions contain caustic ingredients that can destroy skin tissue. If you must use cuticle removers, take care that they do not come in contact with the surrounding skin, and allow your nails to dry thoroughly before using your hands.

WHAT YOUR NAILS TELL ABOUT YOUR HEALTH

Nails reveal a great deal about your general condition and may indicate undiagnosed diseases.

THICK, YELLOW NAILS: can signal certain thyroid, lymph system, and respiratory diseases. They can also result from long-term use of the antibiotic tetracycline.

BLUE NAILS: can indicate circulatory problems caused by heart disease or Raynaud's disease—a condition characterized by impaired blood circulation in the hands. (See the Encyclopedia.)

WHITE MARKS: may indicate cirrhosis of the liver.

HORIZONTAL GROOVES: also known as Beau's lines, these furrows can be caused by a variety of illnesses, malnutrition, or certain toxic substances.

HORIZONTAL LINES: also called Mees' lines, these white stripes can be caused by heart attacks, kidney failure, Hodgkin's disease, or sickle-cell anemia. Red streaks can signal high blood pressure or heart valve disease.

PITTING: in the nails can signal psoriasis or eczema.

SPOONING: nails with large depressions may indicate anemia.

CLUBBING: curled nails may signal liver, colon, lung, or heart disease.

There are numerous lotions and creams on the market intended to counteract nail damage. These preparations are ineffective because, like hair, nails are dead protein tissue. Nails cannot be "nourished" by topical treatments or diet supplements, such as vitamins or gelatin (even though many women swear by the latter). The best these paint-on or stick-on products can do is act as a physical barrier that may help nails resist damage.

BASIC CARE: HOW TO HAVE A PERFECT 10 The best way to have healthy-looking nails is to treat them with care. To avoid frequent immersion in water and exposure to strong chemicals, wear rubber gloves when washing dishes or doing housework. Having gloves on will help keep you from using your nails to scrape at stubborn spots or to open or cut things.

To keep your nails looking neat:

• Cut or clip them with sharp scissors or clippers after you bathe or shower, when they are soft and less likely to tear.

• Conversely, only file them when they are dry. File in one direction only, from the side to the center. Use the rough side of the emery board for shaping or major repairs, the fine side to smooth out the edges. Repair any tears immediately so the nail does not catch on something and tear more.

• After you bathe, gently push back the cuticles with a towel or orangewood stick. If you do this daily, you should never have to cut your cuticles. Since the cuticle protects the unseen part of the nail that is still growing, your nails will be less prone to damage or infection if your cuticles are intact.

• If you do have a loose cuticle (hangnail), cut it gently with scissors. Do not use cuticle remover.

• If your nails are dry and brittle, you can rehydrate them by soaking your fingertips in warm water with a little bit of detergent or in warm olive oil. Then dry them and rub on hand cream. Another trick is to rub petroleum jelly onto your nails and cuticles each night.

• If you use nail polish, stay away from products containing free formaldehyde (toluene sulfonamide formaldehyde resin seems to be okay). Use polish and remover only in a well-ventilated area to minimize breathing the fumes.

• Far worse than nail polish is polish remover. If your nails chip, touch them up rather than removing the polish too quickly and doing them over. Try not to use polish remover more than every 1 to 2 weeks. When you do, use as little as possible. Soak a cotton ball in remover and hold the cotton against the nail 2 to 3 seconds to loosen the polish before wiping it off. Then use cotton wrapped around an orangewood stick to carefully remove any traces of polish on the cuticles.

TEETH

TLC FOR TEETH Everyone wants a beautiful smile, but teeth should be protected for health as well as cosmetic reasons. Preventive dental care will not only enhance the appearance of a smile, but also ward off tooth decay, gum disease, and even bone destruction.

After age 40, most tooth loss is due to periodontal disease, commonly caused by bacterial plaque, a sticky substance that accumulates on the teeth near the gum line and eventually hardens into tartar. The bacteria release toxins that inflame the gums and begin to destroy the healthy tissue and bones that support the teeth. Gums begin to bleed and detach from the teeth, and pus-filled pockets form. Eventually the teeth loosen, protrude, or spread apart.

Periodontal disease is especially prevalent among people with poor tooth brushing habits. Diabetes, thyroid problems, and other hormonal imbalances can worsen the condition by impairing the body's ability to kill the bacteria. The condition can also be aggravated by grinding the teeth during sleep.

The best defense against periodontal disease is to clean the teeth daily, taking special care to floss between the teeth. Regular visits to the dentist are recommended to remove tartar.

If despite these efforts gum disease does develop, it can be successfully treated in its early stages. Treatment involves scraping under the gum margins to remove plaque and tartar. In successful cases, the gum will reattach itself to the tooth. More advanced cases of periodontal disease may require surgical procedures to eliminate the pockets between the teeth and gum or to remove excessive gum tissue.

BRACES: NOT JUST FOR KIDS Some cases of periodontal disease may be helped by orthodontic treatment, which changes the position of the teeth. Moreover, orthodontics may help prevent an assortment of oral health problems. Crooked teeth are more difficult to clean, which makes them more vul-

nerable to decay. Misaligned teeth put extra stress on supporting structures, which can lead to bone or gum disease. They also contribute to disorders of the joints that connect the lower jaw to the skull, resulting in chronic headaches, earaches, and facial pain.

In the last decade, adult orthodontia patients have more than doubled. Braces have changed, too. New materials and techniques have been developed that make them more comfortable, effective, and attractive. (See Figure 15.17.)

The wires used to connect all the teeth together, for example, are made of more flexible, resilient materials, allowing for easier adjustments, fewer replacements, and less frequent office visits, which cuts down on costs.

The brackets that attach to the teeth to hold the wires in place are available in translucent white material to match the teeth and also in bright colors. Retainers and the small bands used with braces also come in colors ranging from neons to pastels.

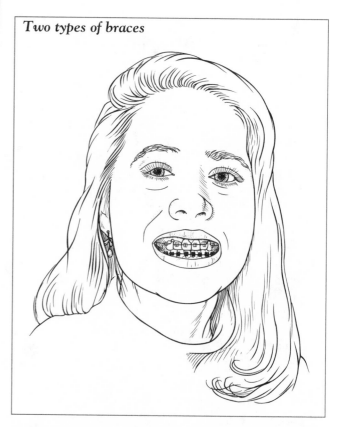

Two types of braces

Fig. 15.17 *Many women who did not have orthodonture problems corrected as adolescents are opting to do it as adults now that new materials have made braces less visible and cumbersome. Shown here are two types of braces; a third goes behind the teeth.*

EYES

Preventive maintenance for the eyes means getting regular checkups and preventing eyestrain and injury. After age 40, regular testing for visual acuity and for glaucoma is recommended at regular intervals (see "Screening Tests" in Chapter 18, "Women and the Health Care System").

Despite what your mother may have told you, you cannot go blind by reading in bad light, but you can strain your eyes by prolonged work in poor light, doing close work for long periods of time without resting your eyes, or working or playing in glaring light, whether reflected off a work surface, snow, or sand.

Eyestrain will not permanently damage your eyes, but it will make them feel irritated. To avoid this, use task lighting—a light source behind the shoulder if possible and far enough away to bathe the entire work surface in light without producing a glare. Rest your eyes at least every half hour by changing focus, such as gazing into the distance if you have been doing close work. This is especially important if you spend long hours at a video display terminal (see Chapter 17, "Women in the Workplace"). Continued eyestrain may be an indication that you need glasses or that your prescription must be changed.

Preventing injury takes some common sense and an investment in the right safety equipment for your activities. The most common injuries are from the sun or foreign objects. Here are some basic rules:

• Always wear sunglasses when you are outdoors, choosing a type that is appropriate to your activities (see box, "Types of Sunglasses"). Gray lenses are best, followed by brown and then green. Phototropic lenses—those that darken in sunlight—can take up to 10 minutes to change and they may not become dark enough for strong sun.

• Do not look directly at the sun, even during an eclipse. Sunglasses, exposed film, and smoked glass, sometimes suggested for viewing an eclipse, are not effective at preventing damage to the retina.

• Avoid sunlamps, which are as bad for your eyes as they are for your skin.

• Sports and home power tools are the two main sources of eye injuries. Always wear sports eye protectors or industrial safety glasses when playing squash or racquetball; operating a lawn mower, trimmer, or power saw; or spraying paint or chemicals. The best safety glasses conform to the National Stan-

TYPES OF SUNGLASSES

The Sunglass Association of America, an industry group, defines sunglasses according to these categories:

COSMETIC: block 70 percent of UVB rays and 20 percent of UVA rays. Offer minimal protection.

GENERAL PURPOSE: block 95 percent of UVB rays and 60 percent of UVA rays. Sufficient protection for most outdoor activities.

SPECIAL PURPOSE: protect against 99 percent of UVB rays and at least 60 percent of UVA rays. For use on ski slopes, beaches, and other places where glare is especially harsh.

dard Practice for Occupational and Educational Eye and Face Protection; the best sports eye protectors are those made of optical-quality polycarbonates. They are available from opticians, sporting goods stores, and safety equipment suppliers.

• To avoid chlorine or saltwater irritation in pools or at the beach, or bacterial infection in fresh water, wear watertight swim goggles.

• Do not overuse eye drops. These nonprescription preparations are good for irritation due to dust or air pollution, but they will not help eyestrain. They can cause allergic reactions and can easily become contaminated with bacteria.

CONTACT LENS SAFETY Contact lenses have undergone technological changes to make them more comfortable and convenient. Soft lenses, introduced in 1970, are now used by half of the 20 million contact lens wearers in the United States. In 1980, extended-wear lenses were developed to allow for continuous 30-day use. They were followed by disposable extended-wear lenses, which are worn for 1 week and then thrown away.

Along with these innovations, however, have come troublesome eye problems, such as irritating protein and mucus deposits, scratching and scarring of the cornea, and corneal ulcers caused by bacterial infection. Left untreated, such problems can lead to loss of vision.

The risks associated with wearing contact lenses can be dramatically reduced by cleaning them regularly, soaking them in enzyme solution, and disinfecting them. Avoid wearing greasy cosmetics like mascara, which can run into your eyes and cloud the lenses. Look for makeup that is especially formulated for contact lens wearers.

BACK

PROTECTING YOUR BACK Four out of five adults will experience back- or neckaches at some point in their working lives. After colds, backaches are the most common cause of worker absenteeism. Contrary to popular belief, backaches occur more often among office workers than heavy laborers, and are caused more frequently by disc degeneration than injuries.

Discs are the "shock absorbers" that sit between each vertebra, or bone, of the spine. They are made of spongy material surrounded by a hard ring that can be damaged each time the back is abused through poor posture or bad lifting habits. This damage gradually weakens the disc. Eventually the weakened disc becomes drier and may no longer function as a shock absorber. It may become flatter and bulge outward. If it impinges on a nearby nerve, pain may travel along that nerve into the spine and even into other parts of the body. For example, a pinching injury to one of the sciatic nerves that serve the buttocks and legs may send pain to that region, a condition called sciatica. A sudden, heavy lift may rupture a weakened disc, causing a dramatic increase in pain.

Other sources of backache include muscle spasms resulting from overuse or emotional stress, and facet-joint problems. The facet joints are the "hinges" between the vertebrae that guide the movement of the spine. When they are sprained by a sudden twist, it can cause pain to the joint as well as the surrounding muscle.

PREVENTING BACK PAIN Certain people are more likely to suffer back pain than others. Especially at risk are those whose jobs require them either to lift heavy objects or to sit for extended periods of time, both of which place stress on the back. Overweight people may be prone to backaches as well.

Some sports pose special risks to the back. Golfers, for example, use a fast, powerful twisting motion that may jar and injure the spine. Racquetball also puts pressure on the spine, with constant twisting movements in a bent position. During downhill skiing, the spine receives repetitive jolts and can be seriously injured in a fall.

While there are no easy treatments for back pain, there are a number of ways to reduce the risk of injury. Warming up before participating in any sport is essential. Stiff muscles and ligaments can be loosened by stretching slowly. The activity itself should begin slowly and gradually raise the heart rate, which improves blood flow all over the body. This is especially important if you have a sedentary job during the week but like to engage in sports on the weekends.

Sedentary jobs can be made easier on the back, too. The first step is to get up from your desk at least once an hour to stretch. (Long-distance drivers also should try to make periodic stops to stretch.) Your chair should be adjustable and not too low or too soft. For extra protection, use a pillow to support the small of your back and a footrest to relieve pressure on the lower back (if your feet aren't long enough to rest flat on the floor comfortably). Position desk materials so as to avoid continual twisting and reaching. (See Chapter 17, "Women in the Workplace.")

To prevent excess strain on your lower back, sleep on your side with your knees flexed rather than on your stomach or back (see Figure 15.18).

To ease the strain on your back caused by constant lifting, keep loads as close to your body as possible. This puts the weight on your leg muscles, not your back. If objects cannot be brought close to the body, kneel first, then lift them using your arm and leg muscles. Avoid bending over or twisting during a lift, and push objects whenever possible rather than pulling them. (See Figures 15.19–15.20.)

Keeping your body strong and fit is the best defense against back pain. Keep your weight within normal limits and do exercises to strengthen your abdominal muscles, which help support your back. Regular stretching will also keep muscles loose and your back flexible. (See Figures 15.21–15.24.)

TREATING BACK PAIN Even with the best preventive program, most people will suffer an attack of back pain, usually due to muscle strain, at some point in their lives. In the past, the recommended treatment included weeks or even months of bed rest, but recent studies show that long periods of reduced movement worsen the condition by allowing the muscles to stiffen and weaken.

Today, doctors recommend a few days of bed rest and prescribe aspirin or other anti-inflammatory drugs to reduce the pain and swelling. Ice compresses also ease the swelling and inflammation during the first 48 hours. After that, you can use heating pads

Best sleeping position

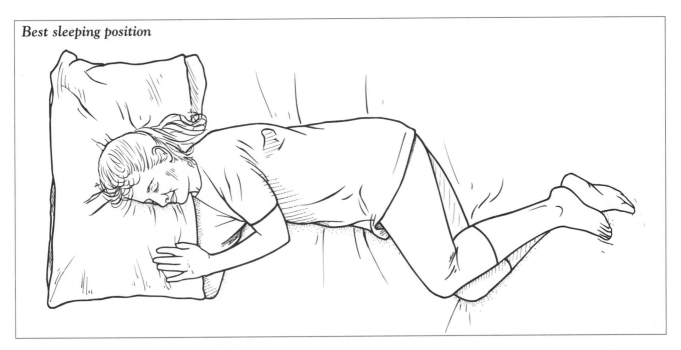

Fig. 15.18 *Sleeping on your side with your knees flexed can take pressure off your lower back. Some physical therapists recommend putting a second pillow between the knees to keep the lower back muscles aligned.*

Proper lifting method

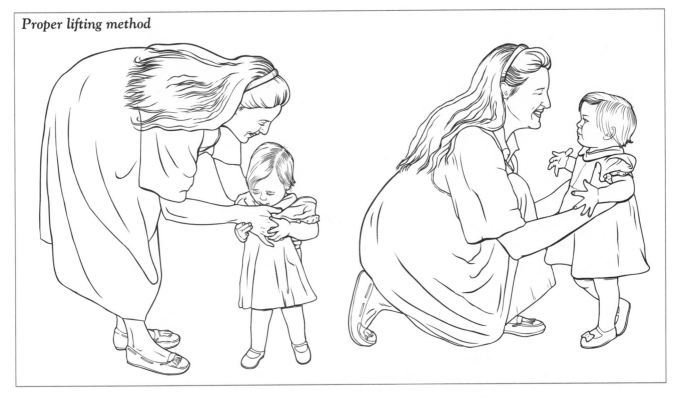

Fig. 15.19–15.20 *Bending over to pick up children and heavy objects forces your back muscles to do the lifting. Kneeling first transfers the strain to your arms and especially your legs, which are less likely to be injured.*

Cat stretch exercise

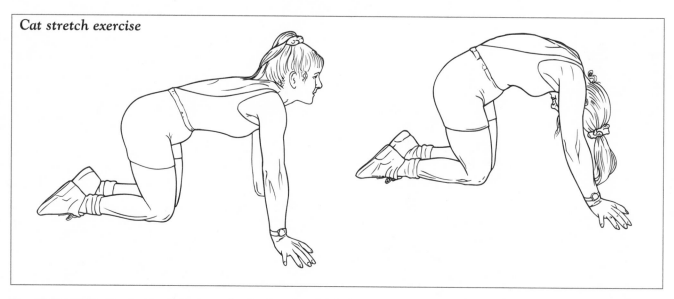

Fig. 15.21–15.22 *Kneel with your back straight. Slowly push it slightly downward, then arch it upward. Repeat 10 times, gradually working up to 20.*

Flexibility exercise

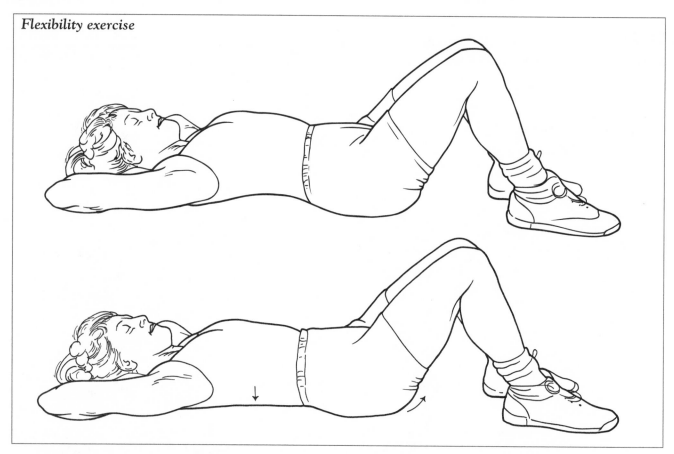

Fig. 15.23–15.24 *Lying on your back with your knees raised, press your lower back against the floor by squeezing your buttocks, tightening your abdominal muscles, and rolling the top of your pelvis backward. Hold for 10 seconds. Repeat 10 times, gradually working up to 20.*

and hot showers to increase your circulation and keep your muscles loose. A gentle exercise program and stress-reduction classes may also help.

If back pain persists, it may indicate a more serious cause, such as a tumor or an infection. Pain that intensifies, wakes you up at night, or is associated with fever or night sweats should be brought to a doctor's attention. One or more tests may be used to diagnose your problem, including X rays, CT (computed tomography) or MRI (magnetic resonance imaging) scans, or a more invasive procedure such as a myelogram.

Depending on the diagnosis, your physician may recommend a combination of rest, medicine, cortisone injections, physical therapy, and a personal exercise program to strengthen the supporting muscles of the back. In most cases, surgery should be performed only after these other options have been exhausted. The goal of back surgery is either to decompress elements that may be pinching nearby nerves or to stabilize elements in the spine. A discectomy, for example, removes the part of a herniated disc—one that has moved out of its proper position—that is pressing on the surrounding nerves.

In a foramenotomy, the bones surrounding a swollen, inflamed nerve are shaved to make space for that nerve. This procedure decreases inflammation and, ultimately, pain. One of the newest procedures is the percutaneous discectomy, in which portions of a herniated disc are removed through an incision small enough to be covered with a Band-Aid.

Surgery alone will not ensure the future health of your back. It must be followed by a rehabilitation program for strengthening the back and a lifetime commitment to staying physically fit.

FEET

Taking good care of your feet is not only good for them, it's good for your whole body, including your back. Wearing shoes with heels more than 2 inches high, for example, can throw your back out of alignment.

Common foot problems include swelling (especially in summer), fatigue, and ingrown toenails, which occur when the nail curves over into the side of the toe and digs into the skin. Feet may also develop patches of rough, hardened skin, particularly around the edges of the soles and heels. With aging, the skin of the feet becomes drier, thinner, and more vulnerable to cracking and infections.

BASIC FOOT CARE

• Wash your feet daily with mild soap and warm water. (Never use very hot or very cold water.) Dry them well, especially between the toes. Dust them with foot powder if you are prone to fungal infections. Change your socks or hosiery daily.

• Check your feet periodically for any rashes, blisters, redness, calluses, etc. See a physician or podiatrist if ailments persist.

• Avoid ingrown toenails by clipping nails straight across once a week, leaving enough nail to protect the tips of the toes. (If a nail does become ingrown, a small V shape cut in the top edge of the nail may relieve pressure on the sides.) If the toe is inflamed and infected, see a podiatrist.

• Soak rough, hardened skin on your feet in the tub to soften it, then scrape it with a pumice stone or hard-skin remover. Moisturizing creams help keep the skin moist and soft, which may alleviate corns and calluses.

• Avoid fungal infections such as athlete's foot by wearing sandals or watersocks at poolside and in locker rooms. If infection does occur, over-the-counter antifungal medications usually provide effective treatment.

• Maintain good circulation in your feet by not wearing hosiery or socks that are tight or have constricting elastic tops. Also avoid sitting with your legs crossed thigh over thigh or with one leg tucked under you.

• Exercise your feet by walking or doing exercises prescribed by a doctor or podiatrist.

SHOPPING FOR SHOES Unfortunately, many women pay far less attention to the comfort of their feet than the appearance of their shoes. Women's shoes are often too pointed and small in front, which squeezes together the bones in the forefoot. Continual wearing of this type of shoe can result in or aggravate bone deformities and calluses or corns, which can cause severe pain.

Some shoes also lack enough cushioning to provide shock absorption, which can lead to heel or knee pain. And those made of synthetic materials may not allow for proper ventilation, which can promote fungal infections and skin irritations.

Even sneakers, which do not pose the same risks as high-heeled pumps, must be chosen with care. Especially narrow or wide feet may be more comfortable in shoes with variable lacing. High tops help support weak ankles. Heavier women should buy shoes with greater shock absorption. If you play sports, choose a shoe that is designed for the specific activity. Manufacturers use different materials and designs based on the type of motion involved in the sport.

The quality of sneakers varies greatly, so it pays to shop wisely. Sneakers that provide adequate support and comfort generally cost $60 to $80. Find a knowledgeable salesperson who can explain the benefits of various materials and designs. Shoes should also be replaced more often than most women realize. The cushion in even the best sneakers flattens out after a while, and the whole shoe may stretch out, which reduces support. When to replace a pair of shoes? When you try on a new pair and notice a big difference in support. Walking shoes usually last about 300 to 500 miles; aerobic sneakers only about 30 to 50 hours of exercise.

ORTHOTICS According to podiatrists, some leg, knee, or hip pain can stem from structural problems or imbalances in the foot that cause it to make uneven contact with the shoe or ground. The solution, say these foot specialists, is orthotics—shoe inserts that are precisely tailored to the individual foot and are designed to "balance" it. For example, an orthotic can help correct supination or pronation—the tendency to turn the ankle outward or inward as you walk. It can also compensate for a discrepancy in the length of your legs, or relieve pressure around a bunion.

Some inserts are available over the counter, but except for simple problems they are usually not as satisfactory as custom-made orthotics. To make these inserts, most podiatrists take a cast of the foot and send it to an outside lab. Orthotics are made of leather, fiberglass, graphite, or other substances, and weigh only a few ounces. The cost is high, several hundreds of dollars in most cases. However, for people in pain, those who exercise a great deal, or spend long periods of time on their feet, the expense can be worth it.

BUNIONS AND HAMMERTOES Two relatively common and painful foot problems that can be exacerbated by ill-fitting shoes are bunions and hammertoes. Bunions, which are much more common in women than in men, are protrusions on the head of the metatarsal bone at the base of the big toe. The problem starts with tenderness and swelling at the toe joint and may involve the bone, which slowly becomes deformed, and the bursa, a soft sac that cushions and lubricates the joint. Roomier shoes and analgesics such as aspirin or nonsteroidal anti-inflammatory drugs may help alleviate mild cases. A splint is sometimes used to keep the toe aligned. In severe cases, a surgical procedure called bunionectomy may be necessary. (See Figure 15.25.) This is done under local anesthesia and may be treated as ambulatory surgery or as an inpatient procedure involving an overnight stay in a hospital. A cast or protective device is usually required during recovery.

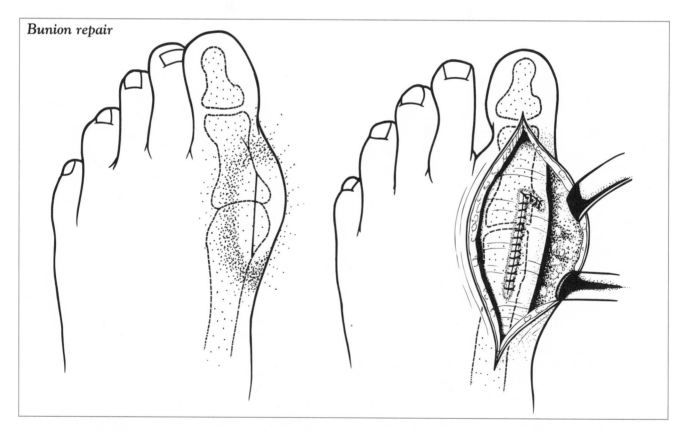

Bunion repair

Fig. 15.25 *In a bunionectomy, a portion of the metatarsal bone is removed to reduce the protrusion that can make wearing even roomy shoes extremely uncomfortable.*

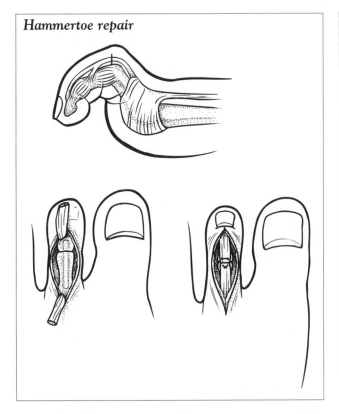

Hammertoe repair

Fig. 15.26 *A hammertoe is repaired by removing a section of the bone or lengthening the tendon or both to allow the toe to lie flat.*

Because this surgery is not always successful, it should be considered carefully and only after more conservative measures have been tried.

Hammertoes usually involve the second toe, but the condition may affect one or more of the smaller toes as well. The toe begins to curl under, taking on a clawlike appearance. (See Figure 15.26.) The underlying problem may be misaligned joint surfaces or shortened and weakened toe muscles. Some people have an inherited propensity to develop hammertoes, and they are also common in people with diabetes.

Many hammertoes require no treatment other than properly fitting shoes; others may result in corns that cause pain when they rub against surrounding tissue or shoes. If the hammertoe produces chronic pain or interferes with walking, surgery may be recommended. In what is often an outpatient procedure, a wedge of bone is removed or the tendon is lengthened so that the toe can lie flat. A thick, sandallike surgical shoe usually must be worn for a few weeks until swelling completely subsides.

CHAPTER 16

Conquering Fatigue

Fatigue is a sensation we all experience, at least in some degree. It may be the feeling of being wiped out at the end of a busy day at work or a long day on the ski slopes. Fatigue of this kind usually responds to a good night's rest and is gone in the morning. More significantly, fatigue may be chronic, the feeling of being mentally and physically tired all the time. Long-lasting fatigue should not be ignored by women or their doctors, who should certainly not brush it off as being "all in your head." At its most severe, fatigue is so overwhelming that sometimes you are all but bedridden. This sort of fatigue is associated with illness, often with severe illness.

Chronic fatigue—a daily lack of energy—is one of the most common reasons why women visit their doctors, and a complaint whose cause is most difficult to diagnose. It may be a symptom of countless medical conditions, such as an underactive thyroid gland, diabetes, mononucleosis, Lyme disease, or anemia. However, chronic fatigue is very often a result of circumstances and life-style choices. If your doctor has found no underlying reason for your fatigue, taking a long, hard look at those circumstances and choices is in order.

EVERYDAY CAUSES OF FATIGUE

According to Dr. Holly Atkinson, author of *Women and Fatigue*, your daily energy capacity is a combination of your natural reserves (the energy you wake up with) and the energy boosters and energy drainers in your life. (See box, "The Energy Equation.") Among the energy boosters, Dr. Atkinson identifies good nutrition, exercise, restful sleep, and taking pleasure in life. Energy drainers include bad habits (smoking, drinking, drugs), mental strain (conflict, loss), overwork, occupational hazards, and illness. Obviously, the more energy boosters in your life, the less tired you will be—and vice versa. Fatigue is a signal of an imbalance: Too much energy is being spent and not enough is being conserved.

It is important to keep track of when during the day (and the week and month) you feel fatigue and to try to pin down which circumstances or behaviors seem to set it off. This will make it easier to schedule important activities at times when you have the most energy. It will also suggest what life-style changes might be most helpful in reducing your fatigue.

THE ENERGY EQUATION

ENERGY BOOSTERS	ENERGY DRAINERS
Good nutrition	Unhealthy habits (alcohol, smoking, drugs)
Exercise	
Restful sleep	Overwork
Pleasure	Stress (conflict, loss, depression)
Mastery of skills	Occupational hazards
	Illness

LIFE-STYLE STRATEGIES TO COMBAT FATIGUE

SLEEPING WELL A good night's sleep leaves you energized and alert in the morning. No one is certain why this is so. Some researchers suggest that sleep gives your body tissues time to recover from daily wear and tear, others that it restores brain function. A bad night, on the other hand, leaves you with slower reaction times, poorer concentration, and a smaller pool of energy from which to draw the next day. People vary widely in their sleeping patterns: Some feel rested after 5 hours' sleep, others need 9 or 10. And sleep-wake patterns change as you age, with elderly people experiencing more wakefulness during the night than they did when younger. Whatever your sleep pattern, if you wake up feeling tired and are not comfortably alert during the day, you are not getting enough sleep. (See box, "A Good Night's Sleep.") Even though people often adapt to inadequate sleep, mood swings, memory lapses, and accidents are more likely to happen.

Many women, because of their busy lives, go to bed late and get up early, and as a result have a chronic sleep debt. Naturally, just being in bed for the traditional 8 hours does not guarantee you will get a good night's rest. A variety of factors can prevent or disrupt sleep, including alcohol, caffeine, eating or exercising too close to bedtime, depression, anxiety, and shift work. (Night-shift workers, on average, get 3 hours less sleep than people working daylight schedules.)

An afternoon nap is an excellent way to counter fatigue. Studies have found that sleeping briefly in the afternoon measurably increases alertness. A nap also improves mood, especially in those who don't get enough sleep at night. There is evidence that, left to themselves without clocks or lights or interrup-

tions, human beings ordinarily have two sleep periods in the course of 24 hours, one considerably longer than the other. The shorter sleep period tends to occur about 12 hours after the middle of the longer one—for example, at about 3 P.M. if you slept from 11 P.M. to 7 A.M. Those whose schedules permit a nap in the afternoon are following the promptings of an internal clock.

EXERCISING Paradoxically, expending energy by exercising increases your energy level. In fact, many experts believe that aerobic exercise is the best way to stave off fatigue. (See Chapter 10, "Keeping Fit.") Many women, too, are familiar with the fatigue-fighting benefits of vigorous activity, and enthusiastically endorse the experts' view.

Vigorous activity is energizing because it wakes up the nervous system and speeds up the metabolic rate. A fast metabolic rate ensures a good supply of energy and less of a feeling of fatigue, not only during exercise but for up to 8 hours afterward. And, over the long term, exercise leads to physical fitness, the stamina to do more and endure more without fatigue.

Exercise also enhances a sense of well-being because it causes the release of endorphins, which produce feelings of pleasure and relaxation. In improving mood, exercise provides an antidote to fatigue. Why this is so is not known, but the link is a strong one: Good spirits go along with more energy (and vice versa).

EATING BETTER What you eat and when you eat it can have profound effects on your energy level throughout the day. Food is our source of fuel and of essential vitamins and minerals. Carbohydrates provide the body's preferred fuel, glucose. A diet rich in complex carbohydrates such as grains, cereals, and starchy vegetables provides the best staying power because these foods are digested slowly. Simple sugars in candy or cookies, on the other hand, cause a sudden surge of glucose in the blood, quickly followed by a drop in blood sugar and a feeling of tiredness.

In addition to providing fuel for the body's cells, food triggers the release of certain chemical messengers, or neurotransmitters, in the brain either to energize or to calm us. High-protein foods stimulate the release of energizing neurotransmitters such as adrenaline. Carbohydrates prompt the formation in the brain of the neurotransmitter serotonin, which is calming and induces sleep. With this information in hand, you can plan individual meals to work in your favor. A good balanced breakfast will boost your en-

A GOOD NIGHT'S SLEEP

If you have trouble falling asleep, here are some tips for breaking the insomnia cycle:

• Establish a regular sleep routine, in which you go to bed at a regular hour and get up at the same time every morning, even if this sometimes means missing a little sleep on holidays and weekends.

• If you cannot sleep, do not lie in bed fretting about it. Instead, get up and do something restful for a while—perhaps read a couple of chapters of a not-too-interesting book—then go back to bed. In this way, bed will be associated with sleep rather than with tossing and turning.

• If worry is what is keeping you awake, get up and put the problem down on paper, along with any possible solutions that occur to you. Then go back to bed, knowing that you have made a start on figuring things out.

• Alcohol may make you drowsy and help you fall asleep, but it is likely to cause you to wake in the small hours of the morning, when it is hard to get back to sleep.

• Coffee, tea, cocoa, and colas all contain caffeine (even the decaffeinated versions may have small amounts) and are best avoided after dinner. For some people, a cup of coffee taken as much as *7 hours* before bedtime is enough to ruin that night's sleep.

• The folk medicine cure for trouble falling asleep—drinking a glass of milk at bedtime—actually has a scientific basis. Milk is a good source of the amino acid tryptophan, which prompts the production of the calming neurotransmitter serotonin. Carbohydrates, too, encourage the transport of tryptophan to the brain. So try a bedtime snack of milk (warm or cold) with some whole wheat crackers.

• Exercise helps you sleep, not only because it leaves you pleasantly tired, but also because it temporarily raises your body temperature. Researchers know that body temperature drops about half a degree shortly before sleep comes. This small drop initiates a string of physiological changes that culminate in sleep. If you time your exercise for the late afternoon or early evening, and give yourself plenty of time to cool down by bedtime, the drop in your body temperature can be a sleep aid. (A hot bath serves the same purpose, although body temperature falls faster after a bath than after exercise. Plan to take your bath an hour or so before you go to bed.)

• Over-the-counter sleeping aids and prescription drugs make it easier to get to sleep at first, but they lose their effectiveness after about 2 weeks. Used long-term, they disrupt sound sleep, especially in the second part of the night. Moreover, the barbiturates (such as Seconal) and the tranquilizers (Valium, for example) that are often prescribed as sleeping aids are potentially addictive. If you stop taking them suddenly, you may experience severe withdrawal symptoms, such as extreme nervousness, agitation, and body aches, as well as serious sleep disturbances. It is best to avoid medicating yourself to sleep.

---

ergy during the morning hours. A high-protein lunch lays the groundwork for a productive afternoon. And a high-carbohydrate dinner prepares you for a sound night's sleep and the replenishment of your energy pool. To keep your energy level up during the day, especially during the notorious afternoon slump, keep a supply of healthful snacks handy—carrot sticks, rice cakes, air-popped popcorn, and fresh fruit.

Dieting is a sure way to invite fatigue. Some weight-loss diets scrap carbohydrates almost entirely. This inevitably leaves you feeling tired and hungry, and craving sweets. To lose weight without feeling fatigued, decrease your calorie intake but maintain a balanced selection of healthful foods and increase the amount of exercise you do. As a rule of thumb, a safe and effective weight-loss diet should derive 50 to 60 percent of its calories from carbohydrates (with an emphasis on complex carbohydrates), 30 percent or less from fat, and the rest from protein. (See Chapter 9, "Healthful Eating for a Lifetime.")

AVOIDING DRUGS AND ALCOHOL Fatigue is a side effect of a great many over-the-counter and prescription drugs. A short list includes analgesics, antidepressants, antihistamines, birth control pills, muscle relaxants, cough and cold medications that contain narcotics, and, of course, sedatives. If you have reason to believe that your fatigue is related to medications you are taking, talk to your doctor about it. Perhaps a lower dosage would be possible, or you could take the medication at a different time so that the peak of your fatigue would come while you sleep. If such modifications are not possible, and you must continue with the medication, then you have to learn to compensate for the fatigue, accepting it, taking naps, and avoiding demanding tasks.

The physiological effects of "recreational" drugs such as marijuana and cocaine are also sources of fatigue. This fact is often overlooked by users of these substances.

Alcohol, too, is a drug and fatigue is one of its side effects. It appears at first to be a stimulant. But the initial high is rapidly followed by slowed-down reflexes, dulled thinking, and drowsiness—the effects of a powerful depressant.

Many women have a drink or two at the end of the day, believing that alcohol's tranquilizing effect will calm their nerves and help them get a good night's sleep. But alcohol does more to hinder sleep than to help it. It disrupts the stages of sleep and is the direct cause of waking during the night. The predictable result is fatigue the following day. Even moderate amounts of alcohol have a depressive effect.

QUITTING SMOKING Anything that affects the delivery of oxygen to the body tissues causes fatigue. Cigarettes do just that. Those who have stopped smoking know, in retrospect, how much cigarettes drain energy.

The nicotine in cigarettes causes a rise in blood pressure and an increased heartbeat, the lift that a smoker craves. With an increased rate, the heart's need for oxygen increases, but more oxygen is precisely what is not available. The carbon monoxide in cigarette smoke commandeers the red blood cells (it binds to hemoglobin two hundred times faster than oxygen does), hampering their ability to deliver oxygen to the heart. In effect, as the smoker inhales, the body suffocates.

Tobacco smoke also contains many toxic ingredients that cause short- and long-term damage to various organs in the body. Smoking may lead to emphysema, bronchitis, or heart disease, with fatigue as a side effect of the illness. In fact, fatigue is likely to be experienced long before unequivocal symptoms of these diseases appear.

REDUCING STRESS There are sources of stress that are unique to women: the struggle of balancing work and family responsibilities, for example, or guilt about not being the perfect wife or mother or daughter. Many women, trying to be everything to everyone, are gravely overextended. Others, attempting to resolve the conflicts in their lives, are mentally exhausted. Still others feel tired without knowing exactly why: Conflict is going on below the surface of their lives and the resultant exhaustion is its overt symptom.

You may not have much control over the sources of stress and conflict in your life (this in itself may be a source of stress). However, there are steps that you can take to keep exhaustion at bay. You can prioritize chores and lower your housekeeping standards to lighten the workload at home. You can learn to communicate effectively with your partner, your children, and your co-workers, to reduce potential sources of conflict. Most important, you can build a little leisure into your life and increase your energy level by taking back some personal time. (See Chapter 11 for specific stress-management techniques such as relaxation exercises.)

COPING WITH LOSS It is absolutely normal to feel fatigue after suffering a loss. Fatigue is also ever-present during the period of grieving. Then, once mourning is completed, one's energy returns. How long the mourning period lasts, and how deep the mourning is, depends on the severity of the loss.

We generally think of loss as the death of a loved one, and, of course, this is one of the most severe emotional traumas. There are others, however, that bring grief and, consequently, fatigue in their wake: a child leaving home, for example, especially if that child is the only one or the last to leave the nest. Divorce is a loss that goes beyond the leave-taking of a live-in partner. There are profound losses involved in the breakup of a marriage even when both partners want out. Entering menopause means the loss of the ability to bear children and, for many women, a felt loss of sexual attractiveness. We may also grieve over the loss of dreams, relationships, ambitions, health, youth, or beauty.

Left alone, the grieving process normally runs its course and the fatigue abates. However, if instead of improving, grieving worsens and comes to include the symptoms of depression (see section on "Depression"), you should consult a mental health professional.

FATIGUE-RELATED MEDICAL CONDITIONS

ANEMIA The first test many doctors give their female patients who complain of fatigue is one for iron-deficiency anemia, which determines your red blood cell count. The root cause of this form of anemia is insufficient iron in the diet or blood loss from, for example, heavy menses or gastrointestinal bleeding. Without enough iron, enough of the red pigment hemoglobin cannot be created. Without enough hemoglobin, the red blood cells cannot carry enough oxygen from the lungs to other cells throughout the body. And without enough oxygen, these cells cannot function at capacity, and our entire body feels the sensation we know as fatigue.

Women lose iron during menstruation. Even normal monthly bleeding can seriously deplete the body's reserves of iron. To replenish these reserves, you must eat plenty of iron-rich foods: low-fat meats, dark meat poultry, dark green leafy vegetables such as spinach and Swiss chard, beans, prunes, dried peaches and apricots, and iron-fortified cereals and breads. If you have heavy periods, or know that your diet is poor in iron, talk to your doctor about taking iron supplements.

Although iron-deficiency anemia is the most common form of anemia, other types can also cause fatigue. These include pernicious anemia, caused by a vitamin B_{12} deficiency, and anemia due to a deficiency of folic acid (another B vitamin). Pernicious anemia is sometimes seen in people who have long been strict vegetarians, or who lack a substance called intrinsic factor and thus cannot absorb the vitamin through their digestive tracts. Although folic acid deficiency is almost always the result of poor diet and often seen in alcoholics, it, too, can be caused by a malabsorption problem, such as celiac disease and other ailments.

DEPRESSION An entire range of blue feelings—from everyday sadness and frustration to the grief of losing a loved one to major depression—is universally characterized by fatigue. This may manifest itself as weakness, drowsiness, lack of energy, loss of interest in the world, or an overall feeling that it is no longer worthwhile exerting yourself about anything.

Clinical depression, the medical term for an unexplained bout of the blues that lasts longer than a month, strikes between 20 and 30 percent of all Americans at some time in their lives. Women are twice as likely as men to be affected. Yet this condition is vastly underdiagnosed and undertreated. Many depressed women think they are just very tired, when in fact they could probably benefit from an antidepressant drug. Others may deny that they are depressed because depression has often been stigmatized as "mental illness." However, this stigma is lessening as it becomes clearer how prevalent—and how treatable—depression really is.

Other symptoms of depression include physical disturbances (changes in sleeping and eating habits, headaches, menstrual problems, impaired sexual functioning), feelings of helplessness and hopelessness, and thoughts of suicide. Depression is much more than a normal mood change; it is a lasting and abnormal mood state.

Researchers are increasingly convinced that depression is a biological phenomenon related to imbalances in certain neurotransmitters in the brain, and that the tendency toward depression may be inherited.

Women can handle some blue moods and mild depression on their own, with the help of their families and friends. However, if your feelings stay low for more than a month, and if they interfere with your daily activities, you should see your doctor for a thorough physical examination to rule out any possible physical causes, such as an underactive thyroid (see section on "Hypothyroidism"). If you are diagnosed with depression, the condition can usually be successfully treated with drug therapy, or psychological counseling, or both. Regular exercise also helps because it raises the brain levels of the neurotransmitter norepinephrine, which are typically low in depressed people. Exercise also boosts energy, raises self-esteem, and decreases anxiety. (For more information, see the Encyclopedia.)

HORMONAL CHANGES Varying hormone levels at different times of the month and at different times of life can make women more prone to fatigue. Although the exact mechanism is not known, hormonal changes before and during menstruation can cause mental and physical fatigue as well as a decreased resistance to stress. Women are particularly vulnerable to fatigue during pregnancy (especially during the first and third trimesters), due both to hormonal changes and to the demands made on their bodies by the growing fetus. At menopause, hormonal shifts can cause hot flashes. If you wake several times during the night, drenched in sweat, you will most probably experience fatigue the following day.

SLEEP APNEA Although this disorder—characterized by brief periods in which breathing stops during sleep—more commonly affects middle-aged, overweight men, it can also occur in obese women. These episodes can sometimes cause you to awaken gasping for breath and feeling frightened, but usually it just produces fitful sleep without awakening. As a consequence, someone with apnea may be tired and drowsy during the day after a seemingly normal night's sleep. Losing weight may help diminish the problem. Mild cases can be treated with medication or special breathing equipment during sleep, while more serious ones may require surgery to widen the airway.

HYPOTHYROIDISM An underactive thyroid, called hypothyroidism and usually due to Hashimoto's disease, slows down many bodily functions and often results in progressive fatigue and lethargy. Among its other symptoms are muscle aches, constipation, increased sensitivity to cold, decreased appetite but continued weight gain, dry skin and facial puffiness, hair loss, decreased sexual drive, and deepened voice. (See the Encyclopedia.)

DIABETES Although some women with Type II, or adult-onset, diabetes may have no symptoms at all, fatigue can be one of its first signals. Fatigue is also a symptom of Type I diabetes, but this type, which usually starts in childhood, also tends to have other, less subtle symptoms. Both kinds of diabetes may result in frequent urination, unusual thirst, weight loss, and weakness. Type II diabetes may produce all of these symptoms as well as frequent infections of the skin, gums, genitals, or urinary tract; blurred vision, or pain or cramps in the legs, feet, or fingers; and slow healing of cuts and bruises. (See the Encyclopedia.)

CHRONIC FATIGUE SYNDROME (CFS) In the spectrum of fatigue severity, chronic fatigue syndrome is the worst, and the least understood. CFS strikes suddenly at healthy, productive people and turns them into virtual invalids; patients report being too weary to get out of bed and go to the bathroom, or being wiped out for days after a routine activity such as showering. They have abrupt mood swings and enormous difficulty with concentration and memory. It is estimated that hundreds of thousands of Americans, perhaps as many as 5 million, may have CFS, three quarters of them women, mostly between ages 22 and 44.

When CFS first appeared in the Lake Tahoe region of California, in the mid-1980s, it presented experts with a mystery. Its symptoms were numerous and varied, and they fitted none of the established diagnoses. Many suspected that it was a newly recognized form of emotional illness. Indeed, one of the most difficult challenges for many CFS patients has been that doctors, families, and friends have not believed that they were suffering from a bona fide physical illness. Today, while many doctors are convinced that CFS is a physical ailment, others still maintain that it is an emotional one and point to the fact that antidepressants are beneficial for many sufferers.

Searching for the cause of CFS, scientists have found evidence that CFS may be an immune system disorder. Some types of immune cells (macrophages and immune killer cells) do not function as well in CFS patients as in healthy people. Also, CFS patients' immune systems seem to have become chronically activated, producing proteins such as interleukin-2 that stimulate immune cells. Other experts believe that CFS symptoms may be related to low levels of two hormones: corticotropin-releasing hormone, which acts on the brain to help increase energy levels, and cortisol. Cortisol is released by the adrenal gland in response to stress, and even mild deficits in this hormone can result in fatigue. Scientists are also still searching for a virus that causes CFS, perhaps one that is dormant in the body until immune abnormalities allow it to be activated.

Although the cause of CFS remains unknown, the Centers for Disease Control and Prevention (CDC) helped establish it as a legitimate illness by setting guidelines for its diagnosis. (See box, "Signs and Symptoms of CFS.") The CDC's criteria, issued in 1988, first require that all other possible physical and psychiatric causes of a patient's fatigue be ruled out. Second, the fatigue must have persisted for at least 6 months (or recurred over that time span) and the patient's activity level must have been reduced by more than half. Finally, the patient must have at least eight of the following signs or symptoms: mild fever or chills, sore throat, swollen glands, joint pain, muscle weakness, muscle aches, headaches, sleep disturbances, neuropsychological problems (confusion, depression, forgetfulness), fatigue lasting at least a day following moderate exercise, and a sudden onset of the condition.

The symptoms of CFS tend to come and go over a period of years. About one third of all patients make a full recovery in less than 2 years. Another third

SIGNS AND SYMPTOMS OF CFS

The following CFS symptoms come on suddenly and last or recur at least 6 months:

- Extreme fatigue
- Mild fever or chills
- Sore throat
- Swollen glands
- Joint pain without swelling
- Muscle weakness
- Muscle aches
- Headaches
- Sleep disturbances
- Neuropsychological problems (confusion, depression, forgetfulness)
- Fatigue lasting at least a day following moderate exercise

show some improvement. The rest, unfortunately, never regain their health. There is, to date, no definitive test for the condition and no effective treatment. Antiviral drugs have been used, but with little success. Treatments are largely limited to relieving the symptoms—pain relievers for headache and muscle soreness, antidepressants to help sleep and decrease fatigue. Unfortunately, many CFS patients fall victim to quack cures, such as hypoallergenic products, detoxification programs, and injections of hydrogen peroxide.

Patients with CFS have started support groups and information clearinghouses—for example, the Chronic Fatigue Immune Dysfunction Association and National CFS Association—which spread the word about new research and potential treatments. (See Resources.)

FIBROMYALGIA Until recently, this condition was known as fibrositis, inflammation of connective tissue, and was thought to be a rheumatic disease similar to arthritis. But doctors have not been able to pinpoint any inflammation in patients suffering from the condition. So they now use a more appropriate term, fibromyalgia, which means, roughly, "pain that affects soft tissue."

Fibromyalgia affects the sexes disproportionately: Eighty percent of sufferers are women, mostly be-

tween the ages of 20 and 50. It displays a perplexing array of symptoms: widespread muscle pain, extreme fatigue, anxiety, depression, headaches, stomachaches, sleep disturbances, and cold hands and feet. (See box, "Multifaceted Fibromyalgia.") However, there is a simple method of diagnosing the condition: Eighteen specific points on the body are tested for unusual tenderness. These points are very precisely located at the front and back of the neck, on the chest and shoulders, on the elbows, hips, and knees. Nearly all patients with fibromyalgia have these unusually sensitive spots, though most are unaware of them until they have been examined by a doctor.

Three out of four women with fibromyalgia are fatigued to the point of exhaustion. Researchers think that sleep repeatedly disrupted by pain may be responsible, at least in part. Strangely, some studies have found that when healthy people are continuously disturbed during deep sleep, they develop sensitivity in the identical tender spots involved in fibromyalgia.

Many women thought to have chronic fatigue syndrome actually have fibromyalgia. Some experts are even beginning to believe that the two illnesses are one and the same. In any case, fibromyalgia may be surprisingly common: A study at the University of

MULTIFACETED FIBROMYALGIA

Symptoms of fibromyalgia include:

- Fatigue
- Chronic headaches
- Anxiety
- Depression
- Irritable bowel syndrome
- Discolored spots on the skin
- Morning stiffness
- Numbness and tingling
- Sensitivity to weather and temperature changes, stress, and physical activity
- Skin-fold tenderness
- Sleep disturbances
- Swelling or numbness in hands or feet
- Reduced blood flow to fingers and toes

Kansas School of Medicine found that 12 percent of all patients in a general-medicine clinic had symptoms of the condition.

Doctors don't know for sure what causes the condition. Although generally it seems to appear from out of the blue, many women develop fibromyalgia after experiencing some sort of trauma—a car accident, the flu, or severe emotional stress. The triggering event is believed to change the normal balance or function of essential body chemicals, although it is not yet known which these are. Some researchers point to abnormally large quantities of a neurotransmitter, called Substance P, in the cerebrospinal fluid of women with fibromyalgia. Substance P helps transmit pain impulses; high levels of it may mean extra sensitivity to pain. Other scientists suspect that the neurotransmitter serotonin might play a part. Imbalances in serotonin levels are involved in sleep disturbances, pain perception, depression, and muscle spasm, all of which are found in fibromyalgia.

As far as treatment goes, patients have been helped most by low doses of tricyclic drugs such as Elavil and Flexeril, to counter sleep disturbance. Simple pain-killers such as acetaminophen are also useful, but the more powerful antiinflammatory drugs have little effect. A program of regular aerobic exercise, begun very slowly and gradually increased in intensity, can ease a patient's pain, improve sleep, and reduce fatigue. For many sufferers, the diagnosis itself brings relief—it confirms their belief that their symptoms are real, not just products of their imaginations.

CANDIDIASIS SENSITIVITY SYNDROME Most doctors are skeptical about the existence of this syndrome, which is also called chronic candidiasis, candida-related complex, and (as the title of a best-selling book has it) the "yeast connection." However, a segment of the public is convinced it exists. The culprit is said to be *Candida albicans*, a type of yeast normally present in the intestinal tract, which supposedly overgrows in response to factors such as antibiotics, oral contraceptives, and pregnancy. The excess yeast is believed to produce inflammation of the mucous membranes as well as a generalized allergic response that shows up as persistent vaginal yeast infections. Other symptoms include severe premenstrual syndrome and menstrual irregularity, fatigue, depression, anxiety, difficulty in concentrating, headaches, nasal congestion, and such gastrointestinal complaints as bloating, heartburn, constipation, and diarrhea.

There have been no good studies to provide a clear definition of chronic yeast infection. There is no definitive test to diagnose it, nor proof that any treatments relieve most of the symptoms.

Candidiasis sensitivity syndrome remains controversial. Patients often accuse doctors of not listening to them or researching the syndrome seriously. Doctors respond that the lack of a working definition of the syndrome prevents serious study.

Patients are usually treated with the antifungal drug nystatin (orally and often vaginally as well). They are advised to avoid oral contraceptives, antibiotics, and a diet high in carbohydrates, all of which are thought to stimulate yeast growth.

Issues in Women's Health

CHAPTER 17

Women in the Workplace

In the 1990s, more women work outside the home than not; only 35 percent are full-time homemakers. Most women will be part of the workforce at some point in their lives.

While 85 to 99 percent of the following job categories are filled by women—secretaries, typists, and receptionists; bookkeepers and auditing clerks; nurses and health care workers other than doctors; child care workers; elementary school teachers; and cosmetologists—each year finds more women engaged in nontraditional occupations.

Not only have women had to win the right to hold nontraditional jobs, but if these jobs were found to be potentially hazardous for pregnant women, they had to fight to continue holding them, whether or not they were planning to become pregnant. In 1991, the U.S. Supreme Court ruled that employers may not exclude women from jobs in which exposure to toxic substances could harm a developing fetus. In writing the majority decision, Associate Justice Harry A. Blackmun declared that "women as capable of doing their jobs as their male counterparts may not be forced to choose between having a child and having a job."

Female workers may be exposed not only to physical hazards but also to stress and the mental anguish of job discrimination and sexual harassment. Because many women enter the workforce later in life, after their children have grown, they may face age discrimination as well.

The workplace is full of potential threats to health and safety: chemical, physical, electrical, biological, and psychological. Although mining and manufacturing are, in general, the most dangerous occupations, even relatively safe white-collar jobs may involve exposure to repetitive strain injuries from working at computer keyboards, and respiratory problems, allergies, and infections such as are associated with recirculated air in poorly ventilated office buildings.

Following are some of the hazards likely to affect large numbers of women. Further information and help in identifying and correcting these hazards, as well as those not covered here, are available from several government and nonprofit sources. (See Resources.)

VDT AND WORD PROCESSOR USERS

REPETITIVE STRAIN INJURIES Disabling job-related musculoskeletal injuries of the wrists, hands, arms, shoulders, and neck are not new to meat processors and packers, assembly line workers, and professional pianists, among others. In the 1990s, however, these repetitive strain injuries (RSIs) have become the fastest-growing category of workers' compensation claims. According to the U.S. Department of Labor, they now account for 55 percent of all job-related injuries. The National Institute for Occupational Safety and Health (NIOSH) reports that RSIs are three to ten times more common in women than in men.

A major reason for the proliferation of repetitive strain (sometimes called repetitive stress) injuries is the computer revolution. More than 70 million video display terminal (VDT) workstations are estimated to exist nationwide in offices, airline terminals, telephone companies, schools, factories, and homes.

Although carpal tunnel syndrome is perhaps the most publicized type of RSI related to computer use, it is only one of several categories of soft-tissue (muscle, tendon, and ligament) injuries that can result from repeating the same motions—sometimes awkward or forceful ones—over and over, usually at a rapid speed and without adequate rest breaks. Various forms of tendinitis and De Quervain's disease, which affects the thumb and inside of the wrist, are probably more common. (See box, "Symptoms of Repetitive Strain Injury.") These injuries can be treated by a combination of physical therapy, pain control techniques and, in some cases of carpal tunnel syndrome, surgery. They can, however, be prevented by modifying the work environment and learning correct movement techniques.

Why are RSIs proliferating now when people have used typewriters for years? For one thing, typewriters are much slower than computer keyboards, so even fast typists were pounding far fewer keys per hour. For another, the repetitive keystrokes are broken up by the necessity to stop after each page and insert a new piece of paper—a built-in break in the action.

PREVENTION Ergonomics, the term for human engineering, is the science of fitting the workplace to the workers for maximum comfort and therefore efficiency. Since experts agree that chronic musculoskeletal injuries are easier to prevent than to cure, many companies are redesigning the workplace. (See box, "The Ergonomic Workstation," and Figure 17.1.)

THE ERGONOMIC WORKSTATION

To prevent strain on your back, eyes, shoulders, forearms, and wrists, your computer workstation should be set up as follows:

- Place the computer keyboard on a flat surface that is no more than 26 to 28 inches off the floor. (Standard desks are 30 to 32 inches high.) If you don't have a typing return or computer stand of the correct height, a keyboard drawer that pulls out from under the desk may solve your problem.

- Adjust the seat height of your chair so that when your feet are flat on the floor in front of you, the angle between your thighs and calves is about 90 degrees. Depending on how tall you are, the top of your seat should be 16 to 22 inches from the floor. If you are short and your feet don't touch the floor comfortably, use a footrest to keep your knees at a 90-degree angle.

- To prevent fatigue and back strain, use a chair with lower lumbar support and adjust the angle between the seat and the back so that it falls between 80 and 110 degrees.

- To avoid cutting off circulation to your lower legs, adjust the chair seat so that it pitches downward slightly (about 3 degrees) from back to front. The ideal chair has a "waterfall edge" that is slightly rounded and drops off sharply to take pressure off the underside of the thighs.

- Place your chair in front of the keyboard so that when your fingers are on the keys, your elbows bend at 90 degrees and your forearms *and wrists* are parallel to the floor.

- Once you have made these adjustments, sit in the chair and position the monitor so the screen is about 28 inches from your eyes.

- Tilt the monitor so that the top of the screen is 10 degrees below eye level when you are looking straight ahead.

Dr. Emil Pascarelli, founder of the Miller Institute for Performing Artists at St. Luke's-Roosevelt Hospital in New York City, recommends the following keyboard techniques in *Repetitive Strain Injury: A Computer User's Guide:*

- Keep your wrists parallel to the floor, with the middle finger at the center of the wrist and in line with the forearm. This means that your wrists should not be bent up or down, nor should they be angled toward the thumb or little finger. (See Figure 17.2.)

• Avoid resting your wrists on something while typing. Ironically, many people buy wrist rests for their keyboards, believing that using them while they type will help prevent RSIs. The wrist rest is just a place to put your wrists *while they are resting*. Trying to type with your wrists pinned to the rest causes dorsiflexion, bending your wrists upward, a major source of strain.

• Use your whole arm to move your hand. If you are holding your wrists in the proper position, your fingers will rest only lightly on the keyboard, so you can easily extend your hand, rather than stretch your fingers, to use the function, numerical, and other keys out of immediate reach.

• Keep your fingers curved. First, let your arms dangle at your side and you will see that your fingers curve naturally. Then bring your hands, fingers still curved, up to the keyboard. Be sure to keep your thumbs and little fingers down also. Holding your little finger aloft will strain the tendons in your forearm, while keeping your thumb rigid can lead to tendinitis of the thumb.

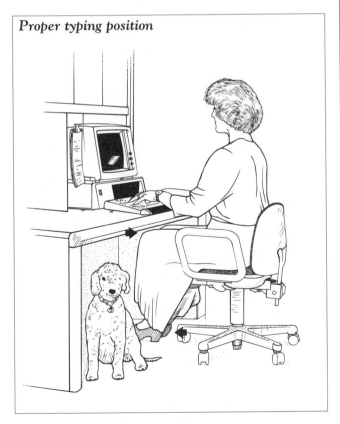

Fig. 17.1 *Placing your chair, keyboard, and monitor at the proper height and distance from your body can help to prevent fatigue, strain, and possible injury.*

SYMPTOMS OF REPETITIVE STRAIN INJURY

Any upper body motion that is repeated over and over again, whether in processing raw chickens, assembling parts in a factory, playing a musical instrument, or typing at a keyboard, to name a few, can result in a repetitive strain injury. The symptoms include:

• Pain in the neck, shoulders, upper back, upper arms, forearms, wrists, hands, or fingers, or a combination of these

• Pain that is aching, burning, or shooting

• Tingling, weakness, or numbness in the fingers or hands

• Tremors or clumsiness, with or without pain

Keeping your fingers curved means that you will be striking the keys with your fingertips, not the flat underside of your fingers. If you have long fingernails, cut them. Long fingernails are not worth the pain that can result from keeping your fingers rigidly flat.

• Rely on your stronger fingers. This may take the most retraining, especially if you learned to touch-type. It means using your index finger alone, or your middle finger together with either your index or ring finger, to hit the CONTROL, SHIFT, ALT, TAB, and ENTER keys. Normally, you would hit these with your little finger, the weakest finger and the easiest to strain.

By the same token, use the fingers of both hands for combination keystrokes.

• Use a light touch. You do not have to hit a computer keyboard as hard as you would an old manual typewriter keyboard—the lighter, the better.

• If you use a mouse, the same rules apply: Don't grip it but hold it lightly, use your whole arm to move it, and keep your wrist in the neutral position.

Even more than good office design and typing technique, the variable that seems to make the most difference in reducing repetitive strain injuries is the amount of time spent at the keyboard. Fortunately, some employers, and even some municipalities, have recognized this and changed routines accordingly.

In San Francisco, "Video Display Terminal Worker Safety Ordinance" calls for a 15-minute alternative work break for every 2 hours of continuous work on a VDT. This break period should be considered a minimum. More frequent breaks are preferable, even if they are shorter—say 5 to 10 minutes every half hour or so. You do not have to be idle, as long as you don't type. Do other office tasks, but also take the time to stretch and move around.

If you do not have discretion over your routine, you should discuss with your employer making a provision for frequent breaks. If necessary, you may want to contact your local office of the Occupational Health and Safety Administration (OSHA) for information and to see what recourse is possible. (See box, " OSHA Assistance and Publications.")

EYESTRAIN While spending many hours in front of a VDT screen will not cause permanent eye damage, many people complain about hot or watery eyes, blurred vision, and headaches caused by eyestrain. Eyestrain comes from sore muscles in the eyes that have to focus for long periods and to compensate for poor lighting conditions. Those affected are likely to be people who must spend long periods of time staring at a screen. Some of the strain can be eliminated by using a good-quality screen that produces clear images without any flickering and that enables you to control brightness and contrast. In addition, be sure to:

• Position the screen so that there is no glare or reflection from other light sources; such as fluorescent lighting, desk lamps, sunlight, and even high-gloss

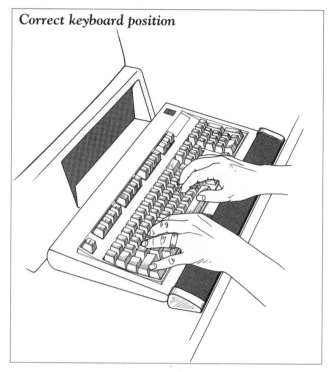

Fig. 17.2 *Wrists should be in a neutral position, parallel to the floor, with middle fingers pointed straight ahead.*

surfaces on desks or floors. If the screen does not have a built-in glare filter, you can add one. If it is not possible to move the monitor, install a glare hood, or fashion one from a piece of nonwhite cardboard.

• Adjust the level of room lighting to cut glare. In many cases, it is too high. Then adjust the brightness and contrast controls on the monitor to a level that is comfortable for you.

• Keep the screen clean with a dust cover when not in use and wipe it regularly with a special screen cleaner.

• Place the screen at the proper distance and angle. (See box, "The Ergonomic Workstation.")

• If you input information, use a monitor copy stand to hold your reference material. These inexpensive plastic clips attach to the monitor and hold material at the same height and distance as the screen. This keeps your eyes from having to change focal distance constantly as they move from copy to screen and back.

• Rest your eyes whenever you take a typing break. Look out the window or at distant objects in the office.

• Have your eyes checked regularly. If you wear glasses, ask your doctor if your prescription should be

OSHA ASSISTANCE AND PUBLICATIONS

Write to the Occupational Safety and Health Administration for free copies of the brochures "All about OSHA" and "Employee Workplace Rights." A complete publications list is also available.

Send your request to OSHA Publications Office, Room N3101, 200 Constitution Avenue NW, Washington, DC 20210. OSHA representatives are also available to check the workplace in response to complaints as well as to help employers with safety and health problems. To locate the OSHA office near you, consult the blue pages in your telephone directory for listings under U.S. Department of Labor.

modified for computer work. Bifocals cause problems because these glasses are designed for closer work, such as reading, and for long distances, but not for the middle distance, where the screen is. You may have to wear trifocals or special lenses just for computer work. When you visit your ophthalmologist or optometrist, bring measurements of the distance from your eyes to the keyboard, from your eyes to the screen, and from the middle of the screen to the floor. If possible, also bring a picture of yourself sitting at the computer or terminal.

RADIATION AND ELF RISKS In evaluating the potential dangers of exposure to radiation from VDTs, health specialists are concerned with the effects of chronic exposure—more than 4 hours a day. Radiation levels vary widely from brand to brand and from model to model. The bigger the screen and the sharper its resolution, the more radiation is emitted. Color monitors are likely to emit more radiation than monochromatic models, and placing the monitor on a metal desk or one with metal parts is said to increase radiation levels. The question is, is the exposure level high enough to pose a health risk?

A 6-year NIOSH study published in the *New England Journal of Medicine* in 1991 indicated that pregnant women who work all day at VDTs were at no greater risk for spontaneous abortion (miscarriage) than women who work at similar jobs without using the terminals.

A Finnish study published in 1992 in the *American Journal of Epidemiology* suggests a link between exposure to VDTs that emit extremely low frequency (ELF) electromagnetic fields and a higher risk of miscarriage, but this study has not been confirmed by others. Similar electrical and magnetic fields emanate from such ubiquitous household appliances as electric blankets. No ELF standards have been set because scientists still do not know what level is safe, but manufacturers have voluntarily reduced the fields in newer VDT models.

The evidence of these risks is not strong enough to recommend that women completely avoid using VDTs during pregnancy. However, given how long it took scientists to establish the health risks of asbestos and smoking, many occupational health experts recommend "prudent avoidance" of possible dangers. You can reduce radiation and electromagnetic exposure by:

• turning off the VDT when not in use

• sitting no closer than 28 inches from any monitor (ELF emissions fall off drastically after 28 inches, according to the Food and Drug Administration, which is monitoring research in this field)

• not sitting near the back of a co-worker's monitor. Radiation and electromagnetic emissions fields are strongest from the back and sides of a monitor

Pregnant women who spend more than 4 hours a day at an active terminal may want to discuss with their doctors whether they should arrange to work only part time at the terminal, especially during the first trimester.

HEALTH CARE PROVIDERS

Working in a hospital or other health care setting can be hazardous to your health! In performing their daily tasks, nurses, lab assistants, hospital pharmacists, paramedics, X-ray technicians, dental hygienists, and other health care workers are exposed to an astounding array of biological, chemical, physical, psychological, and reproductive hazards. Nurses make up the largest category of health care professionals, are overwhelmingly female, and are subject to everything from back injury (from lifting and turning patients) to burnout, as well as a host of infections.

Health care workers can protect themselves by becoming familiar with the basic principles of hazard control as well as with new government regulations intended to reduce risk. To help limit the number of hazards in hospitals and other health care sites, they can request:

• Product substitution—for example, using solvents that are less irritating to the skin or mucous membranes, gases that are less volatile, or chemicals that are less toxic.

• Engineering controls—installing, for instance, well-designed ventilation systems or exhaust hoods over individual pieces of equipment, redesigning equipment or work space so that it is less likely to cause injury, and soundproofing to reduce noise.

• Personal protective equipment—wearing gloves, masks, goggles, gowns, and lead shields to minimize the risk of infection or radiation exposure. Women should be especially careful to wear equipment that is designed for them and small enough to fit securely and comfortably.

• Work practices—disposing of needles and other "sharps" in appropriate containers can cut infection risk substantially. The most effective method of infection control is still a low-tech one: careful hand washing.

• Administrative controls—scheduling regular work breaks and rotating staff in jobs with high-risk exposure are two personnel practices that can help reduce exposure.

Some of these practices are now required under OSHA rulings instituted in 1992 to protect workers from infection by AIDS and other blood-borne viruses. Hospitals and other health care sites must provide gloves, masks, mouth guards, and smocks for workers likely to be exposed to patients' blood. They must also provide for proper needle disposal, thorough cleaning of equipment, and careful storage of medical waste. Employers must create an "exposure control plan" and identify workers at special risk so that they can be trained to protect themselves. Finally, these workers must be offered hepatitis B vaccinations at the employers' expense.

If you are a health care worker and are planning to become pregnant, you should have a thorough discussion with your obstetrician, an employee health physician, or an occupational medicine specialist about the exposure you receive on the job and its potential effects on your ability to conceive and carry a healthy baby to term. A number of studies have been done on the effects on fertility and the incidence of miscarriage and birth defects among hospital personnel (male and female, and their spouses) who are exposed to solvents, medicinal and laboratory gases, ethylene oxide (used to sterilize instruments), and drugs used for cancer therapy. The results of these studies are mixed and offer no definitive answers. In some cases, the evidence seems to be stronger for potential miscarriage than for congenital defects.

Studies on the effects of infection on the fetus are more definitive. Health care workers should always be aware of their immune status for various infectious diseases, but especially if they are planning pregnancy. A simple blood test can verify your immune status. If you have not had, or been immunized against, rubella (German measles), you should be immunized at least 3 months before attempting to become pregnant. You should also consider being immunized against hepatitis B, if you haven't already done so. An HIV test for health care workers prior to becoming pregnant is also a sound idea.

Pregnant health care workers who are at risk for measles, mumps, chicken pox, poliovirus, or hepatitis B should avoid contact with patients who have these infections. Pregnant workers, especially those who have not had cytomegalovirus, should limit contact with patients at high risk of having this infection, such as HIV-infected patients and hospitalized pediatric patients (see next section); if contact is unavoidable, thorough and careful hand washing is advised.

Parvovirus B19 (the only one of these animal viruses known to infect humans) is spread by respiratory secretions and can cause miscarriage in somewhat less than 10 percent of women who contract it during pregnancy. Pregnant health care workers should wash hands before eating and after contact with respiratory or other secretions when B19 is known to be present in a community.

During the third trimester, avoid contact with patients infected with the Coxsackie and echo viruses, and, during the late third trimester, with those who have gastrointestinal infections such as rotavirus. Finally, pregnant workers should wear masks and take other precautions when caring for patients who have infectious tuberculosis.

DAY CARE AND PRESCHOOL WORKERS

The lack of sanitary sophistication among babies and toddlers means that certain infections can run rampant through day care centers and preschools. These youngsters tend to drool, wipe their noses with their hands, and put their hands in their diapers. Then they touch other children and teachers, splash in tabletop water tanks, and drink from the water fountain, thus transmitting infections through saliva, sputum, feces, urine, and blood. Fortunately, the majority of these infections are not serious, but a day care worker can help protect herself from exposure by washing her hands carefully and frequently, especially after changing diapers or wiping runny noses.

One infection that *is* potentially serious for pregnant day care workers or others exposed to small children is cytomegalovirus (CMV). This group of viruses is related to the herpes viruses but can result in illnesses ranging from a mononucleosis-like syndrome (malaise and self-limited fatigue) in otherwise healthy adults to life-threatening disease in those weakened by other serious illnesses. It can also cause severe birth defects in infants born to mothers who contract it during pregnancy.

CMV is excreted in the saliva and urine of infants who carry the virus (and may not have symptoms), and it can be transmitted by repeated or prolonged intimate contact, but not casual contact, with these body fluids. Pregnant day care workers should therefore be especially careful to follow the preceding hygiene guidelines.

PRESCHOOL TEACHERS AND ARTISTS: DANGEROUS SUPPLIES

Nursery school and kindergarten teachers as well as others whose work involves the frequent use of art materials, ceramics supplies, and photographic chemicals may have health problems related to the toxicity and flammability of many of these products. Users may be exposed to fumes, dusts, liquids, and sprays containing benzene, arsenic, toluene, and silica.

The U.S. Consumer Product Safety Commission issued guidelines in 1992 for identifying hazardous art materials that can cause cancer and pose risks to the nervous system, the reproductive system, and the developing child. However, following the guidelines is not mandatory. Manufacturers may decide how detailed the labels should be, so users must assess the true risks. Fortunately, manufacturers are required by OSHA to create Material Safety Data Sheets (MSDSs), which list for each product the ingredients, potential hazards, and precautions for safe use. If a substance in use is not adequately labeled or has been decanted from a container no longer available, the MSDS can be obtained from the manufacturer.

Good judgment is essential in establishing safety rules:

• If the label says "Use in a well-ventilated area," that means not merely keeping the window open, but using an exhaust fan vented to the outside if the material is in constant use.

• If the material contains toxins that can enter the body through the skin, mouth, or respiratory tract, wear gloves and a face mask, and use it in very small amounts.

• Do not eat, drink, or smoke in the work area.

• Never use solvents to clean your skin. Oil-based paints can be removed with baby oil, followed by scrubbing with soap and water.

• Whenever possible, choose water-based paints, food and plant dyes, dustless chalk, white glue, library paste, and wax crayons over more toxic materials.

The Center for Safety in the Arts and ACTS (Arts, Crafts, and Theater Safety) are two New York City–based organizations that provide information on potential dangers in the visual and performing arts. (See Resources.)

A CLOSER LOOK AT COSMETOLOGISTS

Beauty can be a hazardous business for anyone who works in hair and nail salons, and it is especially hazardous for those with breathing problems, back problems, or sensitive skin. Chronic asthma and other respiratory damage can result from constant exposure to the chemicals in hair dyes, bleaches, permanents, straighteners, aerosol sprays, and the acrylics in nail care products.

Repeated use of these materials can cause two types of skin irritation: rashes involving cracking and flaking, and contact dermatitis, an allergic reaction that may take the form of blisters, hives, or itching. Eye, nose, and throat irritation is caused by the chemicals in neutralizers and tints, liquid and powdered bleaches, and artificial nail materials. The chemicals in many of these products can also cause headaches, dizziness, drowsiness, unsteadiness, and confusion.

Occupational health and safety experts offer these suggestions for on-the-job health protection:

• If you are a hairdresser or cosmetologist, you are entitled, under federal right-to-know laws, to information about the potentially harmful effects of the substances you use. Manufacturers must provide essential information to employers, and employers must provide essential information to you. Read the labels of any materials you work with. If substances are not labeled, ask for the manufacturer's data sheets.

• If you own or manage a beauty salon, keep in mind that the most important health safeguard is proper ventilation. Also, be sure that clients and employees alike obey ordinances against smoking on the premises. (Cigarette smoke combined with the fumes from many of the products being used in the salon can be doubly hazardous to everyone's health.)

• Manicuring tables should be fitted with tabletop hoods that collect and filter dangerous dusts away from workers.

• Remember that toxic chemicals can be absorbed through the skin into the bloodstream. Wear disposable gloves and powder your hands frequently to keep them as dry as possible. To keep them from getting *too* dry, apply a lubricating cream before and after work and at bedtime. (Moisture on the hands can act as a conduit for chemicals to enter the skin, but so can dry, chapped skin. The trick is to strike a balance between the two.)

• When you use permanent wave lotion or hair dye, never rub your eyes or any exposed part of your skin.

• If you don't wear gloves, be sure to wash your hands between clients so as not to spread any potential infection. Use an antibiotic spray or salve on any cut or nick that breaks the skin.

• Since manicure instruments can also spread infection, protect yourself and your clients by disinfecting them after each use.

SEXUAL HARASSMENT: AN OCCUPATIONAL HEALTH HAZARD

Law professor Anita Hill's testimony before the U.S. Senate Judiciary Committee in 1991 catapulted the issue of sexual harassment in the workplace into the media spotlight—a position it might otherwise not have achieved. It is too early to tell whether this has made a difference in the number of incidents, but it *has* encouraged more women to speak up about what was happening all along. Within days of the hearings, government agencies reported a dramatic rise in the number of complaints received. Professor Hill herself was flooded with letters from women sharing their own stories. Some, she reports, came from women who had been silent for 50 years.

Despite the tendency of many male employers to deny, dismiss, and discredit complaints from women, sexual harassment in the workplace is astonishingly pervasive: According to various studies, anywhere from 42 to 90 percent of women will experience some form of sexual harassment during their working lives, and 30 to 50 percent of female undergraduates will experience it in school. Although much less frequently, sexual harassment is experienced by men as well.

Nancy Baker, Ph.D., a Los Angeles psychologist who has researched the experiences of women in so-called nontraditional jobs, concludes that women who hold jobs that men consider to be their special turf are far more likely to be harassed than those who do "women's" work. This conclusion appears to hold true whether the women are skilled machinists, firefighters, neurosurgeons, investment bankers, or—as it would seem from the "Tailhook Incident"—naval officers.

SEXUAL HARASSMENT AND THE LAW In the 1970s, suits filed in lower courts attempted to establish sexual harassment as a form of sex discrimination in the workplace and therefore a violation of the antidiscrimination laws under Title VII of the Civil Rights Act of 1964. This concept formed the basis for guidelines issued in 1980 by the U.S. Equal Employment Opportunities Commission (EEOC), which state that:

Unwelcome sexual advances, requests for sexual favors and other verbal or physical conduct of a sexual nature constitute sexual harassment when (1) submission to such conduct is made either explicitly or implicitly a term or condition of an individual's employment, (2) submission to or rejection of such conduct by an individual is used as the basis of employment decisions affecting such individuals, or (3) such conduct has the purpose or effect of substantially interfering with an individual's work performance or creating an intimidating, hostile, or offensive working environment.

In 1986, a U.S. Supreme Court ruling confirmed that sexual harassment in the workplace was indeed a violation of the Civil Rights Act of 1964. It also violates Title IX of the 1972 Education Amendments, and the laws of most states and some cities.

Although previous rulings had declared that pornographic pictures in the workplace contributed to sexual harassment, in 1991, a federal judge ruled that the presence of such pictures is in itself sexual harassment. He reasoned that pictures depicting women as stereotypical sex objects demean them as competent co-workers. It is now the legal responsibility of both men and women in management to see that the pictures are removed.

The latest version of the Civil Rights Act, signed into law in 1991, represents another gain for women who take their complaints to the courts. It gives plaintiffs the right not only to a jury trial but also to compensatory and punitive damages for financial and emotional harm, with awards based on the size of the company being sued.

Sexual harassment takes so many forms that both men and women are often confused about precisely what it means. The EEOC guidelines state precisely: It must be conduct of a sexual nature—either physical or verbal—and it must be *unwelcome*. If, for example, a male colleague shares a bawdy joke with you *and* you are not offended, this does not constitute sexual harassment. Nor is it harassment if he spontaneously hugs you when saying good-bye *and* you interpret his gesture as a sign of collegial affection. If, on the other hand, incidents like this make you uncomfortable, and they continue after you make it clear that they do, or they stop but there is retaliation for your complaints, you have a legitimate grievance.

There are two general categories of harassment: quid pro quo and hostile environment. A quid pro quo case is one in which the employer or professor demands sexual favors as a condition of employment (getting or keeping a job, a raise, or a promotion) or receiving good grades. A single incident is considered harassment.

A hostile environment is one in which a supervisor or academic administrator permits an atmosphere where *unwanted* jokes, innuendos, propositions, "accidental" or deliberate physical contact, sexual threats, pornographic pictures, and the like make it uncomfortable and difficult for you to do your job. There is no precise definition of a hostile environment, but rather the totality of offensive conduct—including severity, frequency, and duration—is taken into account.

SEXUAL HARRASSMENT AND HEALTH For many sexually harassed women, the emotional anguish they undergo spills over into their private lives as well. According to the American Psychiatric Association (APA), "being sexually harassed can harm your psychological health and your physical well-being and interfere with your work and career plans." In its publication, "Sexual Harassment: Myths and Realities," the APA catalogs the psychological effects: depression, anxiety, shock, denial, anger, fear, frustration, irritability, insecurity, embarrassment, feelings of betrayal, confusion, feeling powerless, shame, self-consciousness, low self-esteem, guilt, self-blame, and feelings of isolation.

The APA also lists physical ailments: headaches, lethargy, dermatological reactions, weight fluctua-tions, sleep disturbances, nightmares, sexual problems, and gastrointestinal distress.

HOW TO HANDLE A HARASSER Women who don't want to be whistle-blowers or "troublemakers" should not suffer in silence and allow the situation to escalate to the point where their health is affected. Sometimes the culprit can be made to mend his ways before it becomes necessary to take drastic measures. If you are a target of sexual harassment, try these steps:

• **Speak up, but keep your cool.** Asking the person to stop and letting him know that his words or actions are unwelcome serves two purposes. With luck, he will comply. If not, you have laid the groundwork for further action.

For harassers who are immune to subtlety, you can state your preferences clearly but unemotionally. Try: "I'd rather be called Dorothy than Honey," or "Only my husband is permitted to pat me on the fanny," or "You're not really serious about wanting to go to bed with me. How would you feel if your daughter's boss made that suggestion to her?" Practice your response in front of a mirror or with friends outside of work until you can say it calmly while looking directly at your harasser.

• **Put it in writing.** If you're not getting your message across and you're reluctant to complain to your boss (or if your boss is the harasser), write a letter to the appropriate authority that spells out in great detail the behavior you find offensive and how it is causing your health and your work to suffer. Conclude with a formal request that the obnoxious remarks, or ogling, or touching be discontinued. Have the letter delivered by hand and be sure to keep a copy at home. In a significant number of cases, this type of letter gets results with no unpleasant consequences.

It might be appropriate to add a paragraph stating what you will do if the behavior doesn't stop. Quote your company's policy if there is one (see next section).

• **Know your options.** Find out if your company or academic institution has a stated policy on how sexual harassment complaints are handled. Most larger companies have a clear-cut procedure that allows you to deal with the problem without jeopardizing your job. The policy should be spelled out in the personnel manual. If you are a union member, find out what the grievance procedure is. Even if your company or school has such a policy, you may file a claim with the EEOC without first following the grievance procedure if you feel it would be detrimental to do so.

• **Gather evidence.** In a bound notebook (not a looseleaf), write down specifics: what happened; the date and place; your response, if any; witnesses, if any; the name of anyone you may have told and what you said; and the dates of any time you lost from work as a result of psychological or physical effects of the incident (and any pay you may have lost as a result). Keep the notebook at home, separate from your other personal papers. Also keep any notes or pictures your harasser may send you, or copies of cartoons or pinups that appear in the office.

If your company has regular written performance reviews, ask for copies. Mail them to yourself in a sealed envelope. If the postmark is clear, keep the envelope sealed and in a safe place. If not, repeat the procedure. Favorable performance reviews have been known to be "lost" or changed after the fact to suggest that there were other grounds to dismiss employees who complain or bring suits. Sealed copies may be useful evidence at some point.

• **Get support.** Find out discreetly if any of your co-workers is being harassed (either by the same person or someone else). It is advisable not to ask questions within the workplace itself because others may have been threatened with loss of their jobs if they speak up. Other women who have not been harassed may nevertheless be sympathetic and become your allies.

Contact such organizations as the National Organization for Women (NOW) Legal and Educational Defense Fund and 9to5: National Association of Working Women for guidance. (See Resources.)

Seek out support groups, rap sessions, and workshops sponsored by the local Y, your union or professional organization, or local women's advocacy organizations to boost your morale by taking some actions in your own behalf.

• **Take legal action.** If you have exhausted the formal grievance procedure in your company or academic institution, or if there is no such formal procedure, you may want to file a claim with your state (in a few cases, local) Fair Employment Practices agency or with the EEOC. Sometimes you can file with both agencies simultaneously. A key requirement for filing with the EEOC is that your company have at least fifteen employees; most states have lower minimums, such as three or four.

You can file the claim on your own or with the help of a lawyer. The state or federal agency you choose may be able to resolve the case by negotiating a settlement with your company, often with little involvement from you. If not, your next recourse is to file a lawsuit under the state Fair Employment Practices statutes or the U.S. Civil Rights Act. The NOW Legal and Educational Defense Fund or the Women's Bar Association in your county or city can refer you to a lawyer. Some attorneys take cases on a contingency basis, which means you pay a fee only if you win. You may also be awarded legal fees and court costs.

The Resources section contains addresses of organizations that can help see you through the legal process.

CHAPTER 18

Women and the Health Care System

No one is unaffected by the health care crisis in this country. In early 1994, an estimated 37 million Americans were still without health insurance and the majority of them were women. At this printing, the federal government is grappling with plans to remedy this situation, but most experts expect it to be several years before universal health coverage is a reality.

Obtaining affordable insurance is not the only challenge women face: Even if they can afford to see a doctor, they are not guaranteed the same quality of care as male patients. Women are more frequently misdiagnosed and their symptoms dismissed as emotional or "just part of being a woman." They have been left out of major scientific studies that determine treatment plans for such conditions as coronary artery disease, the number one killer of American women. They receive fewer organ transplants than men with comparable conditions, and they are more apt to receive unnecessary surgery.

However, there are signs of progress. In 1991, the National Institutes of Health formed the Office of Research on Women's Health. Its first major study, the Women's Health Initiative, will track several thousand women for 10 years and address the major causes of female death and disability. Although the results of this study will not be available for some time, it has heralded a greater awareness of women's health concerns and raised the consciousness of physicians and other health care professionals.

As more women enter the medical profession, they are influencing medical school curricula and encouraging a wider perspective on women's health care. Nurses and midwives, who are almost exclusively female, are receiving additional training, gaining more responsibility, and taking on broader roles.

Women patients are also becoming more active participants in their own health care. They are asking more questions, educating themselves about their health concerns, and leading more healthful lives.

DISCREPANCIES IN WOMEN'S HEALTH CARE

Women use the health care system more often than men. They see a health care professional an average of three times a year, usually for routine care or minor illnesses. Women also undergo surgery more frequently than men; in 1988, 23.5 million procedures were performed on women, while 15.7 million were performed on men.

One might expect all this medical care to result in healthier women. Indeed, women still outlive men by several years. However, many of the surgical procedures performed on women—especially hysterectomies and cesarean sections—may be unnecessary. And, while women's life expectancy has increased somewhat in the last decade, it hasn't increased as rapidly as that of men.

Part of the reason for this may be that numerous large-scale studies on the prevention and treatment of coronary heart disease—the number one killer of both men and women—have consistently excluded women. So when physicians recommend that women reduce their cholesterol levels, for example, they are assuming that high cholesterol has the same effect on women that it does on men. This may be true (and lowering cholesterol levels does not appear to have deleterious effects), but few studies have been done to confirm this. Likewise, the differences in how women metabolize medication or respond to surgery are not well researched.

Two studies published in 1991 in the *New England Journal of Medicine* found that women suffering angina (chest pain) and other symptoms of coronary artery disease are less likely to receive appropriate treatment. In fact, one of the studies found that women with angina underwent cardiac catheterization, a diagnostic procedure to determine the necessity for surgery or angioplasty, half as often as men, even when their symptoms were more pronounced.

As Dr. Bernadine Healy, former director of the National Institutes of Health, has pointed out, the fact that women have been left out of major studies cheats not only women but men. For example, because women rarely suffer from coronary artery disease before menopause, it is assumed that female hormones such as estrogen have a protective effect, but this has never been proven. There may be another explanation, one with more potential benefits for men.

In most American medical schools, the study of women's health is not given its share of attention. Male anatomical models are used almost exclusively, while conclusions are extrapolated for theoretical female patients. Obstetrics/gynecology (ob/gyn) has in the past been considered a surgical specialty, with emphasis more on procedures and reproduction than on general female health.

Although there is a strong movement to add specific courses on women's health to medical school curricula and to include a subspecialty in women's health to the practice of family medicine, it will no doubt be a long time before these changes are fully implemented. What should you do in the meantime? The best way to ensure that you receive quality health care is to educate yourself and take an active role in your care by following the steps recommended in this chapter.

THE ROLE OF THE PRIMARY CARE PROFESSIONAL

First, choose your primary care physician or other primary health care professional carefully. Ideally, this person will not only treat your illnesses, but also act as an educator and as a liaison between you and the health care system, making referrals to specialists, coordinating your care, and helping you determine the most appropriate treatment for your needs.

In the past, a general practitioner played this role. He (or occasionally, she) was a physician who served a 1-year internship after medical school before opening a practice. Today, general practitioners are rare. Their role has been partially filled by family practitioners, who are not generalists but specialists, and who account for only about 10 percent of doctors in practice.

While general practitioners often treated their patients from "cradle to grave," nowadays patients often move from one city to another and locate a doctor when necessary, not before. Often it is the patient who decides when a specialist is needed and then finds one. This fragmented approach has several drawbacks: There is no continuity of care and no one to coordinate that care among specialists. This lack of continuity may contribute to a late or missed diagnosis because none of the doctors has an overall picture of your health. It may also mean increased costs due to higher fees for specialists, duplication of tests, and conflicting treatments.

Although ob/gyns are specialists, about two thirds of women use them as their primary physicians. Because women visit their ob/gyn anyway—for regular

Pap smears, birth control, prenatal care, or other concerns—they find it easier to ask a few general health questions than to develop another relationship with a different physician. Some ob/gyns welcome this role of primary physician and offer quality care, whether the condition is vaginitis or mild bronchitis. Others may feel that complaints about an earache or chronic headaches are best handled by someone else.

Other women get their primary care from a family practitioner or internist. Although this may be a good choice, these physicians generally have had little training in women's health (only 3 months of ob/gyn training is required for family practitioners, and internists may not have had any gynecological training after medical school). They may be qualified to diagnose common female problems, such as vaginitis or bladder infections, but both physician and patient may feel uncomfortable with this arrangement.

Some women end up having two primary care physicians—an ob/gyn to handle gynecological concerns and a family practitioner or internist to take care of everything else. Still others choose a health care professional who is not a physician. (See box, "Who's Who in Primary Care.") (Although other health care professionals are playing an increasing role in primary care, the great majority of women still see a doctor. For simplicity, we use that term here.)

CHOOSING A PRIMARY CARE PHYSICIAN Depending upon your financial condition, your insurance plan (if any), and whether the area in which you live is adequately served medically, you may or may not have a choice of primary care physicians. It helps to know the differences among the various health professionals because, even if you belong to a managed care plan that randomly assigns patients to practitioners, you can usually voice your preferences. If the choice is completely yours, here is how to go about your search:

• **Gather recommendations.** Ask friends, co-workers, clergy, or others whose opinion you value for physician recommendations. Be sure to ask what it is they like about the doctor, since people have different priorities: One woman may choose a physician because he or she has evening office hours or prescribes medications over the telephone, while another may value someone who explains each aspect of the examination and discusses different health care options.

Find out whether the doctor is in solo or group practice or works for a clinic, as this may influence your decision (see section on "Primary Care Settings").

Lists of licensed physicians are available from local medical societies and hospitals. Many hospitals now have referral services that attempt to match your requirements with the doctors on their staffs. If not, you can simply call the hospital's department of medicine and ask for the names of three attending physicians. In areas where there is a choice of hospitals, some people prefer to pick the hospital first and then choose from among its affiliated physicians.

• **Check credentials.** Most libraries have copies of the *Directory of Physicians in the U.S.*, published by the American Medical Association, or the *Directory of Medical Specialists*, which list dates and details of a doctor's medical education and training, experience, teaching positions, hospital affiliations, and other accomplishments. Both directories also indicate whether doctors are board-certified or board-eligible, but since listing in the latter directory is voluntary, do not assume that someone who is not listed is not certified. Board-eligible means that the doctor has finished a residency in a particular field but has not completed the other requirements, so it can be tricky to make a determination. Certification usually requires that a doctor not only pass an exam but also practice in his or her field for a specified number of years and present records of a minimum number of cases treated. A young doctor may still be amassing cases; an older doctor may not have passed the exam. You can use the directories to narrow your choices, or you may ask each doctor directly about his or her credentials.

• **Make an appointment.** Some women try out a new practitioner when they need a routine examination or have a specific illness. Others prefer to set up an interview with a potential physician before going for a medical reason. Either approach is valid. However, if you choose to set up a get-acquainted interview, do not expect to get medical advice at this time. In most cases, it is difficult (and in some cases, it may be irresponsible) for a physician to offer medical advice without conducting an examination first. Ask about the doctor's hospital affiliations and experience in certain areas of medicine (such as gynecology) as well as about fees, office hours, policies on telephone consultations and home visits, coverage when he or she is unavailable, when payments are expected, and which insurance plans are accepted. Write down your questions beforehand and take notes during the in-

WHO'S WHO IN PRIMARY CARE

All licensed health professionals receive special training that prepares them for treating patients. The differences among the them depend on the amount and content of that training. More training is not necessarily better if it does not include the study of women's health.

All physicians go through 4 years of medical school beyond their undergraduate education, plus 1 year of postgraduate training, formerly called internship and now known as PGY-1. Most then enter a residency program that lasts 3 or more years. Physicians who pass a comprehensive exam given by their respective specialty board are considered board-certified.

FAMILY PRACTITIONERS AND INTERNISTS. For family practitioners, residency includes training in many aspects of medicine, from pediatrics to geriatrics, including a 3-month stint ("rotation") in obstetrics and gynecology. Internists go through a similar rotational residency, excluding pediatrics, orthopedics, and obstetrics. An internist's training, which may or may not include a short rotation in gynecology, focuses more on internal organ systems, such as the gastrointestinal system, the heart, or the endocrine system in adults. Most internists subspecialize in one of these organ systems by taking an additional year of training. Internists, especially those who have a subspecialty, generally charge more for an office visit than a family practitioner.

OBSTETRICIANS/GYNECOLOGISTS. After their PGY-1 year, ob/gyns also complete a 3-year residency focused solely on the female reproductive system and divided evenly between gynecology and obstetrics training. Some ob/gyns choose to subspecialize in infertility, high-risk pregnancy, or gynecological cancer. Obstetricians pay malpractice fees that are among the highest in medicine and so their fees may be higher than those of internists or family practitioners.

D.O.s VS. M.D.s. Although the overwhelming majority of physicians are medical doctors (denoted by M.D. after their names), some are doctors of osteopathy, or D.O.s. The education and training of these physicians are generally equivalent to those of medical doctors, and they also have specialties, although fewer than those available to M.D.s. They may practice in traditional or osteopathic hospitals. They differ from M.D.s primarily in their philosophy, which emphasizes the ability of the body to heal itself without drugs or invasive procedures, but in some cases with the help of physical manipulation.

NURSE-PRACTITIONERS. Registered nurses who have completed additional education and training in one of thirteen primary care specialties such as midwifery (see next section), nurse-practitioners may work independently, in a clinic, or in a physician's office. They provide counseling and routine health services such as physical examinations, monitor chronic conditions, and administer screening tests, vaccinations, and first aid. In many states they can prescribe medication. Nurse-practitioners play an important role in primary health care, especially in rural areas where medical resources may be scarce.

Because many nurse-practitioners are women, they may take a special interest in gynecological or pediatric concerns. They are an important option for women who want a female practitioner. Generally, it costs less to see a nurse-practitioner for routine care than a physician. Nurse-practitioners may be more willing to make house calls if the situation warrants. They will also make referrals to a physician or specialist if needed, and will usually continue to manage a patient's care even after the physician has been consulted. Medicare and most private insurers cover their services.

CERTIFIED NURSE-MIDWIVES. While midwifery skills have traditionally been passed down informally from generation to generation, today certified nurse-midwives are registered nurses who have received additional training in prenatal care, child delivery, and well-woman care, and have taken a certification exam. Most nurse-midwives are associated with a medical clinic, hospital, or private gynecology practice. They provide maternity care (with emphasis on education, counseling, and nutrition), delivery (possibly at a special midwifery center within or separate from a hospital, or at home), and postpartum care. They cannot perform surgery and do not accept high-risk patients, such as women with uncontrolled diabetes or who have a history of difficult pregnancies or deliveries. If problems arise during pregnancy, they will refer a woman to an obstetrician.

Some women continue to see their midwives for routine gynecological care after delivery. Some midwives offer well-woman care and birth control counseling for women who do not intend to have babies or who have already had their children.

An office visit to a certified nurse-midwife is usually less expensive than an ob/gyn, although nurse-midwives' fees are rising because of higher malpractice insurance premiums. The services of a nurse-midwife who is associated with a physician or hospital are covered by many insurance plans.

Note: Not all midwives are certified nurse-midwives. Lay midwives, who train by apprenticeship to other lay midwives, are generally not licensed by the state or other governing board, and they do not usually offer services beyond child delivery. Although these unlicensed midwives may charge much less than nurse-midwives, most insurance companies do not cover their services.

PHYSICIAN'S ASSISTANTS. Physician's assistants receive postgraduate education in special P.A. training programs. They may specialize in various aspects of medicine or they may become surgical assistants in various surgical specialties. They may work independently, in clinics, or in private practice with a physician. Like nurse-practitioners, their authority to work autonomously and to prescribe drugs varies from state to state.

terview. Some questions, such as those about fees and hours, can be handled by the office staff. (See box, "Questions to Ask When Choosing a Doctor.")

Note: Although some doctors will not charge for these preliminary interviews, many do. Ask about this when you make your appointment. These charges are generally not covered by insurance.

• **Consider personal factors.** During your 10- to 20-minute initial visit, you should get some idea of the doctor's attitude and approach to medicine. If he or she seems impatient with your questions or gives answers that are curt or vague, you may want to go on to the next one on your list. Perhaps you would prefer a female practitioner to a male, especially when discussing gynecological concerns, or it may not matter at all. (See box, "Do Women Make Better Doctors?") You may feel more comfortable with a physician who is close to your age, or has the same religious or ethnic background. While a physician's qualifications should be your primary concern, do not underestimate the importance of comfort level and trust in choosing a doctor. (For information on choosing a mental health professional, see Chapter 11, "Managing Stress and Promoting Emotional Health.")

PRIMARY CARE SETTINGS Primary care is available in a variety of settings, from one-clinician offices to huge university medical centers. Your choice will depend on availability, the type of care you require, the qualifications of the practitioner, the reputation of the institution, your insurance coverage and financial condition, and your personal preferences.

• **Private doctor's office.** The private office—one or two doctors with their own staff—has the potential to offer more continuity of care and personal attention. Each time you come for an appointment, the same receptionist greets you, the same nurse takes your pulse, and the same doctor examines you. The downside of this, of course, is the issue of coverage when the doctor is not available. Although most physicians select their colleagues carefully for this task, it can be disconcerting to have to consult a stranger in times of emergency.

Unfortunately, the age of the solo practitioner may be coming to an end. The costs of running a practice—rent, equipment, staff, and malpractice insurance—are often too high for one person. As a result, the personal attention and care a patient gets at a private doctor's office usually comes at a higher price than at a larger clinic.

A small group practice that includes several doctors combines many of the advantages of a solo practice with those of a larger organization. Sometimes there are several specialties represented on the staff; other practices include several doctors with the same specialty, such as ob/gyn. With this option, you will usually see the same doctor during each visit, but have the opportunity to meet the other doctors who cover for him or her. If you need a specialist, your doctor may be able to refer you to someone in the same office, eliminating the need to transfer records.

• **Clinics.** The term "clinic" encompasses a wide spectrum of organizations, from a private group of primary care doctors and specialists to a health maintenance organization, a hospital-based outpatient clinic, or a government-subsidized health care provider.

A clinic can provide a range of primary care doctors and specialists along with a central records department, high-tech equipment, and a variety of additional services. However, some studies have found that doctors working in clinics that are equipped for medical testing may be more apt to order unnecessary tests, which drives up the cost of health care.

Some clinics are associated with a hospital or medical center, and may be located there or in the community. These clinics are generally staffed by residents or postdoctoral fellows on the hospital payroll (house staff) or by physicians with hospital admitting privileges. If the hospital is well respected, these clinics are often good choices.

However, some clinics can be poorly organized, crowded, or understaffed. If your insurance plan or financial situation limits you to a crowded clinic, it is especially important that you know your rights as a patient. If you think that the care you receive is unsatisfactory, you should not hesitate to notify the insurance company and/or lodge a complaint with the clinic administrator.

Hospitals. Changes in Medicare reimbursement, the rise in outpatient surgery, declining populations in rural areas, and a variety of other factors have led to major changes in hospitals over the past decade. Those that have the resources to meet the challenges have thrived, while poorly funded community hospitals, especially in the inner cities and in rural areas, have faltered.

These changes affect patients by narrowing their choices. For some routine health care, a small community hospital near your home is the best place, even if it does not have the latest high-tech equipment and big-name physicians. For example, an elderly person recuperating from pneumonia may get more personal care and receive more visitors in a facility that is close to home than she would in a large university medical center an hour or two from her community. However, in cases of serious illness or complicated surgery, patients want the latest in technology and the most talented surgeons. Personal touch, although important, is not nearly as crucial.

When choosing a personal physician, it is important to discuss his or her hospital affiliation. Some physicians have admitting privileges at two or more hospitals—one small, community-based hospital and another more prestigious institution. Discuss the advantages and disadvantages of each and how decisions are made on a patient-by-patient basis. Set up tours of each hospital and perhaps attend a patient education program. Although such activities may seem onerous, it is better to know what the local hospital is like before you are admitted.

Hospitals pay a yearly fee to be inspected and accredited by the American Hospital Association. This accreditation means the hospital has met certain minimal standards.

QUESTIONS TO ASK WHEN CHOOSING A DOCTOR

About qualifications:
What is your specialty?
When and where did you get your medical degree?
Are you board-certified?
What is your hospital affiliation?

About his or her practice:
Are you in solo or group practice?
Are you a member of any managed care plans?
Who covers for you when you are not available?
When can you be reached by telephone?
Do you make house calls?

About office details:
What are your office hours?
Are payments expected at the end of office visits or can billing be arranged?
Do you accept Medicare, Medicaid, or insurance assignment (if applicable)?

DO WOMEN MAKE BETTER DOCTORS?

The vast majority of women, as much as 80 percent, prefer a female gynecologist to a male. Women who are looking for someone who listens to and understands their health concerns feel they may be better served by a woman physician than by a man. However, do women really make better doctors?

Researchers at the University of California at Santa Cruz videotaped physician-patient interviews and found that the female physicians spent more time with their patients and interrupted them less frequently. In fact, the male physicians interrupted their patients twice as often as female physicians.

Another assumption made about female doctors is that they will be more conservative, using drugs and invasive procedures less often than male physicians. However, a survey of doctors in Boston found that female physicians were twenty times as likely to prescribe estrogen replacement therapy for menopausal women. This finding indicates that not only were the women physicians surveyed willing to use aggressive treatments, they were less apt to dismiss the complaints of women experiencing severe symptoms of menopause.

Generalizations can limit a woman's health care options. Only about 20 percent of doctors in the United States are female. In medical schools, the percentage is better—women account for about 40 percent of students—but to write off all male physicians, and to assume that all female physicians are understanding and patient, is not realistic. Male or female, medical students go through the same curriculum, developed by men and dominated by men. Although some medical schools offer courses in women's health and in patient communications, their focus is on illness and its treatment, not on health and its maintenance.

Medical education emphasizes objectivity and detachment, qualities that may well be crucial in determining the best treatment plan for patients. (Hence the tradition that doctors do not treat members of their family.) Unfortunately, objectivity can read like insensitivity to a patient, whether the doctor is male or female.

Another factor in this equation is simple human nature. For better or worse, all physicians bring their own individual personalities to their practices. And a pleasant personality is not necessarily an indication of excellence in medicine. A cold, austere doctor may not become your best friend but may be the best in his or her field. It's up to the patient to decide whether that personality is worth putting up with to get the best medical care available.

Of course, with a primary care physician—especially one who will be dealing with gynecological concerns—personality may be the most important consideration. Your primary care physician must be someone with whom you feel comfortable discussing very personal matters, someone you trust to guide you through the health care system. And for many women, talking to another woman is much easier than talking to a man. You do not have to become fast friends with your physician, but when you are very ill, you need to know that you can count on your doctor—male or female.

• **Home Care.** Surveys of elderly and chronically ill people show that most would like to continue living in their own homes for as long as they can. Home care—either by visiting nurses, home health aides, or home attendants—can make that possible. Home care is sometimes necessary for people recovering from major surgery, especially as changes in insurance reimbursement force patients to leave the hospital sooner.

Home care may be provided through a hospital as part of the discharge plan after a hospital stay. Larger hospitals often have home care departments of their own, with registered nurses (who administer prescribed treatment and monitor vital signs), home health aides (who can provide some routine care, such as bathing and supervising exercises), and home attendants (who clean, cook, and provide companionship). Some physicians, nurse-practitioners, certified nurse-midwives, and physical therapists also make home visits when necessary.

The Visiting Nurse Association is perhaps the

best-known private home care agency, but there are many smaller, local companies in communities across the country. Home care agencies are licensed and regulated by most states, which usually require that home health aides and home attendants get special training. Check into the qualifications of your local home care agency and its staff before signing up for services.

As long as 24-hour care is not necessary, home care is usually less expensive than at a nursing home or hospital. Unfortunately, many insurance companies put a limit on the number of days per year or per illness they will reimburse for home care services.

• **Hospices and Nursing Homes.** For elderly people, those with disabilities, or those who have debilitating or fatal illnesses, hospices and nursing homes are an important part of the continuum of health care.

Hospices are usually small, private facilities that offer routine care and treatment for people with terminal illnesses. They provide an alternative to hospital care for those who are too ill to care for themselves or be cared for at home. Hospice care may or may not be covered by health insurance.

Nursing homes are also usually privately run. They offer round-the-clock supervision, regular physician visits, some social activities, and meals for mostly elderly patients who can no longer live by themselves. Some nursing homes are warm and caring and offer creative outlets and intellectual stimulation through arts-and-crafts programs, discussion groups, and lectures. Others are little more than warehouses, providing minimal care and exerting few efforts to make the patients' lives more pleasant. The only way to determine the quality of care of a nursing home is to visit it and talk to the patients and their families as well as staff. If many of the patients seem content, clean, and busy with activities, chances are the facility is a quality home.

Nursing homes are licensed and inspected regularly by the state. When inquiring about complaints lodged against a specific home, focus on the nature of the complaints and how or if problems were resolved.

(Primary care is also available through health maintenance organizations and similar plans, which are described in the section on "Managed Care Plans.")

A HEALTHY DOCTOR-PATIENT RELATIONSHIP

You can play an important role in maintaining optimal health care by cooperating with your primary physician during examination, diagnosis, and treatment, and by taking responsibility for your own care between consultations. Here are some examples of how to work with your doctor and office staff.

• **Appointments and waiting time.** It is up to you to make appointments for routine examinations and when you have a specific concern. Only in rare cases do doctors send out appointment reminders.

If you arrive on time, you should not have to wait more than 15 or 20 minutes to see your doctor. However, emergencies do occur (especially in surgical and ob/gyn practices), and you should be understanding. It might be a good idea to call the doctor before leaving for your appointment to find out if he or she is running late.

If the staff routinely books more than one person for the same appointment slot, which results in frequent long waits, and does not respond to complaints, you may want to consider changing physicians.

• **Detailed history.** A detailed health history is an essential part of medical care and should be taken on the first visit. The doctor or someone on the staff will ask you about previous illnesses and operations, pregnancies, current medications, family history of disease or disability, exercise habits, occupation (as an indication of job hazards you may be exposed to), and alcohol, tobacco, and drug use. Because stress is an important factor in assessing health, you may also be asked about your work, personal relationships, and any recent events, such as the loss of a job or a loved one, that may affect your emotional well-being. The questions may be oral or your physician may ask you to complete a printed questionnaire.

You are responsible for answering these questions as honestly and accurately as possible. Keeping a personal record of past illnesses and surgeries, medications, inoculations, and menstrual periods may be helpful. If your doctor does not ask you about something that you believe may affect your health, then you should bring it up. For example, if you have had unprotected sex in a nonmonogamous relationship, you may be at risk of getting AIDS. This may not be something the doctor routinely asks about.

• **Questions and complaints.** After taking your history, the doctor will ask the reason, or "chief complaint," for your visit. Unless you are there only for a routine exam, you should bring along a list of symptoms, noting when and how they occur, as well as any questions. While you enumerate your symptoms, the doctor should listen to you carefully, letting you explain fully. (If you have a lot of questions and concerns, list them in priority order. Although it is the doctor's responsibility to answer all of them adequately, time may be limited.)

Each subsequent visit should allow time to discuss the purpose of your visit, your symptoms, and any important events or changes in your condition since you last saw the doctor.

• **Confidentiality and medical records.** You have the right to expect that anything you tell your doctor or members of the office staff will be confidential. This includes your medical records, health statistics, any medications you take, and your financial situation. This information should not be given to any person or company without your written consent. Be aware that as part of most insurance claim forms you are signing permission for the insurance company to have a copy of your records or test results. The doctor must obtain your written permission if information connected to your case is to be used in medical or marketing research.

You have the right to see your medical records at any time. If you decide to change doctors, you can authorize the transfer of your files to the new doctor (by simply putting your request in writing) or take them there yourself.

• **Medical testing.** Doctors use medical tests to confirm or rule out potential diagnoses or to detect certain conditions before symptoms appear. Medical tests can be lifesavers—especially in cases of early detection of cancer and other potentially fatal diseases. However, studies have shown that some of the medical testing done today is unwarranted. Some attribute this to a litigious environment in which doctors must always be wary of malpractice suits and may feel that they have to order tests to protect themselves.

Before agreeing to any diagnostic or screening test, you should know what the test will show, why it is needed, and how the outcome will affect your treatment. In some cases, the treatment will not differ whether the results are positive or negative. Although a screening test may detect a disease before symptoms appear, this knowledge may be of little use if no treatment or preventive measure is effective at this early stage.

You should also ask what the test will cost, if there are any risks or side effects, and what the consequences to your health would be if you didn't have the test. You should weigh the cost and risks of the test against the possible benefits to determine if it is really necessary. You have the right to think it over and, if necessary, return for the test at a later date.

• **Informed consent.** Your doctor is responsible for informing you—in clear, easily understandable terms—of the treatment possibilities for your illness and the risks and possible side effects of each. You have the right to refuse to hear all the risks or to ask to hear only the more probable risks. You may be asked to sign a form stating that you understand the risks or have foregone your right to hear the risks before undergoing the procedure. Read the form carefully before signing it and ask that any confusing language be explained.

• **Second opinions and refusal of treatment.** You have the right to seek a second opinion when considering treatment options. (In fact, many insurance companies require it for nonemergency surgery.) On request, your doctor must supply the names of other qualified professionals or you can find one yourself. With or without a second opinion, you have the right to refuse a certain treatment or procedure. If you decide to forego the treatment, however, you are responsible for informing your physician. Otherwise, he or she will assume that you have followed instructions. If you discuss your decision with your doctor, together you may be able to find a mutually acceptable alternative treatment or procedure.

• **Bills and insurance questions.** Some medical offices bill patients for services; others require payment at the time of the visit. Some offices now accept credit cards; others bill the insurance company directly.

With more than 3,000 private insurers in this country, it is impossible for a medical office to be informed on the policies and procedures of all of them. The office staff should answer your insurance questions as best as they can, but it is not up to them to fill out or file forms (except for Medicaid patients). Some doctors' offices accept insurance assignment. This means they bill the insurance company directly and accept whatever the company pays even if it does not cover the whole fee. The staff may offer to file the form for you. When you make an appointment, ask about payment procedures and what forms and information to bring with you.

Throughout all these exchanges, you, your doctor, and the office staff have the right to be treated with courtesy and respect. Medical offices are busy places, and the staff and patients may be under stress. However, a little patience and understanding on everyone's part can go a long way to fostering healthy patient-physician relationships.

BECOMING AN EDUCATED HEALTH CARE CONSUMER

Besides understanding your rights as a patient, you need to know how to make informed health care decisions. The following sections offer guidelines on when to see the doctor for illness and routine physicals, and how to choose the right insurance plan, avoid health care fraud, and evaluate your risks of serious illness.

WHEN TO SEE THE DOCTOR Few physicians still believe in annual physicals for their healthy patients under age 75. The proliferation of screening tests, which detect the risk of many diseases before symptoms appear, and increased sophistication of patients who have learned to recognize warning signs of serious conditions, make regular annual checkups largely unnecessary. However, many experts still recommend a thorough physical examination every 5 years between ages 20 and 60, then every 2 to 3 years until age 75, and annually thereafter. You should have a pelvic exam no later than age 20, or sooner if you are sexually active, have an infection, or if you haven't begun menstruating by age 16. (See box, "The First Gynecological Exam.")

Abandoning the standard annual physical does not mean that you will go for years without seeing a doctor. Some screening tests, such as Pap smears, are recommended to be done annually. (See box, "Screening Tests for Women.") And clearly there are some symptoms that require immediate attention. The problem is to distinguish between true emergencies, urgent conditions, those that bear watching, and things that will probably go away by themselves. Although doctors are reluctant to discourage any visit that might reveal a serious problem, the following are general guidelines for when to call and when to wait. They apply only to adults, and to women who are not pregnant (see Chapter 6, box, "Danger Signs During Pregnancy.") Remember, these are *only* guidelines and they cover only the most common conditions. If you have any doubt about whether to call or wait, CALL.

• **Emergencies.** Some emergencies are obvious: severe head, eye, neck, or back injuries; amputations; third-degree burns; hemorrhage or uncontrolled bleeding, including uncontrolled vaginal bleeding; shock; anaphylaxis (severe allergic reaction); airway obstruction or choking; drowning or near-drowning; seizures that last more than a few minutes or recur; symptoms of tubal pregnancy (sudden doubling over in pain and/or passing out); any acute change in alertness, consciousness, or mental status, especially after a head injury or if you have diabetes; and heart arrhythmias. Others, such as warning signs of an impending heart attack or stroke, may be more subtle but should be treated as serious emergencies. (See box, "Warning Signs You Can't Ignore.")

• **Urgent conditions.** Conditions that require medical attention within 1 to 12 hours include: pneumonia with difficulty breathing; lacerations with intermittent bleeding; persistent pain; persistent vomiting; passing large amounts of blood rectally; second-degree burns that cover large areas of the body; bone fractures; joint dislocations; severe sprains; fever accompanied by severe headache, nausea and vomiting, stiff neck, change in alertness, and hypersensitivity to light (which may indicate meningitis); and animal bites that produce puncture wounds or large gashes, or minor bites if the victim has circulatory problems or diabetes.

• **Conditions that need medical evaluation.** These symptoms do not require immediate attention but cannot be ignored. Call your doctor if you experience: coughing up or vomiting blood; black or bloody stools; sores that do not heal; urinary tract infection that doesn't respond to antibiotics; yeast infection that doesn't respond to over-the-counter medication; any foul-smelling vaginal discharge; postmenopausal bleeding; thickening anywhere on the body, including lumps in the breast; fainting or blackouts; recurrent headaches; any unexplained weight loss; fever of 103°F or higher that is accompanied by recurrent shivering or chills or lasts more than 48 hours.

• **Conditions that are usually self-limiting.** As the late Lewis Thomas, physician and award-winning author, wrote in *Lives of a Cell:* "The great secret, known to internists and learned early in marriage by internists' wives, but still hidden from the general public, is that most things get better by themselves. Most things, in fact, are better by morning."

You can probably treat the following conditions yourself, but pay attention to the exceptions:

THE FIRST GYNECOLOGICAL EXAM

Your first visit to the gynecologist is something of a rite of passage. It is a first step toward taking responsibility for your reproductive health and the ticket of admission to adulthood. For some women, the occasion may also be embarrassing and perhaps anxiety-provoking. Approached with caution and knowledge, however, the first gynecological exam can set a model for a healthy relationship with the health care system.

Most young women see the gynecologist for the first time when they have a minor ailment, such as vaginitis or a bladder infection, or when they become sexually active and need birth control counseling. It is also reasonable to make an appointment just to ask questions and assure yourself that everything is developing normally. In any case, every young woman should have a full gynecological exam (also called a pelvic or an internal exam, although it includes the breasts) by the time she is 20 years old.

CHOOSING A PRACTITIONER. You can see a gynecologist, a family practitioner, an internist, or a nurse-practitioner who has special training in gynecology. (For simplicity, the term "doctor" is used here.) Your mother may have a doctor she recommends, but if you don't feel comfortable seeing that person, don't be afraid to look into other choices. Sometimes a school health clinic will recommend someone or have someone on staff whom you can see. Planned Parenthood has birth control clinics across the country that offer gynecological care to women of all ages.

MAKING AN APPOINTMENT. When you call for an appointment, the receptionist will ask if this visit is for a specific concern and if it is your first visit to that office. You may want to mention that this will be your first gynecological exam. Make your appointment for a day when you are not menstruating.

Ask the office staff about fees and if you must pay on the day of your appointment. Sometimes clinics offer sliding-scale fees and charge lower-income people less. Ask also if they accept assignment from your insurance company (see section on "Bills and Insurance Questions.")

PREPARING FOR THE APPOINTMENT. Although your mother or father may want to accompany you to the office, it is all right to say no if you prefer to go alone. However, having an older sister or a friend along may be a comfort. It could be someone who has already experienced her first exam, or a friend who wishes to make an appointment for her first exam at the same time. Your friend can be with you in the examining room, but remember that *you* are the patient. She will get a chance to ask questions when it's her turn.

Before you see the doctor, write down any questions you may want to ask. Don't be afraid to ask "dumb" questions—if they concern you, they're valid. Everything you tell the doctor or nurse is strictly confidential.

You will also need to gather information about your family. Ask your parents about any illnesses or disabilities that run in your family. If you haven't started menstruating yet, ask your mother and any older sisters about their menstrual experiences: what age they started and whether they had any problems.

Don't douche or tub bathe for 2 days before the examination, or use a vaginal deodorant on the day of the exam. If you are sexually active, do not have intercourse for at least 24 hours before your appointment. These activities may wash away, cover up, or otherwise interfere with cells and vaginal discharge that are important for your Pap test or for detecting or diagnosing any infection.

THE DAY OF THE APPOINTMENT. You should arrive at the office or clinic at least 10 minutes before your appointment so you have time to fill out any forms before seeing the doctor or nurse. Give the receptionist your name and the name of the doctor you are seeing. Fill out the forms as best you can. If you don't understand a question, ask the receptionist or nurse to explain it to you.

When the nurse calls your name, she may ask you to go into the bathroom and urinate into a cup. This will be used as a sample to detect certain conditions, such as diabetes. If you are seeing the doctor because you suspect you have a bladder infection, be sure to mention that to the nurse. The procedure for giving a urine sample may be slightly different when it will be tested for infection.

You may then be asked to return to the waiting room to wait for the doctor or you may be shown directly to the office. (If you have a long wait to see the doctor, it's probably a good idea to ask if you can urinate again—you'll be much more comfortable during the pelvic exam if your bladder is empty.)

You should have a chance to talk to the doctor before you undress for the examination. He or she may ask about your medical history, your family and whether you have started menstruating. If you have started menstruating, your doctor will want to know how old you were when you started, the date your last period began, how long your periods usually last, whether they are regular, and if you have cramps or other problems. If you have not started menstruating, the doctor may ask when your mother or sister started.

The doctor may also ask if you are sexually active and if you have been using birth control. Answer the questions to the best of your ability. Hiding facts can only prevent the doctor from giving you the best care possible. (See box, "What Does a Pelvic Exam Show?")

Take this opportunity to ask the questions on your list. Don't worry that you're taking up too much of the doctor's time. It's much more difficult (although certainly not impossible) to call the doctor and ask questions later.

THE EXAMINING ROOM. After you have talked, the doctor will show you to the examining room and ask you to undress and put on a cloth or paper gown. The nurse will take your blood pressure, weigh you, measure your height, and perhaps take a blood sample.

Next comes the physical exam. If your doctor is male, a female nurse will remain in the examining room with you. The doctor may first examine your face and neck for signs of hormonal imbalances or other conditions. Then he or she will examine your breasts for lumps or growths and show you how to examine your own breasts. (Although it's not necessary to start examining your breasts monthly until you are in your twenties, it certainly doesn't hurt to get into the habit early.)

THE PELVIC EXAM. Now comes the moment you may have been dreading. The doctor will ask you to lie down on an examining table that has supports for your feet that are called stirrups. These allow you to keep your legs raised, your knees bent, and your thighs spread comfortably. You may have to slide down a bit so that your lower back is at the end of the table. If you relax, the exam won't be uncomfortable, although the feeling may be disconcerting at first. Take a few deep breaths. Close your eyes. Ask to hold the nurse's or your friend's hand, if that helps. Your doctor should let you know what he or she is doing at each step.

First, the doctor puts on rubber gloves and checks your external sexual organs: the vulva, labia majora and labia minora, and clitoris. If you want to know where each of these is, ask the doctor to show you in a mirror.

Next, he or she inserts a lubricated metal or plastic instrument, called a speculum, into your vagina. (Most doctors warm a metal speculum in their hands first; if it feels cold, ask to have it warmed.) This instrument has paddles that spread apart the walls of your vagina so that the doctor can see the upper vagina, cervix, and cervical os (the opening of the cervix that leads to the uterus). It is normal to feel some pressure during this procedure, but let the doctor know if it hurts. With the speculum still in place, the doctor uses a swab to dab the cervix in order to take a sample of cells. This painless procedure, called a Pap test or Pap smear, is used to detect early signs of cervical cancer. If you have mentioned symptoms of an infection, or if the doctor sees signs of one, a sample of your vaginal discharge may be taken for analysis.

The bimanual examination comes next. In this procedure, the doctor inserts one or two lubricated fingers into your vagina and uses the other hand to press down on your abdomen. (See Figure 18.1.) This helps detect abnormalities of the internal organs, such as the ovaries and uterus. The doctor may also do a rectovaginal exam by inserting a lubricated finger into your rectum while at the same time inserting a lubricated finger into your vagina. This allows a closer examination of the area between the vagina and the rectum. (See Figure 18.2.) You may be asked to bear down (as if you were moving your bowels) as the doctor's fingers enters your rectum. That completes the pelvic part of the exam, which takes a total of 5 to 10 minutes.

If you are seeking birth control counseling, the doctor may discuss birth control pills with you, fit you with a diaphragm, or show you how to insert a contraceptive sponge. (For more on birth control, see Chapter 3, "Contraception, Sterilization, and Abortion.")

POSTEXAM INTERVIEW. After you are dressed, you will meet with the doctor once more to discuss the exam's findings and, if necessary, treatment options. If any medication is prescribed, make sure you know exactly when and how much to take, how to administer it (if it's a vaginal cream or suppository), and how long to take it. If the exam brought up any more questions, feel free to ask them now.

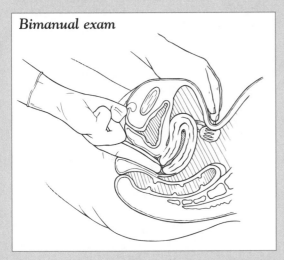

Bimanual exam

Fig. 18.1 *By inserting one or two fingers of one hand into your vagina while pressing down on your abdomen with your other, your doctor can detect any potential problems such as structural anomalies in your organs or abnormal growths.*

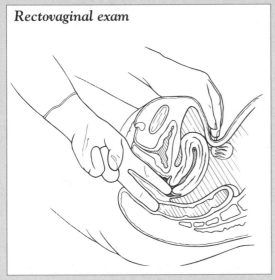

Rectovaginal exam

Fig. 18.2 *In a rectovaginal exam, the doctor inserts one finger into your vagina and a second into your rectum, which also helps detect any abnormalities in structure.*

WHAT DOES A PELVIC EXAM SHOW?

The pelvic exam is a crucial part of the gynecological workup. It can tell the doctor a lot about your health, but it doesn't tell your whole history, nor is it sufficient to make many diagnoses. Some of the things that can and cannot be detected from a pelvic examination alone are:

DETECTABLE	NOT DETECTABLE
pregnancy (sometimes, 6 weeks or more after last period)	virginity (not reliably)
	sexual preference
	masturbation
recent intercourse (within 24 hours)	fertility
	gonorrhea
previous childbirth	previous miscarriage or abortion
	ability to deliver baby to term
	need for cesarean section

Headaches—Run-of-the-mill headaches usually respond to aspirin or acetaminophen, or to relaxation techniques if they are caused by tension. Sometimes massage is helpful. If the headache is sudden, very severe, does not respond to analgesics, is associated with a blow to the head, or is accompanied by a change in behavior, such as irrationality or confusion, call the doctor immediately.

Sore throat—Most sore throats go away in a few days. In the meantime, home remedies like lozenges, warm salt-water gargles, and hot tea with honey can help. If you have a fever, take an analgesic as well. However, if the fever is higher than 100.4°F and lasts more than 8 hours, call the doctor because you may have a strep-throat infection, which can lead to serious complications if not treated. Even without fever, if your throat does not improve after 2 to 3 days of self-treatment, or if it worsens and is accompanied by headache, earache, cough, and enlarged lymph nodes, call your doctor.

Backache—Most backaches are caused by muscle strain or spasm and will respond to analgesics, moist heat, gentle massage and, if necessary, bed rest. If the backache does not improve after 2 days, call the doctor.

Colds—There is not much your doctor can do for a cold except offer sympathy and reassurance. It will all be over in 4 to 7 days, no matter what you do. In the meantime, you will feel better if you increase your fluid intake to at least double, take aspirin or acetaminophen for achiness and fever, and use a vaporizer for nasal stuffiness. If the cold lasts longer than a week, call your doctor because you may have a bacterial infection that can be treated medically.

Itchiness and skin irritation—Bathe sparingly and use soap sparingly. Apply moisturizers (those containing 10 percent urea are particularly effective) and lotions liberally. Use a humidifier in winter if your house and/or office is dry. If these measures don't help, you may have an allergy and should see a doctor.

GETTING THE RIGHT INSURANCE

Until universal health care insurance is available, the following brief overview of various insurance plans available now may be helpful if you want to purchase insurance or are offered choices by your employer.

If you must purchase insurance yourself, be sure to research the company offering it as well as the specifics of the policy itself. Insurance companies are rated annually by A. M. Best. Insurance buyers can look up the ratings in *Best's Insurance Reports—Life/Health*, available at most public libraries. Insurance companies are also regulated by individual states, and you can call your state insurance board to determine whether there have been any complaints lodged against a company.

Because most insurance companies do not permit you to examine an actual policy until you pay the initial premium, many states allow you a specified period of days to examine the policy. If you decide it is not what you expected, you can return it for a refund. Here is a summary of the range of health care insurance options:

MAJOR MEDICAL INSURANCE Major medical insurance is designed to cover the costs of medical care in case of illness. It is the most comprehensive and usually the most flexible type of health insurance—and one of the most expensive.

After you meet a deductible (which typically ranges from $200 to $2,000, depending upon the plan), the insurance company pays for a percentage of health care costs (usually 80 percent). You pay the remaining 20 percent until an "out-of-pocket cap"

WARNING SIGNS YOU CAN'T IGNORE

According to the American Heart Association (AHA), the following warning signs of heart attack and stroke require immediate emergency attention. If you experience any of these signs, call 911 or your local emergency rescue squad right away. If you can get to a hospital faster by not waiting for an ambulance, the AHA advises that someone drive you there.

HEART ATTACK

- Uncomfortable pressure, fullness, squeezing or pain in the center of the chest that lasts more than a few minutes, or goes away and comes back
- Pain spreading to the shoulders, neck, or arms
- Chest discomfort with lightheadedness, fainting, sweating, nausea, or shortness of breath

(Not all of these warning signs occur in every heart attack. If some appear, however, don't wait.)

STROKE

- Sudden weakness or numbness of the face, arm, or leg on one side of the body
- Sudden dimness or loss of vision, particularly in only one eye
- Loss of speech, or trouble talking or understanding speech
- Sudden severe, unexplained headaches
- Unexplained dizziness, unsteadiness or sudden falls, especially along with any of the previous symptoms

---

(usually $1,000 to $5,000) is reached. Then the insurance company pays the full remaining cost of treatment. Some companies put a lifetime cap of anywhere from $100,000 to $2 million on benefits. Others offer unlimited lifetime benefits. Unlimited benefits are best, but a cap is acceptable if it is at least $1 million.

Major medical covers both in-hospital and outpatient care, as specified in the policy. It may or may not cover preventive care, routine pregnancy, or well-baby care. Generally, it covers a limited amount of home care following surgery. Read the policy summary carefully to determine whether it covers all nec-

SCREENING TESTS FOR WOMEN

The following is a compilation of screening recommendations from voluntary health organizations such as the American Cancer Society, government agencies, and physicians' organizations such as the American College of Obstetricians and Gynecologists. It is intended for healthy individuals without symptoms. Women at high risk for particular disorders may be advised by their physicians to begin certain tests earlier, have them more frequently, or supplement them with other tests:

Ages 20 to 40

Every 6–12 months:	Dental exam (X rays every 2–3 years)
Annually:	Pelvic exam
	Pap test (can be every 2–3 years after two consecutive negative tests)
	Breast exam by physician (monthly self-exams)
Every 2 years:	Blood pressure
Every 5 years:	Fasting HDL/LDL cholesterol, triglycerides
Once at age 20:	Electrocardiogram

Ages 41 to 50

Every 6–12 months:	Dental exam (X rays every 2–3 years)
Annually:	Pelvic exam
	Breast exam by physician (monthly self-exams)
	Pap test
	Digital rectal exam
Every 2 years:	Blood pressure
	Blood test for hyperthyroid after menopause
	Mammogram, if recommended by physician
Every 3 years:	Eye exam (visual acuity and glaucoma)

Every 5 years:	Fasting HDL/LDL cholesterol, triglycerides
Once at age 40:	Baseline electrocardiogram
	Occult-blood stool test
Once at age 50:	Sigmoidoscopy

Ages 51 to 64

Every 6–12 months:	Dental exam (X rays every 2–3 years)
Annually:	Pelvic exam
	Breast exam by physician (monthly self-exams)
	Mammogram
	Digital rectal exam
Every 2 years:	Blood pressure
	Blood test for thyroid function after menopause
Every 2–3 years:	Pap smear
Every 3 years:	Sigmoidoscopy, if tests at 50 and 51 are negative, every 3–5 years
	Eye exam (visual acuity and glaucoma)
Every 5 years:	Fasting HDL/LDL cholesterol, triglycerides
Once at age 60:	Electrocardiogram

Ages 65 and over

Every 6–12 months	Dental exam (X rays every 2–3 years)
Annually:	Pelvic exam
	Mammogram, to age 75
	Digital rectal exam
	Blood pressure
Every 2 years:	Blood test for thyroid function
	Eye exam (visual acuity and glaucoma)

essary hospital and physician services, and consider any exclusions carefully.

Some policies will not pay more than "reasonable and customary charges" for medical care, based on health care costs in your area. Before you consult a specialist or choose a hospital, find out what amount your insurer considers "reasonable and customary" so you will know whether you have to make up any difference, or have to choose another doctor. This is especially important if you live in an urban area where health care costs may be significantly higher. Find out also if the coverage is good for treatment outside of the United States.

You should also compare premiums for different deductible amounts. If you are generally healthy, you will usually save money on a policy that has a higher deductible but lower premiums. Some of your out-of-pocket costs may be tax deductible. (See box, "Tax Deductions for Medical Expenses.")

Preventive care, discount prescriptions, and other benefits can sometimes be added on to a base policy. If the additional premium cost is lower than the amount these services will likely cost, add-ons may be worth the money. However, check to see if the add-on covers the full cost or only a small percentage of the service or if it is a fixed amount that is much lower than the actual cost of the service.

Other questions to ask: Does the deductible apply per illness or per year? (Generally, a per-year deductible is better.) Is the policy guaranteed renewable? Are preexisting conditions covered? Is there a discount for paying the premium yearly or quarterly rather than monthly? Will the premium go up each year?

HOSPITALIZATION INSURANCE A hospitalization policy covers services provided by a hospital on an inpatient basis. Sometimes a policy covers services provided on an outpatient basis in a hospital-affiliated clinic. Some policies pay only a specified amount per day after a certain number of days in the hospital ("indemnity benefits"). Others limit the number of hospital days covered or the total amount of the benefits. Generally, these policies will not protect you from financial distress in the event of a long illness.

Find out if the hospitalization policy covers specialists and specialized care (such as intensive care costs, which can run $1,000 or more per day), emergency room visits, operating room expenses, prescription drugs received at the hospital, medical tests and

TAX DEDUCTIONS FOR MEDICAL EXPENSES

If you have heavy medical expenses that are not covered by your health insurance policy, you may be able to deduct them from your taxes. Unreimbursed medical expenses in excess of 7.5 percent of your adjusted gross income are tax-deductible. For example, if you had $3,000 of unreimbursed expenses and your adjusted gross income was $30,000, you can deduct $750 on Federal Form Schedule A—Itemized Deductions.

Unreimbursed medical expenses may include payments made before the deductible was met, coinsurance payments (the percentage you pay of medical costs, usually 20 percent), and uncovered benefits, such as psychotherapy, substance abuse counseling, chiropractor services, etc., depending on your health insurance policy.

X rays, and preexisting conditions. Some policies cover only care provided at a specific hospital. Hospitalization policies do not cover office visits to a private doctor and any care that is not directly associated with a hospital.

MEDICAL-SURGICAL INSURANCE Medical-surgical insurance is divided into two parts, covering (1) in-hospital physician costs, laboratory tests, anesthesia, and prescription drugs and (2) surgical fees and follow-up visits. Together these coverages approximate major medical insurance, with some significant limitations. Regular doctor visits (not associated with surgery or hospitalization), home care, and tests performed in an independent lab or doctor's office may not be covered. The policy may cap the number of in-hospital doctor visits covered and may not include an assistant surgeon's or consulting surgeon's expenses.

Medical-surgical insurance may require a deductible and copayments similar to a major medical policy. In general, if you can afford major medical insurance, it is a better choice than medical-surgical insurance. However, only by carefully reading the policy exclusions and inclusions and comparing premium costs and out-of-pocket expenses can you determine which is actually better for you.

MEDICARE AND MEDICAID Medicare and Medicaid are the two government-sponsored medical plans. Medicare is provided to people with disabilities or those over age 65. Medicaid is for low-income people who meet various eligibility requirements.

Medicare reimburses physicians at 80 percent of a prescribed rate for care provided to older Americans. The patient pays the remaining 20 percent. Because this rate may not cover the physician's regular fee, some physicians choose not to accept Medicare patients. Some patients buy supplementary insurance to cover the difference; others choose another physician who does accept Medicare patients. Premiums for Medicare coverage are minimal and are based on income.

Medicaid covers very low-income Americans who would not be able to receive medical care otherwise. People covered by Medicaid generally must seek treatment at special community-based clinics and public hospitals. All expenses are covered, but there may be long waits for nonemergency care.

For more information on Medicare and Medicaid, contact the state health department or the agency on aging in your area.

MANAGED CARE PLANS

A managed care plan finances and delivers health care services through an organized system of providers. These plans seek to rein in the spiraling costs of medical care by controlling access to health care services. The two most common plans are provided by health maintenance organizations (HMOs) and preferred provider organizations (PPOs).

HEALTH MAINTENANCE ORGANIZATIONS An HMO is a prepaid plan in which individuals, independently or through their employers, pay a predetermined monthly fee (for example, $100 per month) for all medical care. In some cases there may be a minimal fee (say $2.00) for an office visit, but otherwise all expenses are covered. In exchange for this service, HMO members give up some of their health care choices. For example, in what is called a staff-model HMO, they are assigned to a staff doctor who provides primary care at a clinic. In an independent practice association, or IPA model, patients choose from a list of doctors who work in their own offices and may see other patients on a fee-for-service basis. In either case, the doctor acts as a "gatekeeper" to the medical care system. Any medical tests, surgical procedures, or referrals must be approved by the primary care provider.

HMOs vary greatly in quality. Before joining one, talk to an account representative (one is usually assigned to an employer offering enrollment in the HMO) and visit the nearest facility. Ask how the HMO works: Are the doctors paid a salary or an amount based on the number of patients enrolled (a capitation fee)? Are all the providers board-certified? What services are included in the monthly fee? If other services are required, how will they be covered? What happens in case of emergency? How are services obtained outside the local HMO area covered? Is emergency service in another country reimbursable?

Because you will be dependent on this organization to provide all medical care, it is essential to know that the company is stable and reputable. Ask the following questions: How long has the HMO been in business? Is it nonprofit or for-profit? How many members does it have? Has the enrollment dropped or grown in recent years? Has the organization been involved in malpractice suits?

State insurance commissions and health departments also have records of any complaint that has been lodged against an HMO. Although there is no formal accreditation board for HMOs, some choose to become accredited through associations such as the American Association of Ambulatory Health Centers. The U.S. Health Care Financing Administration's Office of Prepaid Health Care may also be able to offer information about larger HMO chains.

PREFERRED PROVIDER ORGANIZATIONS A PPO negotiates discounted fees with certain providers (doctors) and then offers greater coverage to patients who choose these providers. Unlike HMOs, however, PPOs are run on a fee-for-service basis, so doctors are reimbursed only when specific services are rendered. If you choose to see a nonparticipating doctor, you will have to pay a larger portion of that doctor's fee. If, for example, the preferred doctor's fee is $100, the PPO might cover $80. If you choose a nonparticipating doctor, the PPO might cover only $50.

OBTAINING INSURANCE

If you are not employed, are self-employed, or if your company does not offer insurance, there are still several ways in which you can obtain coverage.

INDIVIDUAL POLICIES Some insurance companies offer policies to individuals. They are likely to require you to have a physical exam or at least to fill out a detailed questionnaire before they accept you for coverage. The reason is that, without a group, they lack the ability to spread the risk over a number of people. If you have a chronic illness, you may not be accepted, or you may be accepted but any subsequent illness related to your existing condition may be excluded.

Individual policies can also be extremely expensive; premiums of $5,000 annually for a family are not unheard of. Some companies avoid this by pooling individuals according to profession. For example, they put all individuals in the accounting field in one risk pool and calculate a premium based on that. This yields a premium closer to that offered to a group, but without some of the additional benefits groups may receive. Individual policies tend to have higher deductibles and higher out-of-pocket expense limits.

Blue Cross and Blue Shield, nonprofit insurance companies overseen by state insurance boards, must offer coverage to individuals regardless of medical history. Unfortunately, despite state controls, the cost of these insurance policies have risen dramatically in recent years, and companies in some states are experiencing severe financial problems.

COBRA If you are enrolled in a plan through your job or your husband's job, the Consolidated Omnibus Budget Reconciliation Act of 1985 (COBRA) enables you to keep that insurance in the event of a layoff or divorce. COBRA requires an employer to offer insurance to former employees or former spouses of employees for 18 to 36 months after termination or separation. You pay the premium plus an administrative fee (no more than 2 percent) but retain the group rate. After 18 to 36 months (depending on the size of the company and other factors), you are usually offered an individual policy from the same insurer. At this point you may want to comparison shop for similar coverage at a lower rate.

Employers of fewer than thirty people, churches, and federal government plans are exempt from COBRA requirements.

PROFESSIONAL ASSOCIATIONS AND OTHER GROUPS Group insurance is also available through professional associations, alumni associations, church groups, small-business organizations, and organizations for the self-employed. The National Organization for Women (NOW) offers insurance to its members in many states.

OBTAINING CARE FOR AGING PARENTS

In our society, it usually falls to women to care for aging parents, whether they provide care in their own homes or make arrangements with third parties, sometimes from thousands of miles away. If you are facing health care and housing decisions for a parent, here is some basic information to help begin the process:

• On turning 65, all United States residents automatically qualify for Medicare and some for Medicaid (see earlier section).

• Private insurance is available to pick up the deductible and 20 percent of medical costs not covered by Medicare. Policies vary as to what else they cover, such as drugs.

• Medicare, Medicaid, and some private insurance plans cover some of the costs of home health care services, especially those prescribed by a doctor and performed by a nurse.

• The American Association of Retired People (AARP) is open to everyone age 50 or over for a nominal fee. The AARP has information about health care services and types of insurance coverage.

• Religious, fraternal, and community organizations often offer services for the elderly, such as adult day care or meal delivery, and some run nursing homes.

• In many communities, you can hire a professional to help you assess, identify, and coordinate care for a relative. This is especially useful if you must do so at long distance. These care managers are usually geriatric social workers and, sometimes, nurses. There are also eldercare lawyers (check with your county bar association), who can help in making financial decisions, especially regarding financial assets and nursing homes.

• The following organizations may be able to help you locate services: the county, state, or municipal

Office for the Aging; veterans' organizations; some labor unions and large corporations; the American Red Cross; the YWCA; the Visiting Nurses Association; and the Veterans Affairs Administration.

• The U.S. Administration on Aging sponsors the Eldercare Locator, a toll-free referral line (see Resources) that has information about services throughout the country.

• The American Association of Homes and Services for the Aging and the American Health Care Association have information on choosing a nursing home or other housing alternatives (see Resources).

PROTECTING AGAINST HEALTH AND NUTRITION FRAUD

Perhaps because women often feel frustrated by the established health care system, they may become targets for health fraud, ranging from misleading advertising claims to questionable or even dangerous medical treatments. Older women in particular are a prime target because they tend to suffer chronic and debilitating illness such as diabetes and arthritis. Some individuals or corporations may also try to take advantage of women's concern for their appearance with fad diets, devices to improve their figures, and risky plastic surgery techniques.

Diets that emphasize a single food (rice or grapefruit), prohibit certain food categories (nothing white), or have specific rules about when to eat what (only fruit before noon) should likewise be avoided. (See Chapter 9, "Healthful Eating for a Lifetime.")

The back pages of certain magazines are full of mail-order ads for creams, special exercisers, and similar devices that purport to increase your bust and tone your muscles. Since your breast size depends upon heredity and the amount of fat on your body, these products have no value. Likewise, you cannot lose weight or build muscles without effort. Machines that vibrate, use rollers, or electrically stimulate your muscles (called continuous passive motion tables or toning tables) while you recline and relax are useless for body shaping and muscle toning. Bodysuits, rubber corsets, and other gadgets designed to sweat off fat are other examples of quackery.

Plastic surgery should be approached like any other elective procedure: Weigh the risks and benefits, research the possible side effects, and talk to other people who have had the procedure. A diet regimen that guarantees quick weight loss (30 pounds in 30 days) or relies heavily on nutrition supplements, herbal mixtures, or vitamin potions should be suspect.

The following clues may help you detect medical charlatans and nutrition quacks:

• **Bogus Credentials.** Watch out for phony degrees in nutrition, "naturopathy," or "metaphysics," which may have been obtained from an unaccredited institution or simply by filling out a form and paying a fee. (Only degrees from institutions accredited by the Council on Postsecondary Accreditation are considered legitimate.) Ask specific questions about the education, training, and background of a practitioner. Unfortunately, even some doctors with legitimate credentials may practice questionable medicine, so this should not be your only criterion for deciding on a treatment.

• **Promises of Quick, Full Recovery.** For many conditions, such as arthritis, AIDS, and cancer, there is either no cure or treatment is not always totally effective. A doctor who *guarantees* a cure for any disease should be suspect.

• **Unusual Diagnostic Techniques or Diagnosis of a Condition for Which You Have No Symptoms.** Hair analysis to detect "hidden" nutritional deficiencies is a common example of fraudulent diagnosis. It is usually accompanied by a sales pitch for expensive vitamin supplements. You should also be suspicious of anyone who immediately diagnoses vague symptoms (headaches or stomach upsets) as due to a condition you have never heard of. Likewise, you should be wary of warnings of an imminent deterioration of your condition.

• **Secret European Formulas, Medical Breakthroughs, Accidental Discoveries, and Miracle Cures.** Your antennae should be raised by these unlikely claims, as well as any vague or simplistic explanations of the disease and the "cure."

• **Testimonials from Patients Who Were "Cured."** Their condition may actually have improved or disappeared. The problem is, without documentation of their diagnosis, you have no idea what they were cured of or whether the condition would have gone away by itself.

• **Lack of Published Data.** The sine qua non of medical research is a controlled, double-blind study that is published in a peer-reviewed medical journal. Be wary of any practitioner who cannot substantiate a treatment with such a published study. Check the library for additional research on the topic. Note: Be cautious about books, magazines, and articles available in health food stores. Because the Food and Drug Administration prohibits specific, unsubstantiated claims on the labels of various herbal and vitamin potions, manufacturers often get around this by providing the store with written materials, protected by First Amendment rights, that "sell" their products for them.

• **Claims of No Risk.** There is almost always some risk involved in any treatment, especially of chronic illnesses. As with any other treatment, a second opinion—from a doctor of your own choosing—is recommended.

• **Refusal to Discuss the Proposed Treatment with Your Doctor.** A practitioner offering legitimate treatment will have no objection to discussing your case with your primary care doctor.

• **Charges of Conspiracy.** Medical charlatans often claim that the "medical establishment" is jealous of their success, "out to get them," or otherwise conspiring against the acceptance of their techniques or the dissemination of information about their treatments. This is rarely the case. It is more likely that there has never been any convincing evidence that the treatments work. Medical journals have everything to gain by publishing news of a true breakthrough.

• **Requests for Payments Up Front.** Quacks often insist on full payment or a large down payment before beginning treatment. Legitimate health care providers do not usually require deposits, although physicians, such as obstetricians and orthodontists, who offer well-defined care for a specific period of time may request payment in installments.

ASSESSING HEALTH RISK

Sometimes it seems that each daily news report reveals another health risk—from the ingredients of sunscreens to the alcohol content of mouthwash, from electric blankets to cellular phones. Even more perplexing are the conflicting studies and the competing risks: Drinking a moderate amount of alcohol may raise the risk of breast cancer, but it seems to decrease the risk of coronary heart disease; large amounts of regular coffee may affect your heart, but decaf may be worse; pesticides sprayed on produce may increase the cancer risk, but so will a diet poor in fruits and vegetables.

To use this information when you make life-style and health decisions, here are some general guidelines:

• **Do Not Make Changes on the Basis of One Study.** In 1981, great alarm was caused by a study suggesting that perhaps one half of all pancreatic cancers might be due to drinking as little as two cups of coffee a day, even though the results were preliminary. No other study ever confirmed the link; in fact, the authors of the study themselves found no association in their follow-up study.

A number of studies by different researchers on different populations must all reach the same conclusion before a specific risk factor is accepted by scientists. Smoking, for example, is generally accepted as a high-risk activity because its effects on the risk of cancer, lung disease, and heart disease have been shown in scores of studies over more than 30 years.

A single study (which is likely to be small as initial studies usually are) may have been poorly designed and may show an association that is actually due to chance. A finding is generally considered significant if there is a probability of less than one in twenty that the findings could have happened by chance.

• **Remember That Association Is Not Cause.** A link between events does not necessarily show cause and effect. The fact that people who use artificial sweeteners tend to be heavier than those who do not does not mean that sweeteners cause weight gain. Rather, it probably means that overweight people use these sweeteners to limit their calories.

• **Keep in Mind the Magnitude of Risk.** A 50 percent increase in risk may sound like a lot, but not if the risk is very small to begin with. If your risk of developing a rare form of cancer is 1 in 1,000, then a 50 percent increase raises it to 1.5 in 1,000. A 50 percent increase in your risk of heart disease is a much more meaningful number. Yet most epidemiologists consider anything less than a 100 percent increase (or doubling) to be a weak association.

• **Put the Risk in Perspective.** Your risk of developing breast cancer over your lifetime may be 1 in 9, but if you are an average 40-year-old woman, your risk of developing it this year is 1 in 1,000. While this should not make you complacent, it may help you get over the fear of getting a mammogram lest a lump be found.

• **Don't Be Prey to "Gambler's Fallacy."** This is the myth that lightning doesn't strike twice, that a hurricane won't hit next year because you've just survived the storm of the century. Whatever the statistical odds are for a given event, they are the same for each potential occurrence. For example, if the odds are one in four that a child will inherit a genetic trait, *each* child has a 25 percent risk of inheriting it. This means that if your first child inherits it, your next three children are not necessarily home free.

How do these risks relate to life choices? Say you are going through menopause and you have a strong family history of osteoporosis as well as several personal factors that put you at risk: You have small bones and pale skin, have only recently quit smoking, and have always disliked milk. Your doctor has recommended hormone replacement therapy but you have heard that it increases your risk of breast cancer, which recently caused your aunt's death.

After you learn more about it, you find that there is stronger evidence that hormone replacement will reduce the risk of osteoporosis than that it will increase the risk of breast cancer. Further, new studies show that family history is not as strong a factor in breast cancer as once thought. There is also evidence that it will decrease your risk of heart disease. The risk of any woman dying of heart disease is more than three times as high as that of dying from breast cancer. In addition, your personal risk of developing osteoporosis is great. You conclude that for you, hormone replacement therapy makes sense.

CHAPTER 19

Women and Violence

Domestic violence is the number one cause of injury to women in this country. It accounts for more injuries than muggings, rapes, and auto accidents combined, according to the Centers for Disease Control and Prevention.

Violence against women in their homes covers a wide spectrum of behavior. In its broadest definition, it is a pattern of abuse men use to establish power and control over women through fear and intimidation, often including the threat or use of violence. (See Figures 19.1–19.2.) The abuse can be primarily psychological—name-calling, forced social isolation, economic deprivation, emotional degradation, spitting, destroying personal property or harming pets, physical displays of violence such as putting a fist through a door or playing with guns or knives, intimidation, and threats of violence or death. It can include minor assaults, such as pushing, shoving, slapping, restraining, or pinching.

The abuse may escalate to include biting, kicking, punching, throwing a woman to the ground, or hitting her with objects. In the extreme, it may mean repeated beating, burns, broken bones and life-threatening injuries, and it can be fatal. Thirty percent of the women who are homicide victims are killed by their husbands, ex-husbands, or boyfriends, according to the Federal Bureau of Investigation.

Domestic violence involves more than just men who batter their wives. It is the abuse inflicted upon each other by family members, or by people who live together or formerly lived together. It is also the violence inflicted on women by husbands or ex-husbands, on husbands by wives, on women by boyfriends, on children by parents, and on elderly parents by grown children. However, some experts argue that the term "domestic violence" is a misnomer because the vast majority of victims are women.

Traditionally, society has turned a blind eye to this dark side of family life. The family is still considered sacrosanct by many people. Neighbors may feel that they shouldn't interfere in an abusive situation, even though the sights and sounds of violence are too plain to miss. Often co-workers may pretend to believe that a colleague's black eyes and bruises are the result of a fall. Teachers and police may sometimes hesitate to get involved in "family matters." Doctors may overlook marks of abuse and prescribe tranquilizers to calm their female patients.

There are some signs of change. More and more, violence is being reported and abusers are being punished. Women are speaking out about the violence in their homes. There is increasing social support for women who choose to leave—and want to prosecute—violent men.

Negative and positive behavior

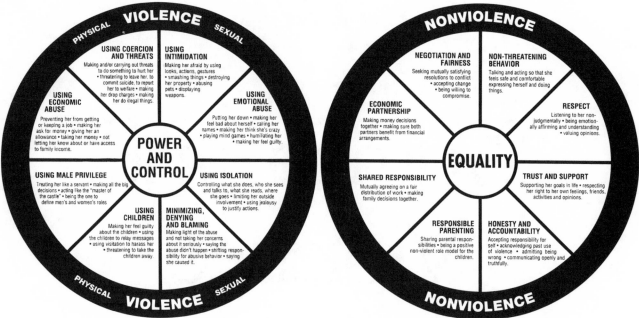

Source: Domestic Abuse Intervention Project, Duluth, Minn.

Fig. 19.1–19.2 *Listed on the left are some of the behaviors exhibited by abusive men to achieve power and control in their relationships with women. Abuse diminishes as behavior is changed to promote equality through the actions listed in the wheel on the right.*

For all of that, however, domestic violence remains largely a closet issue. The pervasiveness of the problem and the wide spectrum of abuse make it difficult to discuss each aspect of violence in detail. This chapter is therefore limited to a discussion of the physical abuse of women at home. It concludes with a section on rape by both known and unknown assailants.

BATTERED WOMEN

There are battered and emotionally abused women at every social and economic level of society and in every ethnic group. While low-income women are somewhat more likely to be on the receiving end of physical abuse, and abuse appears to be more common under conditions of economic stress, it is by no means unknown among the prosperous and well educated. Various studies attempting to define and describe a "typical" abused woman have not been successful. Research is fraught with problems: bias, difficulty in standardizing definitions or obtaining records, societal notions of propriety, the unwillingness or inability of many victims to report acts of violence, the ability of batterers and battering victims with financial means to protect themselves from exposure. Yet there seems to be little that distinguishes the personality traits of battered women, or

those who will become such victims, from other women.

There are, however, some demographic and situational factors that increase a woman's vulnerability to abuse, according to a review of various domestic violence studies by Drs. Evan Stark and Anne Flitcraft. It should be stressed that these factors are not causes of abuse. The majority of women who fit some or even all of the categories are not abused. The following are simply risk factors that increase the possibility that abuse will occur:

• **Age.** Violence occurs more often in couples under 30 than in older couples. However, it may continue indefinitely. Women, because they outlive men and perhaps because they are less able to defend themselves, are the main recipients of elder abuse. Although adult children, often overworked as caregivers, have been identified as the prime abusers of their parents, more recent studies find that elderly women are more than twice as likely to be abused by their husbands as by their children (58 percent versus 24 percent). Some experts find that this statistic is not startling at all; it merely reflects a continuation into the geriatric age group of the same abuse that plagues younger wives.

• **Marital Status.** Women who are separated from their husbands are the most likely to have histories of abuse. Divorced and single women are also more apt to have been abused than married women.

• Income, Occupation, and Status. Numerous studies have found that abuse is substantially higher among poor and working-class couples, but the most exacting statistics show that this difference may be no more than 3 percent. There is some evidence that a woman is at higher risk if her education or occupational status is higher than her husband's, or if there is an inconsistency in her status (as when she is well educated but has a low-income job).

• Race. Black women are more likely to be abused than white women.

• Pregnancy. According to the American College of Obstetricians and Gynecologists, 25 to 45 percent of battered women are beaten while they are pregnant. Battered women have higher rates of pregnancy, miscarriage, stillbirths, abortions, and low birth weight babies than women who are not abused.

• Violence in the Family of Origin. A woman who witnessed or received abuse in her family as a child is more likely to be abused as an adult. While this early experience increases the possibility of future violence, it should be remembered that most abused women (and their abusers) were not beaten as children, nor do most people who were beaten as children become involved in violent adult relationships.

• Social Isolation. Violent couples are consistently more socially isolated—cut off from family, neighborhood, or institutional support—than nonviolent couples, but the isolation can also be a consequence of ongoing abuse. This may be a particular problem for military families and others whose frequent moves may leave them without a social support system.

Some studies have concluded that women in abusive relationships may suffer from low self-esteem, which can cloud their judgment of men and marriage. It may prevent them from realizing that battering is both wrong and undeserved. They may feel that if they were "good" or "deserving" enough, or if they worked hard enough at the relationship, they would be able to turn things around and stop the violence. In contrast, battered women in other research studies have described themselves as stronger and more independent than women who are not battered. Some researchers conclude that low self-esteem is a *result* of repeated abuse (especially psychological abuse), not a factor in its cause.

While there may be no specific personality characteristics that predispose women to being battered,

studies do show that those who endure years of severe mistreatment may develop similar symptoms and behavioral traits. They are more likely to abuse drugs and alcohol, to suffer anxiety and depression, and to attempt suicide than other women. This despairing mental state, along with headaches, backaches, sleeping and eating disorders, abdominal complaints, and chronic pain, make up what is referred to as battered syndrome.

Recognized since 1979 as an official medical diagnosis, battered syndrome is not considered a "set of symptoms" per se, but rather a group of conditions that includes a history of physical injury (often including sexual assault), general medical complaints, psychosocial problems, and unsuccessful help-seeking efforts. It may explain why some women feel unable to leave their batterers (or voluntarily do not leave them) and why a few feel that their only means of saving themselves is to kill their abusers.

Women with battered syndrome sometimes encounter institutional victimization when they attempt to get help. The legal system may not prosecute their batterers, the medical system may fail to identify the cause of their injuries or dismiss their physical and psychological symptoms, the social welfare system may punish them for abandoning their children when they flee the abusive situation.

Women who resort to killing their abusers have specific characteristics in common. They usually have been beaten more severely and frequently, and are more likely to have endured sexual abuse than women who do not kill their batterers. Plus the men whom they kill tend more to be alcohol and drug abusers and are more likely to have abused their children (sometimes sexually) than batterers who are not killed.

MEN WHO BATTER

Male batterers have been described by their women as being angry, suspicious, tense, moody, and, when they want to be, extremely charming. These men may feel frustrated and powerless in a society that glorifies success and power in men. (However, complicating matters, male batterers are often rich and successful, leaders in their communities.) Typically, a man who abuses his wife has a powerful need for physical, psychological, even financial control. He may "keep the upper hand" in the marriage by using force and by ordering every detail of his wife's life. He watches her closely, isolating her from friends and family. He may forbid her to work outside the home or, if she does have a job, constantly call to check up on her.

As with battered women, studies have failed to show many traits that consistently predict which men will become violent toward their wives or girlfriends. Several studies have described batterers as having low self-esteem; feelings of helplessness, powerlessness, or inadequacy; and traditional attitudes, particularly about sex. They exhibit pathological jealousy, fear of abandonment, lack of assertiveness, and conflicts over being dependent. The problem is that these qualities may also describe men who are in troubled domestic relationships, but who do not resort to abusive behavior.

A few factors seem to place men at risk of becoming abusive. As children, witnessing violence in their own families (for example, their fathers beating their mothers) seems to increase this possibility, and is more predictive of future violence than their having been abused personally. Men who abuse women also tend to abuse alcohol or drugs. Substance abuse does not cause violence, but it distorts and magnifies the feelings that feed it. Violent men may claim a "time out" from the normal rules of behavior because they have been using alcohol or drugs.

THEORIES OF DOMESTIC VIOLENCE There are a number of theories on why domestic violence occurs and how it evolves. Some scientists have tried to identify personality factors in violent men, while others have looked at interactions between men and women in intimate relationships.

One theory that has received wide attention is the "cycle of abuse." It postulates that physical abuse is not inflicted at random times, but typically follows a three-phase cycle. The first phase, the "tension building" phase, includes verbal abuse, minor physical abuse, and increasing friction between the couple. (See box, "Signs of Impending or Escalating Domestic Violence.") The woman tries to be nurturing and compliant in order to keep small incidents from escalating.

This phase may last for days, or weeks, even years. But eventually mounting tensions explode into the second phase, the "acute battering" incident. This is not usually triggered by the woman's behavior but rather by some minor event, often when the man has been drinking. The assault is characterized by extreme rage and destructiveness. The man may seem out of control, or he may have enough control to hit only where the bruises will not show, on the torso, for example. The phase usually lasts 2 to 24 hours,

SIGNS OF IMPENDING OR ESCALATING DOMESTIC VIOLENCE

According to the National Coalition Against Domestic Violence, you should beware that there may be impending violence at home if you notice that your partner:

• Drinks increasing amounts of alcohol or increases his drug use, finds petty things to complain about, or noticeably changes his habits. For example, he normally wants to go out every night, but now prefers to sit at home gravely watching television.

• Exhibits changes in his tone of voice, habits, or behavior toward the family, or overreacts to little problems and frustrations.

• Uses force or violence to "solve" problems.

• Is jealous of your friends and family or keeps tabs on you and wants to know where you are at all times.

• Plays with guns, knives, or other lethal weapons, and talks of using them against people to "get even."

• Treats you roughly or uses physical force.

and ends only when he is exhausted and drained of emotion, by which time she may have been severely beaten.

The third phase—the "honeymoon" phase—follows immediately. The batterer is contrite and loving. He may bring the woman extravagant gifts, beg her forgiveness, and promise never to hurt her again. At this stage, he may truly believe that he will never again treat her badly. And usually she wants above all to believe him, to forgive and forget. She cares for him despite the battering, is ashamed of having been so treated, and is afraid of his anger. But soon the tension starts to build again and a new cycle of abuse begins. As the relationship continues, the third phase may no longer be characterized by contrition on the part of the batterer, but only by a lessening of tension.

There are variations on the cycle theory. One expands the cycle from three to seven stages, but makes the important distinction that the event that sets off the violent phase, the "last straw," may never occur. Instead, the man will continue to use verbal abuse and threats.

There are also social-learning theories, one of which suggests that when a man has witnessed violence between his parents, has an aggressive personality, and uses alcohol, he is likely to become violent if there is already dissatisfaction with the relationship and there is some cause of stress.

Finally, there are sociocultural theories that examine the historical, legal, cultural, and political factors that contribute to wife beating. These propose that violence pervades many aspects of our society, and there is also a traditional assumption that men have the right to control their wives by any means necessary, including force.

STAYING IN ABUSIVE RELATIONSHIPS When there is so much violence and unhappiness in their relationships, the obvious question is: Why do battered women stay? Or why, having succeeded in leaving their abusers for a few days or weeks, do they return? The answer is not so obvious; the reasons are many and complex and not always within their control.

A popular belief is that women stay in violent relationships because they are helpless victims of their batterers and have unrealistic views of their situations and their options. While this may be true for some, particularly those who have suffered severe and prolonged abuse, it is not true of all. Some women have examined their options realistically and realized that it is not possible or advisable to leave, at least for a while. These women may be strong and in control of their lives.

Some professionals involved in efforts to help battered women fear that they may become victims of their victim status. Brooklyn Law School professor Elizabeth Schneider points out that many battered women lose custody of their children because judges see them as "helpless, paralyzed victims who can't manage daily life." Conversely, if a woman seems too capable to be a victim, she may not be believed.

Many women stay in violent situations because they have no place to go: They are geographically isolated from family and psychologically isolated from friends; there is no shelter in their community or the shelter is full. Most shelters are forced to turn away five women for every two they accept, and only 5 percent of shelters can accommodate women with their children.

Many women stay because they do not have the financial resources to leave. Often they are unemployed, sometimes because their men have forbidden them to work, or because they cannot keep a job (a key factor here is absenteeism as a result of injuries at home). Often, too, they have young children to support. It is virtually impossible for them to set up and maintain a new household. In leaving their husbands or boyfriends they would lose their only source of food and shelter. In many communities, there is a wait for public assistance, which may require proof of permanent residence.

Other women stay because running away greatly increases the danger they face (more than half of those who are killed by their abusers die in the course of trying to leave the relationship). They fear that the men may track them down, and threaten them or their children if they do not return. The threat of extreme violence from a violent man forms a significant barrier to leaving. (See box, "Leaving a Violent Relationship: Some Suggestions for Safety.")

Some women may stay because it is important to them that their children do not suffer the trauma of a "broken home" (although a violent home is at least as traumatic). Or they are afraid that their partners will abuse the children in their absence, or will get custody of the youngsters if they leave. Their fears are not unfounded. Men who batter their wives are much more likely to abuse their children than are nonbatterers. The Gender Bias Study of the Supreme Judicial Court of Massachusetts, published in the *Suffolk University Law Review* in 1989, found that 70 percent of wife abusers who attempted to get legal custody of their children when their wives were forced to leave were successful.

Women also endure the brutality for complex emotional, psychological, and cultural reasons. Some hope that they can reform their partners—or, somehow, themselves. Many women have been brought up to believe that marriage is the best life for a woman, and that they are responsible for the welfare and happiness of their partners. A woman may blame herself for the failure of the marriage, even as she clings to the hope that somehow her partner will change.

Moreover, the "honeymoon" stage of the cycle of violence holds some women in the relationship. The abuser's tender behavior provides positive reinforcement for staying with him; his promises that there will be no more violence offer hope. Having become isolated from friends and family, a woman may be emotionally dependent on her batterer. She may stay with him out of love and concern, a desire to give him another chance—or out of guilt. Her man may have threatened to kill himself if she leaves (this is not always an idle threat: almost 10 percent of the batterers in one study killed themselves after their women left).

LEAVING A VIOLENT RELATIONSHIP: SOME SUGGESTIONS FOR SAFETY

• Do not mention your plan to leave, but anticipate violence early enough so that you can slip away before a crisis erupts, preferably while your partner is out of the house.

• Know where you are going and how to get there. Suggested places to go: a friend's or relative's house, where there's room for you, and people who care about you; a battered women's shelter or a safe house, if there is one close by and if they have a bed; a motel. To find a shelter, look in the telephone directory under Battered or Women. If yours is a small town, and there's nothing listed in the book, try the nearest city.

• Keep enough money on hand to pay for a cab to a safe place, and for one or more nights in a motel if necessary. Keep small change for calls from pay phones.

• Know where the closest pay phone is located and plan what to do if your home phone or electrical wires are cut.

• Hide an extra key to your house and the car.

• Work out a signal system with a neighbor in case you need help.

• If you have a car and depend upon it for transportation, get into the habit of backing it into the driveway and leaving the driver's door unlocked so that you can quickly get in and leave. Don't let the gas tank get too low.

• Remove any knives, scissors, letter openers, or sharp objects from easy-to-reach places in the house.

• Try to not wear scarves, long necklaces, loose clothing, or jewelry that can be grabbed and used to strangle you.

• Leave *with* the children, if you can. If you can't, go back for them as soon as possible, with the police—or pick them up at school.

• Keep a list of telephone numbers in your wallet to call in case of an emergency. The list should include the numbers of the police, the hospital, the battered women's shelter, your lawyer, your social services worker.

• Stash food and a change of clothes for yourself and the children at a neighbor's or at your workplace.

• If possible, leave nothing behind in the house that would cause you anguish if the man threatened to destroy it—your cat, for example, or your jewelry.

Adapted from *Getting Free: A Handbook for Women in Abusive Relationships*, 2nd ed., Ginny NiCarthy, Seal Press, Seattle, 1984. Used with permission.

Women who have developed battered syndrome may not believe they are capable of making it on their own. Others suffer the effects of denial to the extent that they may be unaware of the seriousness of their situation.

PROTECTION, PUNISHMENT, PREVENTION However instructive it may be to be aware of and to understand why women stay in abusive relationships, it does not address the real issue. Counsels Sara Buel, a former Massachusetts prosecuting attorney and leader in the movement against domestic violence, "We need to acknowledge that it is the wrong question to ask 'Why do women stay?' We need instead to ask 'Why do we, as a society, tolerate such extraordinary amounts of violence, primarily by men against women?'"

To address that issue takes a multisystem approach, a commitment to education, protection, and legal, medical, and social services. The following are some of the areas that need to be examined:

• **Shelters.** Although shelters for abused animals have existed for years, shelters for battered women are a relatively new phenomenon. They have grown over the past two decades from 2 in 1974 to more than 1,200. Yet, in a country of more than 20,000 towns and cities, they only begin to fill the need.

Most shelters are privately financed; a few have some additional public funding. All offer short-term protection and refuge. Other than that, there is no typical shelter with typical services. Some offer personal, legal, and occupational counseling, and can help someone negotiate the maze of the welfare system. Others have the more general goal of providing the emotional and psychological support a woman needs to leave the abusive relationship permanently.

Shelter regulations vary as to how long a woman can remain, and how many times she can return.

Unfortunately, a woman's stay in a shelter may trigger retaliation from an angry partner. However, if she is able to use time in the shelter to take control of her life, and perhaps permanently leave the relationship, the likelihood of new violence may be dramatically reduced.

Shelters do not simply provide refuge for battered women. By creating shelters, society recognizes and legitimizes the right of women to be safe from violence in their homes, and thus sends violent men the message that their battering behavior will not be tolerated.

Besides shelters, there are community groups that offer assistance. The YWCA or YWHA, the National Organization for Women (NOW), victims' services organizations (private or governmental), religious organizations, the Junior League, and other women's groups have set up crisis centers, hot lines, and referral services for victims of violence.

• **The Legal System.** Traditionally, the police have been trained to defuse a domestic violence incident as quickly as they can—to calm things down by listening to the couple's account of what happened, by trying to mediate the quarrel, or by ordering the violent spouse out of the house for several hours. But a woman who calls the police only to see her partner returned home after a while has in effect been victimized again. And the man has learned that there is no real punishment for domestic violence.

In recent years, many police departments have adopted mandatory arrest policies to deter wife beating. Mandatory arrest requires police officers to make arrests in all cases of probable domestic assault, even when the victim is unwilling to sign a complaint. Domestic assault is thus treated in the same way as criminal assault between strangers. With arrest and the possibility of a court appearance and time in jail, a man faces social stigmatization as well as fines and the deprivation of rights and privileges.

Some communities have set up special units for handling marital violence, and increasingly a woman can obtain an immediate emergency restraining order against her abusive husband. The order—which may also be called a no-contact order or order of protection—can afford a woman considerable protection against an abusive husband because it will be backed up by police intervention if needed.

Only a fraction of the incidents of marital assault ever reach the courts. Some police, district attorneys, and judges claim that this is because women almost always drop charges and fail to prosecute. Women, on the other hand, maintain that the police and the prosecutors do not take them seriously, but just urge them to "kiss and make up." In some jurisdictions, no-drop policies have been instituted, requiring women to carry through with their complaints. In other areas, the prosecutor pursues the case, regardless of the woman's wishes.

There has also been progress in the most serious cases. Women on trial for the murder of their partners usually plead that the killing was in self-defense, or that it was a result of the psychological damage done by years of battering. Some lawyers expand the self-defense defense to argue that battered women who kill do so in *psychological* as well as physical self-defense. A few jurisdictions still refuse to allow expert testimony on the battered woman syndrome as part of a defense, but this is becoming the exception rather than the rule. In addition, more women are successful in appealing their murder convictions. One study found that 40 percent of women who appeal succeed in having their sentences thrown out (the reversal rate for homicides as a whole is under 10 percent).

A far better course, however, would be to train everyone involved in the legal system—police, parole and probation officers, judges, district attorneys, private attorneys, victim-witness advocates, and child protection workers—to recognize signs of abuse, understand the issues women in abusive relationships face, and deal with abuse before it escalates to murder. One startling statistic that shows how utterly our society has failed to deal with domestic violence: Sixty-three percent of young men between the ages of 11 and 20 who are imprisoned for homicide are there because they have killed their mother's batterer.

• **Medical Services.** The medical system should play a major role in the identification and prevention of wife battering. The worst injuries come to the attention of doctors and nurses in hospital emergency departments. Unfortunately, only a small percentage of these cases are recognized for what they are, or recorded as such on patients' records. The U.S. Office of Domestic Violence reports that as few as 1 percent of cases are identified as due to abuse; other studies have shown 5 to 10 percent. In part, this is because women have been ashamed to volunteer this information or have denied it when questioned; in part, it is because they were never asked.

Other research shows that battered women are frequently regarded as being emotionally disturbed, their injuries are overlooked or minimized, and their distress and disorientation treated with a prescription for tranquilizers.

Fortunately, this picture may be changing. In 1991, the American Medical Association recommended that all medical professionals routinely screen their female patients for abuse, that record keeping be improved to facilitate treatment plans, and that health care providers make quick and appropriate referrals to specially trained personnel, such as those available at battered women's shelters. It also calls for training on domestic violence at all levels of medical education.

The American College of Obstetricians and Gynecologists has also urged its members to become involved in efforts to identify and stop domestic violence against women.

As of 1992, all accredited hospitals are required to have protocols describing how to respond to battered women and how health professionals are being trained to deal with this issue. That these protocols, *if enforced*, can make a difference is evidenced by a study at the Medical College of Pennsylvania. Before the protocol was introduced, only 5.6 percent of injured female patients seen in the emergency department were identified as victims of battering. After introduction of the protocols, this number jumped to 30 percent.

•**Prevention.** If domestic violence is to be stemmed, society must deal with the roots of the problem. Experts believe the following changes must be made:

• Abuse in the family must be regarded not as a private matter but as a matter of public concern in which the victim requires protection and the family needs support.

• Society must focus on changing those attitudes that legitimize voilence. In America today, violence is condoned as a viable solution to life's problems; it is glamorized on television and in the popular press. The process of reeducation to change these perceptions must start in childhood.

• If, as many believe, conflict is an inevitable part of intimate relationships, information on nonviolent ways to deal with it must be made widely available.

• Men and women should be encouraged to seek marital as well as individual counseling, geared toward learning how to communicate with each other and solve problems without using violence.

• Traditional gender roles and responsibilities must be challenged and redefined. Men may need guidance in seeing that women can be independent as well as responsible for maintaining a marriage; women may need help in accepting their dual roles as caretakers and independent wage earners.

• There must be public education and awareness campaigns about domestic violence. Such campaigns should include public service announcements and listings of domestic violence hotlines and other resources, such as shelters. It should also be emphasized that domestic violence affects all classes and socioeconomic groups—that becoming a victim is no cause for embarrassment, shame, or silence.

• Professional schools that prepare people to work with children and families should include instruction on family violence in their curricula.

• Every community should have a shelter or safe home available for battered women and their children. Every community should also have a full range of health, mental health, legal, and social services for victims and abusers.

• Police, prosecutors, and judges should respond to domestic violence just as they do to violence in the streets. Arrest, prosecution, conviction, and sentencing should be consistent, regardless of the relationship of the victim and the offender.

RAPE

Rape, forcing sex on a person against his or her will, is a criminal act. It almost invariably involves a man forcing a woman or female child, although the incidence of men and boys being raped is much higher than once thought. The man may be a stranger, but much more often he is someone the woman knows. He may threaten her with a knife, or merely overpower her with his weight. She may submit or fight him off. No matter the amount of violence involved, or the degree of submission, it is rape, and it is criminal if the victim does not consent.

Victims of rape come from every ethnic group and social class. They are rich and poor, students, housewives, and professionals. Thousands are young girls, others are elderly women.

There are no accurate figures on the incidence of rape, but the consensus is that it is vastly underreported—because in most cases women are reluctant to report it and because official definitions of rape have been very narrow (i.e., forcible penile penetration of a vagina). While most rapes are perpetrated by known assailants, reported incidents disproportionately involve rape by strangers. This may be because women are reluctant to report family members or other men they know and/or because they may not consider forced sex with these men to be rape, especially if the relationship has also involved consensual sex.

The National Women's Study, funded in part by the National Institute on Drug Abuse and released in 1992, shows that rape is much more prevalent than had been previously reported. The study asked a representative national sample of more than 4,000 adult women if they had ever been raped and whether they had been raped in the past year. Extrapolating from the results, more than 12 million women have been raped at least once and more than 680,000 women over age 18 are raped each year. This does not include children and adolescents who, according to the survey, account for more than half of the victims.

Years ago, rape was believed to be an expression of lust. More recently, it has been seen as acting out anger toward women through sexual violence. New research suggests that these are oversimplifications, that there are several different types of rapists, and that the mix of violence and eroticism differs from one type to another.

Most rapists are thought to be men with otherwise normal sexual feelings and behavior who rape impulsively when the opportunity presents itself—often on a date. More often than not, both they and the women involved have been drinking. They do not show anger unless a woman resists and are not likely to use unnecessary force. Almost one fourth of all convicted rapists fall in this category, according to the research, but there are probably many more "opportunistic" rapists among those who are never caught or convicted.

Another one fourth of convicted rapists are preoccupied with a sexual fantasy that they try to act out in the rape—for example, the rapist imagines that the woman will fall in love with him after he has forced her to have sex with him. These men are the least violent; some have even been known to place a coat on the ground before forcing the woman down. About one third of convicted rapists, whose attacks are physically harmful, are characterized as being clearly out to take revenge on women and to degrade and humiliate their victims. Another 11 percent are angry at the world in general, and 8 percent are sadists who are aroused by their victims' fears.

What triggers such attacks? The idea that women "ask for it" by dressing or behaving provocatively was thoroughly discredited long ago, though it is a common theme among rapists. It seems that in many cases the rapist feels angry or depressed or worthless in the days before the rape. The assault is triggered by a woman angering him, usually by rebuffing a sexual advance. This is perceived as a slight on his manhood, intensifying his feelings of misery. The rape is the end result.

RAPE BY KNOWN ASSAILANTS Less than one in four rapes involves a stranger, according to the National Women's Study. Almost one third of the women in the study reported that the rapist was a nonrelative whom they knew; the rest were raped by their fathers, stepfathers, or other male relatives, their boyfriends or former boyfriends, or their husbands or ex-husbands.

Other studies have found that as many as one woman in four or five has experienced "date rape," in which the man persisted in trying to force sex on her in spite of her verbal resistance, tears, screams, and attempts to fight him off. For most of the men in this category, the episode probably represented "just sex"; for most of the women, it was an unpleasant experience for which they felt partly to blame.

Date rape exemplifies the sexual double standard under which "nice women don't say yes and real men don't listen to no." Men who rape tend to see all protests as token. They refuse to believe that no most often means no. They also tend to misinterpret actions on a woman's part that are simply friendly—smiling, joining them for a drink—as indicating an interest in sex. Nevertheless, every woman has the right to say no, even if she has said yes in the past or has engaged in sexual behavior short of intercourse. No man is ever justified in forcing sex on a woman. Most date rapes are never reported, and few men admit to it, even though these encounters usually meet the legal definition of rape.

For three centuries, under common law, there was an exemption to the crime of rape: A man could not be convicted of nonconsensual sexual intercourse with his wife. Now the laws are changing. About one third of states have abolished the marital exemption completely. Most of the others have either partially abolished it or have created a special legal category for marital sexual assault.

Gang rape is a rare event that occurs disproportionately on college campuses. Studies indicate that because the men involved usually considered the women to be promiscuous, this perception legitimized the rapes. As each man took his turn, the victim was increasingly seen as a whore who deserved the abuse.

AVOIDING RAPE Sociologists and others who study rape ask why we don't spend as much time teaching men not to rape as we do teaching women how to avoid being their victims. Their point is valid, but until the attitudes that produce rapists can be changed, women need to know what they can do to protect themselves.

Unpleasant as it may seem, the best way to avert a rape is to be ready for one. If you think about and rehearse what you would do in case of an attempted rape, you will be better prepared to react.

The American College Health Association offers this advice to women who want to avoid acquaintance rape: "Believe in your right to set limits, and communicate these limits clearly, firmly and early. Say 'no' when you mean 'no.' Be assertive with someone who is sexually pressuring you. Often men interpret passivity as permission."

There is no one right way to react to an attempted rape—only what seems right for you and the circumstances. If the would-be rapist is armed (fewer than 30 percent are), compliance may be the best course. As bad as rape is, it is not worth risking permanent injury or death. The fact that you submit does not minimize the crime. Even if the rapist is not armed but you feel that resisting will not help or may get you badly hurt, you should not feel guilty if you submit.

Nevertheless, experts say that women who resist in any way, from talking back to attacking, have a better chance of deterring their assailant than women who do not resist. Statistics from the U.S. Bureau of Justice bear this out. Studies that compare cases in which women avoided rape and those in which they did not reveal that:

• The more strategies a woman uses—including fleeing, shouting for help, verbal resistance, and physical resistance—the better the odds that she will not be raped.

• Fleeing, screaming, and using physical resistance are individually more often successful than verbal resistance or no resistance.

• Several kinds of verbal strategies have been successful. In some cases, a woman says no, insists that the man stop, tells him what she thinks of him and his actions. In others, she pleads with him or gives him her name or talks about her children so that he will think of her as an individual. Some women (lying if necessary) tell the attacker that they are pregnant, sick, have their period, have a sexually transmitted disease, or anything else that may turn him off.

• Physical resistance is more likely to be successful if it is used immediately. The element of surprise seems to work in a woman's favor.

• Women who fight back are more apt to be injured but not seriously (in general, 90 percent do not require hospitalization). Women who submit are not immune from injury, even serious injury.

• It appears to be a myth that rapists become sexually aroused by women's attempts to resist.

You do not need to be trained in martial arts or even to be strong to protect yourself from a rapist. (See box, "Protecting Yourself Against Rape.") Your attitude is one of your best defenses. Unfortunately, traditional female socialization sets women up to be raped because they are often taught to acquiesce, to be trusting, not to "make a scene." If you fall into this category, it is important to understand that no one has the right to hurt you; you must learn to trust your gut feelings. If you believe that you can control the situation—even if control means deciding to submit—you will stay calmer and recover faster.

AFTER A RAPE Experts agree that a woman who has just been raped should call someone—911, a rape crisis or victim-assistance counselor, a friend or family member—to talk it through.

Many communities have a rape-crisis center with a hotline number (there are about 700 of these nationwide). Specially trained counselors can explain the medical and legal procedures after a rape and can help a woman deal with her feelings of shock, fear, and helplessness. She may be embarrassed and reluctant to report the rape, but reporting it is a way to strike back, a form of therapy. Ideally, a rape victim can help put her assailant behind bars. If she prefers, however, she can report the crime without having to press charges. Giving details about the event could help the police and might ultimately protect other women.

The first decision a woman must make is whether to get medical attention. Even if injury is not obvious, there are several reasons to seek help: she may be in shock and thus be unaware of an injury; she may need advice on dealing with a possible sexually transmitted disease or pregnancy; and, should she decide to report the rape to the police, necessary evidence must be taken in the first few hours after the rape. Going to a hospital emergency room does *not* mean having to report the rape; evidence can be taken and stored until a decision is made. (See box, "In the Hospital Emergency Department.")

The fear of AIDS complicates care after a rape, and adds to a woman's distress. In those states that have confidentiality statutes, some rape suspects have capitalized on this fear, trading their cooperation in medical testing for lesser criminal charges. If the rapist is known to be HIV-positive—or if his status is not known—the victim should be tested at the time of the initial medical evaluation, and she should consult her doctor about follow-up testing to see whether she has developed antibodies. Fortunately, HIV infection is unlikely following a single sexual exposure.

PROTECTING YOURSELF AGAINST RAPE

The following defense strategies have been compiled from various sources, including law enforcement officers, self-defense experts, rape-crisis counselors, and rape and violence prevention organizations. Although these strategies have worked for other women, only you can decide if they are right for you and the situation.

• You are less likely to be a victim if you don't act like one. First, you need to be aware of your surroundings, not lost in thought. Stand straight, stride confidently, look around as you walk. Give the impression that you can't be easily intimidated.

If you must walk alone at night, walk down the center of the sidewalk, not near parked cars or bushes or dark doorways. Keep your car or house keys handy, but not in view (a sign that you are near home).

• If you think someone is following you, assess your options. Your best bet may be to flee. If there is a safe haven (such as a busy store) or a crowded corner nearby, and you can run easily, you probably should run. If you are wearing high heels, or there is no one in sight, your best move may be to turn around and walk toward him. Knowing that you got a good look at him may be enough to deter him.

• If you are taken by surprise, take a deep breath and quickly assess the situation. If your assailant is not armed and you think you can get away, run. If you can't run, refuse to comply. Be firm, but not hostile. Just say, "Stop bothering me." Then, if you are in an area where someone will hear you, yell. Make a scene. Ask someone to call the police.

• If you decide to fight, fight hard. You are defending yourself against getting hurt, and your goal is to disable your attacker. React with anger, not fear.

• Use your hands, your feet, and whatever you have handy—keys, loose coins (to throw in his eyes), hair or breath spray, a pen, a book, an umbrella. If he throws you to the ground, grab a handful of dirt to throw at his eyes.

• The most vulnerable spots are the eyes, nose, chin, windpipe, kneecaps, shins, and insteps. Although the groin is an obvious target, he may be expecting it and may grab your knee and push you to the ground. It is a good second move, however, after you begin to disable him as follows:

• Poke him in the eyes with your fingers or keys.

• Cup your hands and slam them into his ears.

• Jab at the base of his throat with a pen, your fingertips, or the v between your thumb and forefinger.

• Chop at the side of his neck with the edge of your hand.

• Keep your fists in the center of your chest as you twist your torso and swing one elbow up into his chin.

• If you are grabbed from behind, swing one elbow back into his stomach or step back and stomp down hard with your heel on his instep.

• If you're thrown to the ground, roll onto your back, bend your knees, and get your feet up ready to kick his shins or kneecaps.

Before you have to use any of these strategies, consider taking a self-defense course. Many rape-crisis centers, YWCAs, and other community organizations offer courses in physical and psychological preparedness. Even if you don't take a formal course, plan how you would defend yourself. Visualize yourself performing the moves listed above and practice them in front of a mirror. Be angry. Yell "no" with each move. Get comfortable with the idea that you won't allow yourself to be a victim.

IN THE HOSPITAL EMERGENCY DEPARTMENT

After a rape, you need to get prompt medical attention. Usually, this means going to the emergency department at the nearest hospital. There are some things that you should do at this point, and some that you shouldn't. It may be difficult to deal with these details right after a rape, but in the end they will prove helpful.

• Your first impulse may be to get cleaned up. *Don't.* Better evidence of the rape can be obtained if you haven't showered, douched, urinated, used mouthwash, had a drink of water, combed your hair, or washed your hands.

• Take extra clothes with you when you go to the hospital. What you were wearing may be taken by the police as evidence.

• Also take along insurance information. Reimbursement for medical care is available in most states through crime victims' assistance programs, but the hospital will follow its usual check-in procedures.

• Remember that you can insist on being questioned by a female police officer and that you can have a friend with you the entire time that you are in the hospital emergency department.

• The doctor who examines you and takes samples should explain what he or she is doing as well as the medical and/or legal reasons for the procedures. If you don't get an explanation, ask.

• Depending on the circumstances (where you are in your menstrual cycle, what kind of birth control you are using, whether there was penetration and ejaculation), you may be offered short-term hormonal therapy to prevent pregnancy.

• If it is not offered, ask about follow-up testing and/or prevention for sexually transmitted diseases, including hepatitis B and HIV.

• If you are at the hospital helping a friend who has been raped, be supportive of whatever she has done since the assault. She may not have handled things as you might have—perhaps she showered or may still be reluctant to notify the police. Nonetheless, she deserves emotional support and sensitive medical care.

AFTEREFFECTS OF RAPE Immediately after the rape, with its pain and fear and degradation, some women develop rape-trauma syndrome. This is a confusing and recently recognized psychological disorder in which the victim seems calm, relaxed, and unconcerned to the extent of not reporting the rape. It can lead others to suspect that she consented to sexual intercourse, or may not have been raped at all.

Long-term, common problems are depression, nightmares, fear of being alone, loss of interest in sex, distrust of men in general, and fear that the rapist will attack again. Rage at being a victim may transfer itself into intense anger expressed toward family members and other people who try to help. Often, rape victims feel that they have been damaged permanently, that no one will ever again think them attractive. Research studies suggest that it may take from 6 months to 6 years for rape victims to recover, and that some never do.

PROSECUTION One reason that women hesitate to report a sexual assault is that they believe that all rape cases go to trial. At the trial, so the myth goes, the victim will have to testify and present evidence of her injuries. Her sexual history will be the subject of examination and attorneys representing the rapist will victimize her again. The fact is, however, that 90 percent of rapists plead guilty or no contest *without* a trial. Moreover, in most states, "rape shield" laws bar attorneys from questioning rape victims about their sexual history unless it can be proved relevant. Several states have also revised their laws to make it easier to convict rapists, and most states no longer require resistance as proof of rape. These and other reforms give rape victims greater protection against harassment and humiliation. Consequently, more are now willing to press charges. The rape conviction rate has risen to 80 percent or better in some communities.

In addition to the criminal cases, more and more women are bringing civil suits against those who may share liability for the rape: landlords who are responsible for maintaining safe conditions; colleges and universities where students raped classmates; hotels and hospitals whose employees were the rapists. Seeking recourse in the civil system can be part of the healing process after a rape. It can empower the victim and give her a measure of control over her life.

PART V

Encyclopedia of Common Ailments, Tests, and Treatments

ENCYCLOPEDIA CONTENTS

Note: All references in small caps refer to other entries in the Encyclopedia. In addition, please consult the Index.

AIDS (acquired immune deficiency syndrome) is a disorder that attacks the body's immune system, leaving it unable to fight other illnesses. As a result, even mild infections are potentially fatal for people with the disorder.

Symptoms: Many people experience no symptoms at the time of infection, but some may develop a flulike illness within 2 to 6 weeks. They may have fever, joint and muscle aches, abdominal cramps, diarrhea, fatigue and, possibly, a rash; symptoms usually disappear within 2 weeks. There is a symptom-free period (although some people have swollen lymph nodes in the neck and armpits) for 2 to 5 years after infection. Five to 10 years after initial infection, such symptoms as night sweats, swollen lymph glands, unexplained weight loss, diarrhea, lethargy, head-aches, intermittent fevers, and frequent infections are likely to develop.

Within 10 years after infection, about half develop full-blown AIDS. Many people with AIDS develop an otherwise rare type of pneumonia known as *Pneumocystis carinii* pneumonia (PCP), and/or a type of skin cancer known as Kaposi's sarcoma. They are also at greater risk of: tuberculosis; thrush, a fungal infection that causes white spots and ulcers on the tongue and mouth; chronic herpes simplex, a virus that causes blistering sores around the mouth; toxoplasmosis, a parasitic infection that can invade the brain; cryptococcosis, a fungus that attacks the nervous system, liver, bones, and skin; and cytomegalovirus, which causes pneumonia, encephalitis, and blindness. Women with AIDS are prone to CERVICAL CANCER.

Cause: AIDS is caused by the human immunodeficiency virus (HIV). About 1 million Americans are now infected with HIV, and perhaps 50,000 more become infected each year.

Diagnosis: Blood tests can determine whether you have been infected with HIV. Antibodies to the virus develop within 3 months to a year after exposure and are detected in testing. Many city and state health departments offer free, anonymous HIV testing. A positive HIV test does not mean that you have AIDS, however, because it takes many years for infection to lead to illness. You will not be diagnosed as having AIDS until you develop a constellation of characteristic illnesses, such as those listed above, or immune system damage falls below a certain point, which is determined by the level of T4 helper cells in your blood.

Treatment: While there is no cure for AIDS, a number of antiviral drugs help slow the progress of the disease. These include AZT (Retrovir), DDI, and aerosolized pentamadine, which can prevent PCP. To help strengthen your immunity, try to stay as healthy as possible by eating a balanced diet, getting adequate rest, and exercising regularly, which can reduce stress. Avoid contact with anyone who has an infectious illness, even a cold.

Outlook: Although AIDS is ultimately fatal, improved treatment is extending life for many people with the disease. About 30 percent of infants born to HIV-infected mothers are usually infected, but new research suggests that prenatal and immediate postnatal treatment may lower babies' risk of infection to only 8 percent. Your outlook will be better if you avoid smoking, drinking alcohol, and taking drugs, all of which can further damage your immune system or make you vulnerable to other infections.

Tips: HIV is transmitted by contact with body fluids, primarily blood and semen. If you are not in a mutually monogamous relationship, use a condom and spermicide during all sexual encounters. Both male and female condoms are now available. Never share unsterilized needles. If you suspect that you have been infected with HIV, get tested immediately. The sooner you know that you are infected, the more quickly you can receive life-prolonging treatment.

Although blood transfusions were a source of AIDS transmission in the 1980s, this risk has become very small now that donated blood is carefully screened. HIV cannot be transmitted by working, eating, or being in the same room with an infected person unless there is direct contact with the infected person's blood. Household transmission is extremely rare; two recent cases of transmission between children in the same home both involved contact with blood. For this reason, sharing razors or toothbrushes with an infected person should be avoided.

AMNIOCENTESIS is a prenatal diagnostic test that is used to detect chromosomal abnormalities in a fetus. It can also tell the sex of the fetus. The test, which is usually performed between the 14th and 18th weeks of pregnancy, involves withdrawing a sample of the amniotic fluid that surrounds the fetus. This fluid contains cells that have been shed by the fetus, which are then cultured in the laboratory. Amniocentesis is recommended for women over age 35 and for others who have a family history of certain genetic diseases or chromosome defects. If there is such a history in the family, other tests may be available for specific hereditary genetic diseases.

Procedure: Before amniocentesis, you will have an UL-TRASOUND evaluation to locate the fetus and identify a good spot for inserting a needle—a clear space between the wall of the uterus and the fetus. The skin in this area is cleansed with a disinfectant and a local anesthetic given in the area where the needle will be inserted. The doctor then inserts a long, hollow needle through your abdomen into the uterus and withdraws some of the amniotic fluid. You will feel a pulling sensation for a minute or two as amniotic fluid is drawn into the needle.

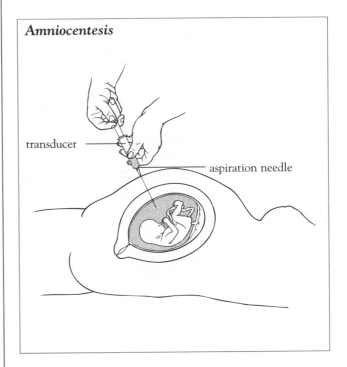

Amniocentesis

transducer

aspiration needle

Risks and complications: Insertion of the needle causes somewhat more discomfort than having blood drawn, but it is not as painful as menstrual cramps. Afterward, some women temporarily experience profuse sweating, faintness, or nausea. The test is generally safe, but there is a small risk of MISCARRIAGE, infection, or damage to the fetus.

Results: It usually takes several weeks to culture the cells for the chromosome analysis. If other genetic tests are being performed, the timing of the results may vary according to the test. A genetic counselor will call within 3 to 6 weeks to discuss findings. If abnormalities are detected, it is probably wise to meet with the counselor to discuss your options.

Tips: You should not have any lingering discomfort. Call your doctor if you experience any pain, cramping, bleeding, fluid leakage, chills, or fever.

ANXIETY is a natural response to real danger or stress. In normal situations it can help you respond more effectively to crises. However, when anxiety and worry are persistent and unrealistic or excessive, the condition is called a generalized anxiety disorder.

Symptoms: Anxiety disorder manifests itself as constant feelings of anxiety or irrational anxiety attacks, such as worrying about a child who is in no actual danger. You may feel restless or irritable or on edge, have difficulty concentrating, suffer from insomnia, or have an exaggerated response when startled. In addition to psychological symptoms, anxiety can produce such physical signs as trembling, twitching, or shakiness; muscle tension or aches; fatigue; shortness of breath; palpitations; sweating or clammy hands; dry mouth; dizziness or lightheadedness; gastrointestinal problems, including upset stomach, nausea, or diarrhea; hot flashes or chills; frequent urination; or feeling a lump in the throat, which makes it difficult to swallow.

Causes: Any difficult problem, from physical illness to a divorce or death of a loved one, can cause you to feel a normal amount of anxiety. However, like most psychological disorders, it is unknown what are the causes of continued generalized anxiety in the absence of a realistic threat. Childhood problems or excessive secretion of stress hormones may be at the root. Sometimes persistent anxiety may be a warning sign of DEPRESSION or psychosis.

Diagnosis: First, a complete physical examination is performed to rule out any underlying disease, such as HYPERTHYROIDISM. While no special tests can identify anxiety, a psychotherapist can usually make an assessment after a short discussion. A key component of diagnosis is a determination that the anxiety has persisted for several months and is linked to more than one concern, as well as the number and type of psychological and physical symptoms present.

Treatment: Therapy is the usual course, although medication may be appropriate. Psychotherapy involves talking about feelings and experiences so that the therapist can help the patient understand the problems that have caused the anxiety. Behavior modification therapy can help treat anxiety triggered by specific circumstances. In some cases, short-term treatment with tranquilizers or other drugs can help the patient calm down and focus more effectively on therapy.

Outlook: Anxiety may come and go, depending on the level of stress in life. If it persists for long periods, it can become disabling if not treated. The frequency and duration of psychotherapy depends on the causes and severity of the anxiety disorder.

Tips: Regular physical exercise can help alleviate stress and assure a good night's sleep, which often has beneficial effects in lowering anxiety. Learning relaxation and self-hypnosis techniques also can help you cope with difficult situations with less anxiety. Avoid substances, such as caffeine, that may increase anxiety.

BREAST BIOPSY is a diagnostic test performed to confirm or rule out breast cancer when an abnormal mass is found by manual examination or mammography. Because nearly 90 percent of all breast lumps are not cancerous, before your doctor recommends a biopsy, he or she will take into consideration many factors, such as the size, location, and texture of the lump as well as your age and family history.

Procedure: Several options are available. Frequently, a needle aspiration is performed first. In this office procedure, you may first receive an injection of a local anesthetic and then a hollow needle will be inserted into the lump. If the lump is a fluid-filled cyst, the doctor is able to withdraw the fluid and the cyst collapses. The fluid may be sent to a laboratory for examination. If the cyst grows back quickly, the lump does not yield fluid during the aspiration, or laboratory examination of the fluid indicates an abnormality, then a needle or surgical biopsy will be needed.

The needle biopsy, also an office procedure with local anesthesia, involves the insertion of a corkscrew-shaped needle that carves out a small part of the lump for laboratory examination. A sophisticated new variation of this procedure, sometimes called stereotactic biopsy, uses mammography to help the doctor locate a mass that cannot be felt. ULTRASOUND can also be used to locate a nonpalpable mass.

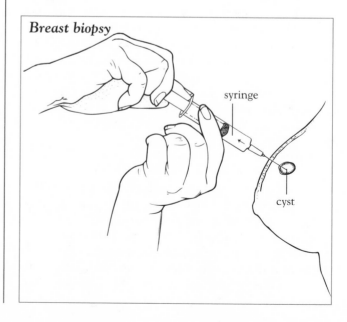

Breast biopsy

syringe

cyst

Surgical biopsies may be done with local or general anesthesia, depending on the size and location of the lump and your own preferences. They may be performed in the doctor's office or as an outpatient procedure in a hospital's ambulatory surgery department. The biopsy may be incisional, removing only part of the lump, or excisional, removing all of the lump and a margin of normal tissue around it. Stitches are used to close the incision.

Risks and complications: Needle biopsies and incisional biopsies may not be fully reliable because some lumps are cancerous in one spot and noncancerous in others. All invasive procedures carry some risk of infection.

Results: Laboratory findings are available within 2 to 3 days. Before the biopsy, ask that estrogen- and progesterone-receptor assays be done immediately on the sample. These tests can significantly affect treatment options.

Tips: In the past, women were required to sign a release for MASTECTOMY before a surgical biopsy, which was performed under general anesthesia. During surgery a tiny part of the lump was sent to the pathology laboratory for a "frozen section" analysis. Now most women refuse to have this done because frozen sections are occasionally inaccurate and they prefer to consider other, nonmastectomy treatments.

BREAST CANCER is the most common malignancy in women. About one in every nine women in the United States develops breast cancer at some point in her lifetime. There are actually many types of breast cancer, but the most important distinction among them is whether they are invasive or noninvasive. Noninvasive breast cancers grow only within the breast, while invasive types have the ability to invade other cells and, traveling through the bloodstream or lymph system, spread elsewhere in the body.

Symptoms: A small lump or thickening in the breast, often discovered during breast self-examination, is usually the first symptom. Other signs may include a change in breast shape; dimpling, puckering, or an inflamed reddish appearance of the breast skin; retraction of the nipple; or nipple discharge.

Causes: Although the cause of breast cancer is unknown, it occurs more commonly in women whose mothers or sisters had the disease, in women of high socioeconomic status, and in women who have never had children or had a first child after age 30. More than 70 percent of breast cancers occur in women who have no identifiable risk factors.

Diagnosis: If you or your doctor find a suspicious lump, you will first have a mammogram if you are over 35. ULTRASOUND may also be performed to see if the lump is cystic (fluid filled) or solid. If these tests do not rule out the possibility of cancer, you may have a needle aspiration, in which a hollow needle is inserted into the lump. If fluid is withdrawn, it is probably a harmless cyst. Fluid or cells from the lump can be sent for microscopic analysis. If the cells are suspicious of cancer or the analysis is inconclusive, a BREAST BIOPSY may be necessary. Examination of the biopsied tissue can help determine if the cells are malignant and if the cancer is an invasive or noninvasive type. If the lump is a cyst that goes away after needle aspiration, cancer can be ruled out.

Treatment: For small and localized cancers, you can usually choose between two equally effective treatments: LUMPECTOMY (or a variation) to remove the lump and surrounding tissue, followed by radiation therapy, or a MASTECTOMY, in which the breast is removed. In breast cancers of certain cell types, one treatment may be more effective than the other.

If the biopsy has shown that the cancer is invasive, the lymph nodes under the arm are removed for examination. When the nodes are removed in conjunction with a breast-conserving procedure such as lumpectomy, the procedure is called axillary dissection; if combined with mastectomy, the procedure is a modified radical mastectomy. If the nodes show that the cancer has metastasized (spread), chemotherapy or hormone therapy is usually necessary.

Outlook: More than 80 percent of lumps found during a manual breast examination turn out to be benign. When they are malignant, early diagnosis and treatment mean your chances of cure are excellent.

Tips: Beginning at age 20, you should perform breast self-examination every month, a few days after your menstrual period is over and your breasts are at minimum fullness.

CARPAL TUNNEL SYNDROME is a disorder that affects the hands and wrists. The carpal bones are small wrist bones that, together with a ligament just under the skin, form a tunnel. Through this tunnel passes the median nerve, which provides sensation to the first three and half of the fourth fingers as well as muscle control to the thumb. When inflammation and swelling arise in the wrist joint, muscles, or nearby tendons, nerve communication to and from the hand can be impeded. The resulting discomfort in the hand, wrist, and sometimes the arm is called carpal tunnel syndrome (CTS).

Symptoms: Pain, tingling, or numbness in all the fingers except the pinkie are usually present. Pressure on the median nerve may produce a shooting pain in the wrist and arm. Symptoms usually worsen at night and can awaken you from sleep. Your fingers may swell and you may also experience weakness in the hand and an inability to grasp objects properly.

Causes: Most CTS is not associated with any local or systemic disease. When an illness is present, DIABETES, RHEUMATOID ARTHRITIS, or HYPOTHYROIDISM is often to blame. The syndrome is also seen in pregnancy.

Diagnosis: Carpal tunnel syndrome is diagnosed through your history (including an analysis of what types of movement cause the symptoms), physical examination, nerve

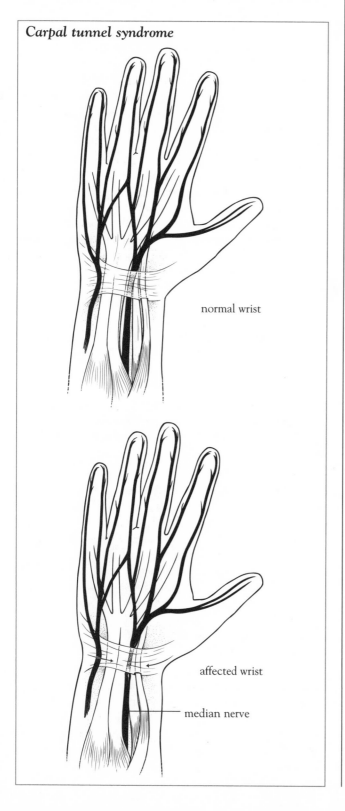

Carpal tunnel syndrome

normal wrist

affected wrist

median nerve

conduction velocity tests, and sometimes other specialized tests to rule out other potential causes of hand or arm pain. It can be diagnosed by a neurologist, rheumatologist, or orthopedist.

Treatment: To reduce inflammation and swelling, your doctor may prescribe aspirin or another antiinflamatory drug, or may inject cortisone directly into the wrist. Wearing a splint can immobilize the wrist and help reduce pain. If an underlying disease is contributing to the problem, controlling the disorder may alleviate or cure carpal tunnel syndrome. If the problem is related to job or home activities, a physical or occupational therapist can help you learn how to reduce wrist stress. If these conservative measures fail, a surgical procedure called carpal tunnel release may be necessary. This is usually done on an outpatient basis.

Outlook: Symptoms may come and go over a period of months or years. If the condition is not treated, the pain may become severe and chronic and weakness may persist. If surgery is performed, special exercises are needed to restore normal hand motion, which usually returns after a few months.

Tips: To prevent or alleviate carpal tunnel syndrome, try to reduce stress and bending of your wrists. Take frequent breaks to exercise your wrists and hands. If symptoms arise, your doctor may recommend using wrist splints.

CERVICAL CANCER is a malignancy that develops in the cervix, the neck of the uterus that protrudes into the vagina. It is the second most common cancer of the female reproductive tract, and usually appears in women age 40 to 55.

Symptoms: There are no symptoms in the early stages. Subsequently, you may develop an abnormal vaginal discharge or bleeding, or pain during intercourse.

Causes: As with most types of cancer, the cause is unknown. However, it occurs more frequently in women who were sexually active before the age of 18, have had multiple sexual partners, have had GENITAL WARTS or HERPES, have not routinely used barrier contraceptive methods, or have a history of cervical dysplasia.

Diagnosis: Cervical cancer can be detected long before symptoms occur, at its earliest and most curable stage, by a PAP TEST during a normal pelvic examination. If the Pap test is abnormal, the cervix may be examined more closely by COLPOSCOPY, after which a tissue sample can be taken for laboratory examination.

Treatment: For the pre-invasive stage of cervical cancer, surgical removal of all or part of the cervix, or laser destruction of the tumor and a small part of the surrounding tissue, may be sufficient. In more advanced cases, radical hysterectomy to remove the uterus, cervix, and tissue adjacent to the cervix, as well as nearby lymph nodes, is

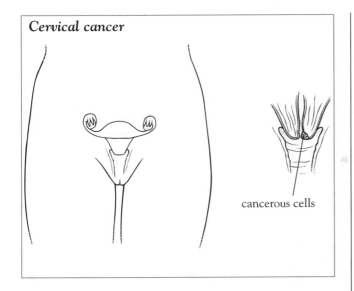

Cervical cancer

cancerous cells

necessary. If the cancer has spread, radiation or chemotherapy may be required to destroy malignant cells elsewhere in the body.

Outlook: The outlook is extremely positive in women who are diagnosed early in the course of the disease, at a stage called carcinoma *in situ*. The survival rate declines when cancers have become more invasive, although the overall rate for cervical cancer in all stages is about 65 percent.

Tips: If you are over 18, or even sooner if you are sexually active, you should have regular Pap tests as recommended by your gynecologist.

CHLAMYDIA is the most common sexually transmitted disease in the United States today. Untreated infections can lead to PELVIC INFLAMMATORY DISEASE, which is responsible for a significant part of the rising incidence of infertility in this country.

Symptoms: In women the most frequent signs are vaginal itching and a foul-smelling, yellowish discharge. As the infection worsens, you may experience abdominal pain, bleeding between menstrual periods, painful or frequent urination, painful intercourse, nausea, and fever. In men the signs are a discharge from the penis, or burning and itching around the opening of the penis, especially during urination. However, many people have no noticeable symptoms of infection until complications begin. In newborns chlamydia contracted in the birth canal can cause infections of the eyes, ears, and lungs, and even death.

Causes: Chlamydia are tiny parasitic microorganisms closely related to bacteria and usually transferred from one person to another by sexual contact.

Diagnosis: In a painless procedure, using a cotton swab, your doctor takes samples of secretions from your cervix for analysis in a laboratory.

Treatment: Antibiotic therapy can treat early infections within 2 weeks. For more advanced infections, treatment may last for up to 6 weeks. If you have a high fever and extensive infection, you may be hospitalized. On rare occasions, surgery may be needed, especially if an abscess forms and ruptures, spreading the infection. Sexual contact must be avoided until you are cured. Your sexual partner should be tested and, if infected, treated simultaneously.

Outlook: If not treated promptly, the infection can spread throughout the urinary and reproductive tracts, causing chronic urinary tract problems, pelvic inflammatory disease, and an increased risk of ECTOPIC PREGNANCY or infertility. Even after seemingly effective treatment, relapses may occur and require retreatment. Many doctors recommend that you undergo retesting a month after therapy.

Tips: Limiting the number of sexual partners, as well as the proper use of condoms, can reduce the risk of infection with any sexual disease. If you are sexually active with more than one partner, or if your sole partner is sexually active with others, you should have regular medical checkups for sexually transmitted diseases. If your partner develops chlamydia, avoid intercourse until treatment is finished and see your doctor at once.

CHORIONIC VILLUS SAMPLING (CVS) is a prenatal diagnostic test that detects chromosomal abnormalities in a fetus. It involves withdrawing some of the hairlike projections, called villi, that compose the chorion, the outer layer of the amniotic sac. The villi contain cells that provide the chromosome information as can the cells in the amniotic fluid, but CVS can be performed between the 9th and 12th weeks of pregnancy. Like AMNIOCENTESIS, it is recommended for women over age 35 and for others whose pregnancies may be high risk.

Procedure: Chorionic villus sampling begins with an ULTRASOUND exam to locate the fetus. Two techniques are available. One is similar to amniocentesis: After a local anesthetic is injected into your abdominal skin, a long, hollow needle is pushed into the abdomen to withdraw the villi. You will feel a pulling sensation for a minute or two as material is drawn into the needle. In the other technique, which is done through the vagina, a very thin catheter is inserted through the cervix into the uterus. Suction is applied to pull the villi into the catheter, which is then removed.

Risks and complications: Insertion of the needle is about as uncomfortable as having blood drawn, and is not as painful as menstrual cramps. In some cases, not enough villi are obtained and the needle must be reinserted. Inserting the catheter may cause some discomfort. There is also a small risk of excessive bleeding and MISCARRIAGE after CVS. The risk of miscarriage seems to be slightly

Chorionic villus sampling

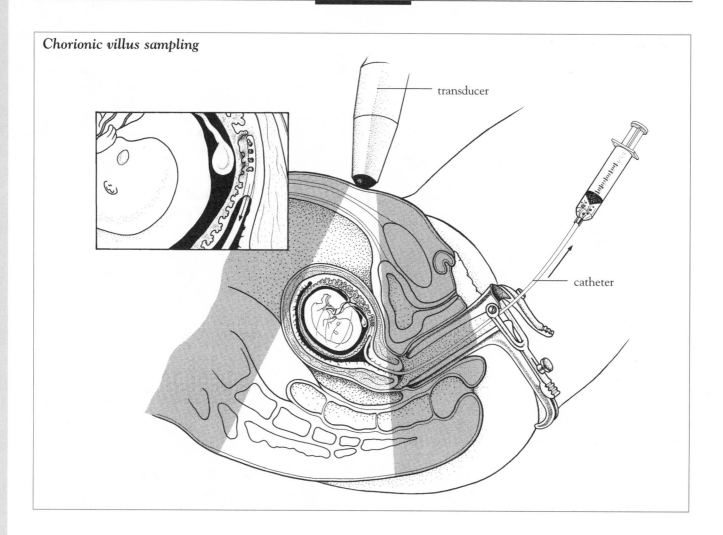

transducer

catheter

higher than with amniocentesis, but this may be because CVS is performed earlier in pregnancy when the risk of miscarriage is already higher.

Results: Findings are available far more quickly by CVS than by amniocentesis. You should receive the results from a genetic counselor within a week. If abnormalities are detected, you should meet with the counselor to discuss your options.

Tips: You should not have any lingering discomfort. If you experience any pain, cramping, bleeding, or fluid leakage, call your doctor immediately.

COLPOSCOPY, a diagnostic test used to evaluate the cervix and vagina, may be recommended if your PAP TEST yields abnormal results.

Procedure: In your gynecologist's office, you recline on the examining table as you would for a routine pelvic exam, and a speculum is inserted in your vagina to expose the cervix. A weak vinegar solution is then dabbed on your cervix, causing a warm sensation. (This highlights the cells and removes any mucus and cellular debris that might impair the examination.) Then the colposcope, which looks like binoculars on a stand, is wheeled into position in front

of the vaginal opening. This specially lit microscope magnifies the cervix ten to twenty times and enables your doctor to locate abnormalities, determine their extent and, in some cases, identify their cause. The procedure takes 15 to 20 minutes and causes no discomfort. Any abnormalities may be further investigated by a PUNCH BIOPSY and/or an endocervical curettage. These tests may cause some cramping, discomfort, and bleeding.

Risks and complications: Colposcopy itself carries no risks, as the instrument never enters your body. The biopsies may cause some bleeding or infection, but these risks are minimal.

Results: Your doctor can tell you the results of the visual examination immediately. Biopsy results may take up to a week.

Tips: Do not douche for at least 24 hours before colposcopy, unless instructed to do so by your physician. To lessen any anxiety you might have during the procedure, bring along a portable radio and headset.

Colposcopy

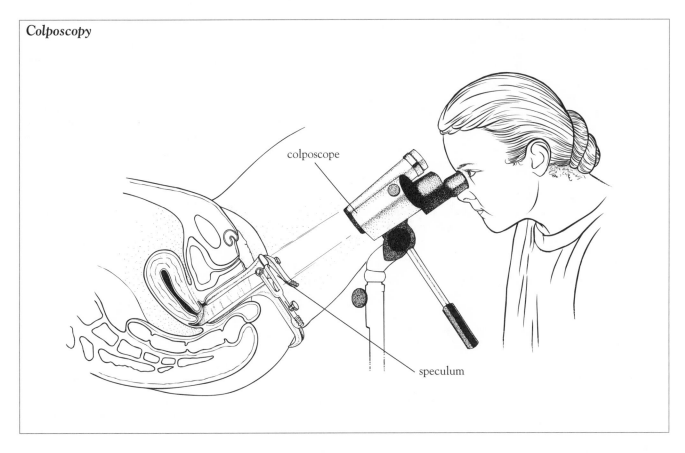

CONE BIOPSY is a diagnostic test used to evaluate abnormal cells in the cervix. Also known as conization, it may be recommended if your gynecologist spots any abnormalities suggestive of cancer during a COLPOSCOPY examination that cannot be defined by PUNCH BIOPSY. The procedure also may be therapeutic because, in some cases, conization removes the precancerous cells completely and no further treatment is needed. Thus, this test can be used to treat severe dysplasia or precancerous cells confined to the cervix.

Procedure: Conization is usually performed in a hospital as an outpatient procedure. Most commonly, it is performed in the operating room with general anesthesia. Your surgeon uses a scalpel to cut out a cone-shaped wedge of the cervix, wider at the cervical opening and narrowing at the base leading toward the uterus. The cone of tissue is then sent to a pathology laboratory for examination. The edges of the wound are then sutured or cauterized to reduce bleeding.

Modifications of this procedure allow the tissue sample to be removed with a laser or an electrocautery loop, sometimes with local anesthesia. With these modified techniques, suturing may not be necessary. These procedures are not all interchangeable. In some cases the location or extent of abnormal cells makes a scalpel cone biopsy necessary.

Risks and complications: You will probably have mild to moderate cramps and bleeding afterward. A small risk of excessive bleeding and infection exists whenever any biopsy is done. If too many of the mucus-secreting glands are removed, a dry vagina or fertility problems may result. If too much of the cervix is removed, you may be at risk of later MISCARRIAGE unless a special procedure is done during pregnancy to close the cervix temporarily with sutures.

Cone biopsy

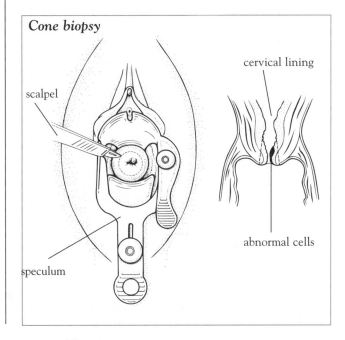

Results: Depending on procedures at the laboratory, results are usually available in 3 to 5 days.

Tips: You may need to wear a sanitary napkin for several days after cone biopsy. Report any excessive bleeding or odor to your doctor right away. To reduce the risk of infection before the biopsy site has a chance to heal, avoid sexual intercourse, douching, tub baths, or using tampons for 5 to 6 weeks after the procedure.

Colposcopy and punch biopsy have replaced many diagnostic cone biopsy procedures, and the laser and electrocautery techniques mentioned above can replace many therapeutic conizations. If cone biopsy is recommended, ask your doctor whether one of these less traumatic approaches can be used.

CORONARY HEART DISEASE, also known as ischemic heart disease or coronary artery disease, is a condition caused by a decreased blood supply to the heart resulting from the narrowing of the coronary arteries. Although the rate of heart disease for women during their reproductive years is lower than for men, it rises dramatically after menopause. One in seven women aged 45 to 64 has some form of heart or blood vessel disease; this figure rises to one in three at age 65 and over. Coronary heart disease is the most common cause of death among American women.

Symptoms: Coronary heart disease takes many years to develop, during which time there are no symptoms. The first symptom women usually experience is a dull chest pain called angina, which tends to occur during exertion or stress. However, there may be no signs at all until a major complication arises, such as a heart attack, congestive heart failure, or abnormal heart rhythms.

Causes: The narrowing of the coronary arteries results from the development of fatty plaques inside the arteries that carry blood to the heart—a process known as atherosclerosis. Although genetics plays an important role in atherosclerosis, four other major risk factors—smoking, high blood pressure, high blood cholesterol, and sedentary life-style—can be treated or modified. Contributing risk factors—diabetes mellitus, obesity, and stress—can also be favorably influenced by life-style modification.

Diagnosis: If you develop angina, you may be diagnosed as having coronary heart disease. In some cases, it is important to know the extent of the disease, which can be revealed by such tests as an exercise stress test; an echocardiogram, which uses sound waves to evaluate heart function; and an angiogram, which produces direct images of the coronary arteries.

Treatment: Life-style modification is the first line of defense to halt or reverse atherosclerosis: eliminating smoking, drastically reducing your intake of fat and cholesterol, and developing a regular exercise regimen. If you suffer from DIABETES or hypertension, these diseases must be carefully controlled. If you are obese, it is essential that you lose weight. If your blood cholesterol levels remain high despite dietary changes, you may need drug therapy as well.

Your doctor may also recommend that you take one baby aspirin every one or two days to help prevent the formation of blood clots that can obstruct narrowed coronary arteries and cause a heart attack. If you develop angina, you will be given medication to relax your blood vessels. If you develop heart failure, which refers to a slowing and weakening of the heart's pumping action, diuretics and other drugs are generally prescribed to strengthen the pumping. If you have a heart attack, you will need drugs to ease the heart's workload, and you may need balloon angioplasty to widen blocked arteries, or coronary bypass surgery to circumvent the blockages.

Outlook: Older women who have a heart attack are twice as likely as men to die within a few weeks of the episode. This is probably because they tend to be sicker than men when the heart attack strikes. It may also mean that treatment was delayed because the disease went unrecognized. In the first 4 years after a heart attack, 20 percent of women have a second attack, compared with 16 percent of men. Women may endure more pain without reporting it to their doctors or may unconsciously modify their activities to prevent angina.

Angioplasty and bypass surgery are, in general, less successful in women than in men. This may be because women have smaller blood vessels, their disease is often more severe by the time of diagnosis, or because they are older when they have such procedures.

Tips: If a parent or other close relative had a heart attack or stroke before age 65, you may be at greater risk. Since it is believed that estrogen protects women against early heart attacks, if you have a family history of premature heart disease or other factors that put you at increased risk, you should seriously discuss estrogen replacement therapy with your physician when you enter menopause.

Learn the warning signs of a heart attack and seek help immediately if you experience any of them. (See Chapter 8, "The Aging Process.")

CYSTOCELE is a prolapse of the urinary bladder that causes it to push against the outer wall of the vagina and protrude into the space occupied by the vaginal canal.

Symptoms: Minor cystoceles usually cause no symptoms. Larger ones may cause a lump or bulge just inside the vaginal opening that is particularly noticeable when you stand or your bladder is full.

Causes: Cystoceles are caused by weakness in the ligaments that support pelvic organs, and by weakness in the vaginal wall. Most prolapse problems stem from damage caused by childbirth. You may also be at greater risk if you are obese or chronically constipated, which strains the pel-

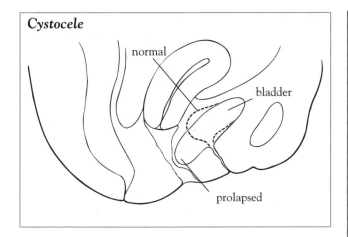

Cystocele

normal

bladder

prolapsed

vic support system, or if you cough excessively from a lung disease or infection. The decrease in hormones after menopause can worsen a previously mild prolapse.

Diagnosis: Your gynecologist can usually diagnose a cystocele simply by observing and feeling the bulge.

Treatment: If the cystocele is causing symptoms, the weakness in the vaginal wall and bulging bladder can be repaired by surgery, which is performed through the vagina.

Outlook: As a cystocele progresses, it can cause diverse urinary problems, including an inability to empty the bladder completely, a need for frequent urination, incontinence, and a greater risk of URINARY TRACT INFECTIONS.

DEPRESSION is much more than simply feeling sad. Doctors use the term "major depression" to diagnose a consistently low mood for at least 2 weeks, accompanied by physical symptoms. People in every age group, from children through the elderly, can develop major depression. Less severe forms of depression are common, can be incapacitating, and may also call for treatment.

Symptoms: Depressed people may have feelings of great sadness, misery, pessimism, low self-esteem, and even undefined guilt. If you suffer from depression, you tend to lose interest in people and activities around you. Your feelings may interfere with your work or social life. You may not be able to see the positive side of any event, and you may even feel suicidal. Depressed people also may experience weight loss or gain, insomnia, loss of appetite, nausea, fatigue, loss of sexual desire, dizziness, and other physical symptoms.

Causes: The cause of major depression remains unclear. It may be due to physiological brain dysfunction rather than just psychological problems. A tendency toward the disorder may be inherited. Major depression may be triggered by real problems in your life or may start for no apparent reason. Even if there seems to be a good cause, the degree of depression may be out of proportion to the problem.

Diagnosis: Your doctor should give you a complete examination to rule out any physical disorder that might be causing your symptoms. In the absence of a physical cause, depression may be diagnosed if the low mood and other symptoms persist more than 2 weeks.

Treatment: Medication can help ease your distress and help you look at your problems more objectively. In many cases, psychotherapy alone or in conjunction with drug therapy can help bring long-term relief.

Outlook: If not treated, depression can persist for months or even years. Although depression can be treated and cured, fewer than half of people with the disorder are properly diagnosed and treated.

Tips: If the initial treatment, whether medication or psychotherapy, does not yield an improvement within 2 months, discuss other options with your doctor or seek a second opinion from a psychiatrist.

DES, or diethylstilbestrol, is a synthetic form of estrogen that was prescribed for many pregnant women between 1941 and 1971 to help prevent MISCARRIAGE. Unfortunately, some babies who were exposed to DES in the womb, as well as their mothers, may have serious problems later in life.

Symptoms: No overt symptoms may be evident. However, DES daughters may develop glandular cells in unusual locations in the vagina (adenosis), occasionally leading to vaginal cancer, and they may have structural abnormalities in their reproductive systems. The latter

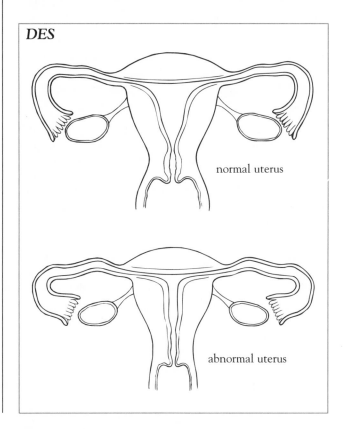

DES

normal uterus

abnormal uterus

places them at greater risk of menstrual irregularities, infertility, ECTOPIC PREGNANCY, miscarriage, and premature delivery. There is also an increased risk of a rare form of vaginal cancer. DES sons may develop benign cysts of the epididymis (a tube through which sperm pass on their way from the testicles to the penis), underdeveloped or undescended testicles, abnormally small penises, and sperm or semen abnormalities that can reduce fertility. As adults, DES offspring may also be at risk for Hashimoto's disease, pernicious anemia, myasthenia gravis, regional enteritis, and MULTIPLE SCLEROSIS. DES mothers may have a greater risk of BREAST CANCER.

Causes: If given during the first 5 months of pregnancy, DES interferes with normal development of the reproductive system of the fetus.

Diagnosis: DES daughters should have a complete gynecological examination annually by a physician experienced in DES screening, with follow-up visits depending upon findings at the first checkup. The exam should include Pap tests of the vagina and cervix, and iodine staining of the vagina and cervix to detect cell abnormalities. Depending on the results, COLPOSCOPY and PUNCH BIOPSY may be advised. DES mothers should practice monthly breast self-examination and have mammograms, as recommended by their gynecologist.

Treatment: DES daughters contemplating pregnancy should consult a specialist to evaluate any structural abnormalities that may cause complications during pregnancy. Once pregnant, they should seek prenatal care immediately because of the higher risk of ectopic pregnancy. Other treatment depends on the problem.

Outlook: The risk of developing vaginal or cervical cancer is very low (1 in 1,000), but extra monitoring is advised. The risk appears to be confined to women under age 32 and, if found early, these cancers can be treated successfully.

Tips: Women who know they were exposed to DES should contact the ob/gyn department of their nearest medical school for referral to a doctor or clinic skilled in DES diagnosis and care. If you remember taking medication during the first 5 months of a pregnancy that occurred between 1941 and 1971, or if you experienced problems during pregnancy, such as bleeding, or if you had DIABETES or any prior miscarriages or premature births, try to find out if DES was prescribed. If your physician is no longer in practice, check with the county medical society for the medical records, or contact the hospital where you delivered to find out whether any prenatal medications are listed in the records.

DIABETES is a chronic disease in which the body does not produce or respond properly to the hormone insulin, which helps metabolize glucose. The main types are:

• Juvenile diabetes, also called Type I or insulin-dependent diabetes, is an autoimmune disease in which islet cells in the pancreas are destroyed so that the body can no longer make insulin; it tends to begin in children and young adults who are of normal weight.

• Adult-onset diabetes, also called Type II or non-insulin-dependent diabetes, occurs when enough or too much insulin is produced but the cells in the body are resistant to the insulin and do not use it properly; it tends to occur in people who are over 40 and overweight.

• Gestational diabetes, similar to Type II diabetes, occurs only in pregnant women but usually disappears after the birth of the baby; although it generally appears in women who are over 30 and overweight, it may occur during any pregnancy.

Symptoms: Type I diabetes usually starts with frequent urination, unusual thirst, weight loss, fatigue, weakness, and uncontrollable food cravings. Type II diabetes may not produce any of these symptoms or may produce all of them as well as frequent infections of the skin, gums, or urinary tract; drowsiness; pain or cramps in the legs, feet, or fingers; and slow healing of cuts and bruises. Gestational diabetes usually has no symptoms but, although the blood glucose levels are not high enough to harm the mother, they are high enough to harm the baby.

Causes: Diabetes tends to run in families, but some environmental agent seems to trigger a genetic predisposition. In Type I diabetes, perhaps a virus encountered in infancy or childhood may set it off; in Type II, obesity may be the triggering factor.

Diagnosis: A series of blood tests can measure the amount of glucose in your blood in a "fasting" state, when you have had nothing to eat or drink for 8 hours, and then again after you have drunk a glass of sugary liquid.

Treatment: A careful diet to control sugar intake, balanced with adequate exercise, is the backbone of diabetes therapy. Many people with Type II or gestational diabetes can be treated by diet and exercise alone. Weight loss can be a very effective treatment for Type II diabetes. Sometimes patients may need oral medication to help their pancreas function more effectively. Others may need insulin injections. All people who have Type I diabetes require daily insulin injections to survive. A woman with gestational diabetes requires special care by a team of experts in obstetrics, metabolism, and nutrition in order to help ensure a healthy baby.

Outlook: When excess glucose builds up in the blood, it damages structures throughout your body. This can cause blood vessel damage, which in turn can lead to heart attack, stroke, kidney failure, blindness, and other problems. High blood sugar levels in pregnancy can jeopardize an unborn baby. Doctors believe that tight control of blood sugar levels can help prevent these complications.

Tips: Learn how to monitor your blood sugar levels at home so you can adjust your food-exercise-medication regimen on a daily basis. Wear a Medic Alert bracelet or carry an identification card in your wallet that indicates you have diabetes so that if you are in an accident or have a high or low blood sugar reaction, you can receive prompt medical attention.

DILATION & CURETTAGE (D&C) is a diagnostic, and sometimes therapeutic, procedure used to obtain samples of cells in the lining of the uterus for examination. It may be performed in cases of repeated bleeding between menstrual periods, as part of an infertility workup, or as a method of abortion. It also may be therapeutic because scraping excess endometrial tissue may restore normal menstrual functioning.

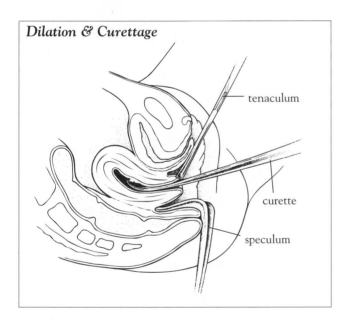

Dilation & Curettage

tenaculum

curette

speculum

Procedure: In the past, a D&C required general anesthesia and an overnight hospital stay. Now it is usually done in the hospital's ambulatory surgery department as an outpatient procedure, and general or local anesthesia may be administered. After you have been given anesthesia, the dilation begins: A series of metal rods of increasing thickness is inserted through your cervix to dilate the opening. When the cervical opening is sufficiently widened, a curved scraping instrument called a curette is inserted through the cervix and used to scrape the endometrium and remove tissue for laboratory examination.

Risks and complications: A D&C carries a small risk of perforation of the uterus and excessive bleeding. There is also a very small risk of infection.

Results: Depending on laboratory procedures, results are usually available in 1 to 3 days.

Tips: A suction ENDOMETRIAL BIOPSY, a less traumatic and less risky outpatient procedure, can often be done instead. After having a D&C, you should report excessive bleeding, fever, or severe abdominal pain to your physician.

ECTOPIC PREGNANCY (tubal pregnancy) is the implantation of a fertilized egg somewhere other than in the wall of the uterus. Ectopics most commonly occur in one of the Fallopian tubes, but they also may occur on an ovary or elsewhere in the pelvis or abdomen.

Symptoms: Minor abdominal bleeding and cramps or a sense of pressure in the abdomen during the early weeks of pregnancy may be the only early warning signals of ectopic pregnancy. Occasionally, the first sign may be severe abdominal pain, shoulder pain, or fainting.

Causes: In nearly half of all cases, ectopic pregnancy is provoked by prior PELVIC INFLAMMATORY DISEASE that has scarred the Fallopian tubes and obstructed the passage of the fertilized egg. Women who have previously used an intrauterine device (IUD) may also be at greater risk. Ectopic pregnancy often occurs for no apparent reason.

Diagnosis: An ULTRASOUND examination can often confirm an ectopic pregnancy by revealing a mass outside of the uterus or the absence of a uterine pregnancy despite a positive pregnancy test.

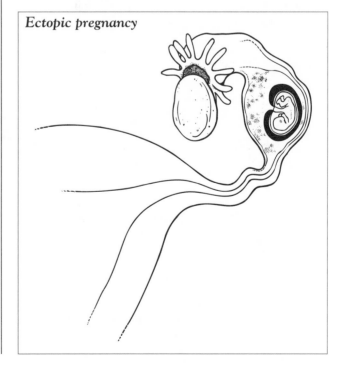

Ectopic pregnancy

Treatment: Surgery is required to remove the tubal pregnancy. Sometimes this can be done by opening the tube and removing the embryo. In other cases, the entire tube must be removed. In some cases, this surgery can be performed with a laparoscope, which may allow a shorter hospital stay than with traditional laparotomy surgery. Some researchers are studying the possibility of replacing traditional surgical methods with a cancer chemotherapeutic drug in combination with laparoscopic surgery.

Outlook: If ectopic pregnancy is allowed to progress, the growing pregnancy may cause the Fallopian tube to rupture, causing internal bleeding, severe pain, and shock. If not treated promptly, ectopic pregnancy can be fatal.

Tips: If you have had PID or used an IUD, try to avoid an unplanned pregnancy, of which you might be unaware during the first month. If you do become pregnant, ask your doctor to monitor you closely for the first month or two.

ENDOMETRIAL BIOPSY is a diagnostic test that obtains samples of cells from the lining of the uterus for examination. It is likely to be performed if you have abnormal menstrual bleeding, or as part of an infertility workup. Many doctors also perform this test on women who take hormone replacement therapy so as to rule out cancerous or precancerous changes in the lining of the uterus.

Procedure: Endometrial biopsy is usually performed as an office procedure that may or may not require local anesthesia. A narrow surgical instrument is inserted into the uterus and a portion of the uterine lining is scraped or suctioned and removed. Even with a local anesthetic you may feel a deep cramping sensation during the procedure. The tissue samples are sent to a pathology laboratory for examination.

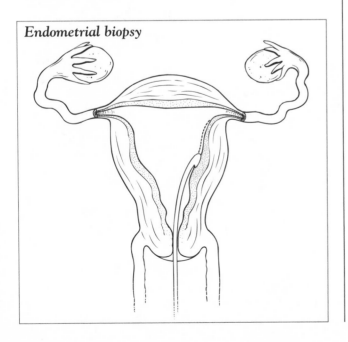

Endometrial biopsy

Risks and complications: The procedure carries a small risk of perforation of the uterus and excessive bleeding. A very small risk of infection exists whenever any biopsy is done.

Results: Depending on laboratory procedures, results are usually available in 3 to 5 days.

Tips: Ask your doctor about taking a mild pain-killer, such as aspirin or ibuprofen, a half hour before the procedure to lessen postbiopsy cramps. Wear a sanitary napkin for 24 hours after the procedure, and report any excessive bleeding or odor to your doctor.

ENDOMETRIOSIS is a disease in which endometrial tissue, normally present only in the lining of the uterus, is found elsewhere, most commonly on the ovaries, Fallopian tubes, bowel, and bladder. Ordinarily, endometrial tissue in the uterus is shed monthly during menstruation. Because any tissue outside the uterus cannot be shed, it causes inflammation and swelling until each menstrual cycle ends, followed by scar formation in the inflamed area. The condition occurs primarily in women between the ages of 25 and 44, especially in those who have delayed childbearing, and it may run in families.

Symptoms: You may have no symptoms or you may experience severe, incapacitating pain that worsens during the last few days before your period and, with time, begins progressively earlier in your cycle. Depending on the site of the abnormal tissue, you may feel pain deep in your pelvis during intercourse, during bowel movements or urination, or elsewhere in your abdomen. Or you may have rectal bleeding during menstruation. Also, the scars that form on your reproductive organs may cause infertility.

Causes: Although the exact cause is unknown, it is thought that endometrial tissue may be transported out of the uterus through the Fallopian tubes, possibly during menstruation, or through the circulation of the blood or lymph in the body.

Diagnosis: A complete gynecological examination, imaging studies (such as ULTRASOUND or magnetic resonance imaging), and direct examination of your pelvis by LAPAROSCOPY may be necessary to confirm the diagnosis.

Treatment: Therapy depends on your age, how severe the condition is, and other factors. If you want to become pregnant, you may be given hormones or other drugs temporarily in order to halt ovulation and enable the abnormal tissue to shrink. Or surgery may be necessary to remove as much of the abnormal tissue as possible. While these approaches do not cure endometriosis, they often provide significant relief and may enable pregnancy. However, the problem is likely to return. If you have severe endometriosis and symptoms that are unresponsive to these techniques, and if you do not intend to become pregnant, total HYSTERECTOMY and OOPHORECTOMY can cure the disease permanently.

Endometriosis

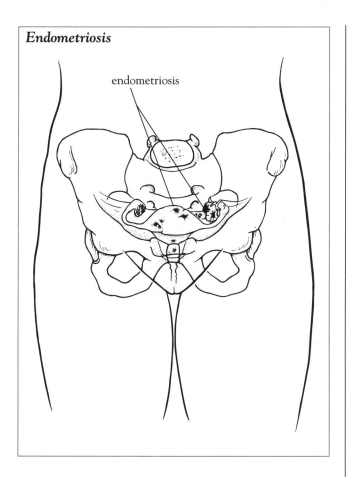

endometriosis

Fibroadenoma

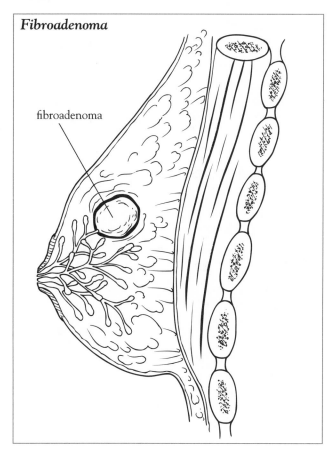

fibroadenoma

Outlook: If left untreated, endometriosis usually gets worse and can cause damage to other pelvic organs and permanent infertility. The only natural cessation of endometriosis occurs during pregnancy and after menopause.

Tips: In addition to taking aspirin or ibuprofen, applying a heating pad or hot water bottle to your pelvis may help ease discomfort. The use of oral contraceptive pills may halt the progression of endometriosis.

FIBROADENOMA is the most common type of benign, noncancerous breast tumor. It is more likely to occur in women between the ages of 14 and 40.

Symptoms: Fibroadenoma generally appears as a single, firm, round lump. When manipulated, it moves freely under the skin but causes no pain.

Causes: Although the cause is unknown, development of fibroadenoma may be hormone related because the tumors tend to occur only after puberty and before menopause.

Diagnosis: Most likely, your doctor will first recommend that you have a mammogram. If your personal history or age put you at high risk for BREAST CANCER, or if the mammogram findings are questionable, a BREAST BIOPSY may be performed.

Treatment: If the tumor is not growing or causing any symptoms, treatment may not be necessary. In some cases, the tumor may even shrink and disappear after menopause.

However, if it is growing or causing other problems, it is usually removed surgically. The surgery requires only local anesthesia and involves taking out only the lump. Small tumors can be removed with little impact on overall breast appearance.

Outlook: These tumors normally grow very slowly although, in rare cases, they may enlarge rapidly during pregnancy. It is not unusual for someone who has had one fibroadenoma to develop a second one months or years later. However, the occurrence of these benign breast tumors does not increase the risk of breast cancer.

Tips: If you have a fibroadenoma that is not removed, monthly breast self-examination is particularly important. Call your doctor promptly if you notice any change in the size and shape of the tumor.

FIBROCYSTIC BREAST DISORDER is the medical term for lumpy breasts. It is not a disease, but a benign breast syndrome in which changes that normally occur due to female hormone fluctuations are exaggerated. More than half of all premenopausal women experience the problem at some time in their lives.

Symptoms: If you have fibrocystic changes, you will have one or more lumps of various sizes, which may give your breasts a "pebbly" consistency. The lumps may be felt all the time or may come and go, arising 1 to 2 weeks before menstruation and disappearing after bleeding ends. Lump-

Fibrocystic breasts

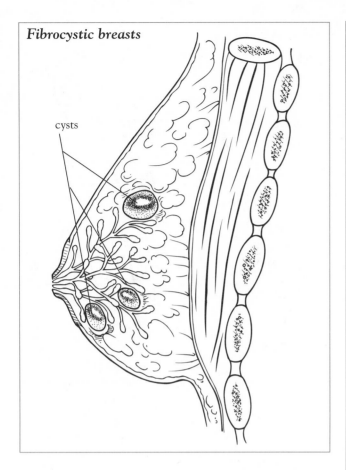

cysts

iness is usually accompanied by breast swelling, tenderness, or pain.

Causes: During the menstrual cycle, changing hormone levels help the breasts prepare for milk production by increasing the number of cells in the milk-secreting glands and the fibrous tissue that surrounds them. When conception does not occur, the excess fluid is normally reabsorbed by the body and the fibrous tissue recedes. If this mechanism fails, excess fluid accumulates in small sacs called cysts. With time, the sacs may fill with fibrous tissue, leading to permanent lumps.

Diagnosis: Your doctor uses a hollow needle to draw fluid from the lump, which confirms that it is a cyst. If no fluid is withdrawn, a biopsy may be needed to determine the contents of the lump.

Treatment: Self-care, not medical treatment, is usually best (see **Tips**). If your breasts are very painful, your doctor may prescribe a diuretic or vitamin E supplements. If the problem is severe, hormonal drugs may be prescribed, but most have significant side effects.

Outlook: Symptoms may last throughout your menstruating years or come and go with no particular pattern, only to disappear after menopause. Problems usually cease during pregnancy and breast-feeding, and may or may not return thereafter. Fibrocystic breasts do not predispose you to developing BREAST CANCER, although they make it more difficult to diagnose any tumors that do occur.

Tips: Examine your breasts regularly to learn your own pattern of lumpiness. Make a chart of your findings (location, size and number of lumps, degree of discomfort) and compare it with your menstrual cycle. By knowing your own pattern, you will be in a better position to spot variations that could warrant medical attention. To prevent breast discomfort, reduce salt intake to decrease fluid retention, and avoid coffee, chocolate, tea, colas, and some aspirin compounds. To alleviate pain, take aspirin or ibuprofen, wear a slightly larger bra when swelling occurs, and avoid jogging or aerobic exercise that jars the breasts.

FIBROID TUMORS, also called uterine fibroids, myomas, and leiomyomas, are benign (noncancerous) growths in the uterus that occur in about 20 percent of women over the age of 30. Fibroids range in size from microscopic to growths the diameter of grapefruits, and they usually grow in clusters.

Symptoms: Most fibroids cause no symptoms, although some women may experience heavy and painful menstrual periods or "spotting" between periods, a sense of fullness in the abdomen, and painful intercourse. A fibroid attached to the uterine wall occasionally becomes twisted (strangulated) and loses its blood supply, causing sudden sharp abdominal pain. Less commonly, a fibroid that grows rapidly during pregnancy may cause pain. MISCARRIAGE or obstruction during delivery may also be caused by fibroids, although these complications are rare.

Causes: Although the cause is unknown, there may be a genetic link, because fibroids tend to run in families. For women who are susceptible, taking birth control pills may precipitate or worsen fibroids.

Diagnosis: Fibroids are usually found during a normal pelvic examination. Their size and location can be confirmed by ULTRASOUND.

Treatment: When fibroids remain small and cause few or no symptoms, they require no treatment. If you have heavy menstrual periods, you may need to take iron supplements to prevent anemia. If large fibroids cause severe pain or result in very heavy menstrual flow, surgery may be advised. If a fibroid causes sudden pain due to strangulation,

Fibroid tumors

tumors

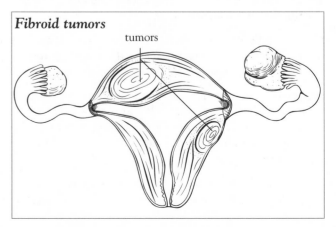

emergency surgery may be required. In young women, my-omectomy is commonly performed. This procedure removes only the fibroids, leaving the rest of the uterus intact. In women close to or after menopause, HYSTER-ECTOMY is usually performed.

Outlook: Most fibroids remain small and grow very slowly. However, they may grow more rapidly during pregnancy, or when you take birth control pills or postmenopausal hormone replacement, all sources of extra estrogen. If a fibroid causes obstruction during delivery, a cesarean section may be necessary. If it obstructs the Fallopian tubes, it may affect fertility.

GALLSTONES are crystalline formations of cholesterol or bile salts that form in the gallbladder. They may be as small as grains of sand or as large as walnuts.

Symptoms: About half of people with gallstones have no symptoms, a condition called silent, or asymptomatic, gallstones. Others suffer attacks called cholecystitis, which cause sudden, severe pain in the upper abdomen, usually on the right side. Pain most often begins after a meal (particularly one high in fat) but can occur spontaneously. Attacks often last several hours and may be accompanied by fever, chills, and vomiting.

Causes: An imbalance in bile composition, usually caused by excess cholesterol, contributes to stone forma-

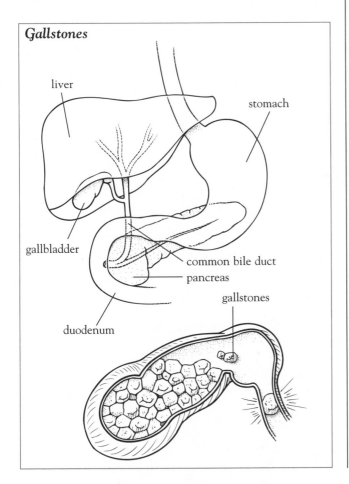

Gallstones

liver

stomach

gallbladder

common bile duct

pancreas

gallstones

duodenum

tion. The tendency to form stones often runs in families. Stones also tend to be more common in people who are overweight or who eat a high-fat diet. Attacks occur when a stone that had been floating in bile fluid becomes lodged in the duct leading from the gallbladder to the intestines.

Diagnosis: Gallstones can be identified by a sonogram or other special imaging studies.

Treatment: If you have frequent attacks, the preferred treatment is cholecystectomy, or surgical removal of the gallbladder (which is not necessary for normal digestion). Although a drug is available to dissolve stones, its effectiveness is uncertain and, because it must be taken indefinitely to prevent the formation of new stones, the risk of side effects is high.

Outlook: In some people, attacks become progressively more severe or frequent. If recurrent gallstone attacks are not treated, stones can lodge in the bile duct, leading to inflammation and infection of the gallbladder, liver, or pancreas. Involvement of the gallbladder may cause it to rupture, resulting in potentially life-threatening complications.

Tips: Try to reduce the frequency of attacks by avoiding high-fat foods, large meals, and any food that may have provoked a previous attack. If you are overweight, reduce. Women should be aware that oral contraceptives and other types of estrogen therapy may increase stone formation. Call your doctor if you have frequent attacks or if any attack lasts longer than 3 hours. Prolonged attacks indicate that the stone may have become lodged in the bile duct, requiring immediate surgery.

GARDNERELLA (also called bacterial vaginosis or nonspecific vaginitis) is one of the three most common causes of VAGINITIS (see also YEAST INFECTION and TRICHOMONAS).

Symptoms: Gardnerella produces a creamy white or grayish discharge and a fishy odor. The vaginal irritation causes an inflammation, which may result in mild to severe vaginal or vulvar itching, burning, redness or swelling, and pain or stinging during intercourse.

Causes: The vagina normally cleanses itself continuously with secretions that bathe its mucous membrane lining. The bacterium that causes gardnerella is among the many microorganisms that naturally live in the vaginal flora and may be sexually transmitted. Gardnerella may overgrow when the normal self-cleansing process breaks down, such as through excessive douching. Stress, poor blood sugar control by people with DIABETES, and the use of oral contraceptives also increase susceptibility.

Diagnosis: Your doctor can usually diagnose gardnerella simply by the appearance and odor of your vaginal discharge. In other cases, a smear of the discharge is taken for laboratory evaluation.

Treatment: Sometimes prompt use of an acidic douche can help halt a gardnerella infection. Look for over-the-counter douche products containing acetic acid, boric acid, citric acid, lactic acid, sodium borate, tartaric acid, or vinegar. Do not use the douche more than twice in 1 week. If the infection does not improve by the end of the week, call your doctor.

Gardnerella may be treated with an oral antibiotic, such as tetracycline or ampicillin, a cephalosporin, or metronidazole (Flagyl), or with a vaginal antibiotic gel.

Outlook: If you are sexually active, your partner must be treated at the same time. During treatment genital contact should be avoided to prevent reinfection.

Tips: If your doctor prescribes a vaginal therapeutic cream or suppository, use it just before getting into bed to help keep the medicine in place as long as possible. Wear a panty shield or thin sanitary pad and underpants to bed to prevent staining the sheets. Never self-treat vaginitis if you also have a fever, pain anywhere in your body (especially the abdomen), or a foul-smelling vaginal discharge, which may indicate a more serious problem that requires medical diagnosis and therapy.

GENITAL WARTS are benign (noncancerous) growths, also called condylomata. Although the warts themselves are usually totally harmless, they can increase the risk of cancer of the cervix and vulva.

Symptoms: Genital warts are pink or flesh-colored growths that range from isolated bumps to elongated ridges to cauliflowerlike clusters. They may grow externally around the labia, vulva, or anus, or inside the vagina or rectum. Although most genital warts are painless, some may itch.

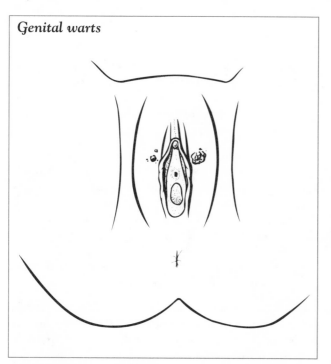

Genital warts

Causes: Warts are caused by papilloma viruses, which are spread by direct contact. Genital warts are highly contagious and transmitted during sexual intercourse.

Diagnosis: You may notice vaginal warts or they may be discovered during a pelvic examination. Your gynecologist can usually differentiate warts from other growths. However, sometimes a sample of the wart may be taken for laboratory examination.

Treatment: Genital warts can be removed with applications of a chemical (either podophyllin or trichloroacetic acid) or by liquid nitrogen, lasers, or surgery.

Outlook: Many warts that have been removed recur within a year. Eventually, the body's immune system helps to prevent recurrences. Although the increased risk for cancer of the cervix and vulva is small, you should have regular PAP TESTS as recommended by your gynecologist.

Tips: Never use over-the-counter wart removers on tender genital areas because this may cause severe skin damage. If you or a partner have genital warts, use a condom during sexual relations to help avoid spreading the virus.

GONORRHEA is one of the most common sexually transmitted or venereal diseases.

Symptoms: Most women have no significant symptoms and can have the disease for months without knowing it. Others may have a slight vaginal discharge or some burning in the vagina. In contrast, men usually develop a thick puslike discharge from the penis and a burning sensation during urination within a week or two of infection.

Causes: Gonorrhea is caused by a type of bacteria that is almost invariably spread through direct sexual contact. You cannot catch gonorrhea from toilet seats.

Diagnosis: Your doctor will take a sample of your vaginal discharge and send it to a laboratory for analysis.

Treatment: Antibiotic treatment, either by pill or injection, is used to treat gonorrhea. Any recent sexual partners also should be tested and, if necessary, treated to prevent reinfection. Avoid all sexual contact until the infection is cured.

Outlook: If left untreated, gonorrhea can cause serious problems. In women, PELVIC INFLAMMATORY DISEASE can cause permanent damage and infertility. Pregnant women can infect their babies' eyes during birth, causing serious eye problems or even blindness. In both sexes, long-term untreated gonorrhea can cause debilitating arthritis or bacteremia, a potentially life-threatening blood infection.

Tips: Using a condom can reduce, but not eliminate, the risk of contracting a sexually transmitted disease. Never have sexual relations with a man who has a penile discharge.

HEMORRHOIDS are structures containing blood vessels and other tissues, located in the lower rectum and anus. They are also known as piles or anal varicose veins. When hemorrhoids cause pain, it is usually because of ulceration or blood clot formation.

Symptoms: Hemorrhoids may cause rectal pain, rectal bleeding, protrusion of the veins from the anus, mucus discharge, or a sensation of incomplete evacuation after a bowel movement.

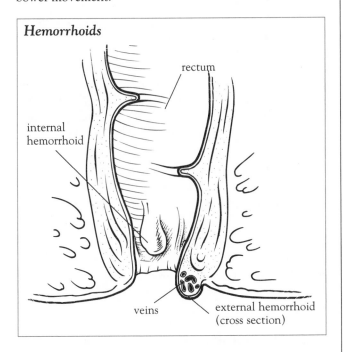

Hemorrhoids

rectum

internal hemorrhoid

veins

external hemorrhoid (cross section)

Causes: Painful hemorrhoids are usually caused by straining to move the bowels, which often occurs when you are constipated, obese, or pregnant. External hemorrhoids also may be provoked by a sedentary job, prolonged standing, or frequent diarrhea.

Diagnosis: Hemorrhoids can be identified by physical examination. If external hemorrhoids are found, your doctor may insert a hollow tube into your rectum to check for internal hemorrhoids as well.

Treatment: Many hemorrhoids can be treated by rubber-band ligation, which has eliminated most hemorrhoid surgery. A small elastic band is slipped around the internal hemorrhoid, cutting off its blood supply. With little or no pain, the hemorrhoid falls off in 4 to 14 days. Other hemorrhoids may be treated with injections or destroyed by freezing. Surgery is usually reserved for prolapsed, strangulated, and swollen hemorrhoids that cause severe pain.

Outlook: If left alone, some hemorrhoids heal themselves. Severely painful hemorrhoids can be removed. However, if the underlying cause is not alleviated, they often recur. A healthy diet, including plenty of fiber from fruits, vegetables, and grains, as well as 6 to 8 glasses of fluid daily, can relieve constipation, which helps to alleviate or prevent hemorrhoids.

Tips: To ease minor hemorrhoid discomfort, sit in a warm bath, apply witch hazel compresses, and use stool softeners to prevent constipation. Over-the-counter preparations containing cortisone may alleviate itching and pain.

HERPES refers to two common viral diseases. Herpes 1 commonly occurs around the mouth, where the blisters are called cold sores or fever blisters. Herpes 2 causes sores in the genital area.

Symptoms: In herpes 1, painful, itchy blisters or small bumps usually appear on or near the mouth. They may also occur on the eyelid, causing the lid to swell, or in the eye itself, which results in eye discharge, light sensitivity, and decreased vision. In herpes 2, sores appear inside the vagina or on the labia, on the penis, and/or in or around the anus, thighs, or buttocks in both sexes. If you have had oral sex with a person infected with herpes 2, you may develop blisters around your mouth that can be difficult to differentiate from those of herpes 1.

Within one to several days, blisters erupt into open sores; those around the mouth form yellowish crusts. With a first attack of herpes, fever, enlarged lymph nodes, and flulike symptoms may occur. Sometimes attacks may be preceded by a "prodrome," tingling or burning sensations that may or may not lead to a full-blown attack. Sores eventually heal by themselves, usually within a few weeks. But the virus remains in the body. Some people may never have another attack; others may suffer repeated eruptions, though much less severe, every few weeks or months for years.

Causes: Herpes 1 is caused by the herpes simplex 1 virus, and more than half of all Americans have been infected with it by the age of 14. Herpes 2 is caused by the herpes simplex 2 virus. Both viruses are highly contagious and are spread by physical contact. It is believed that the viruses spreads very easily when the sores are open.

Diagnosis: Herpes can be diagnosed by its characteristic appearance. Laboratory evaluation of a smear taken from the base of one of the sores can confirm the diagnosis. A blood test for herpes antibodies may be helpful in some cases.

Treatment: There is no known cure. Most herpes 1 sores disappear within a few days. In more severe cases, or in recurrent herpes 2, a drug called Acyclovir, which helps control recurrences and shorten attacks dramatically, is given topically or orally. Another drug, idoxuridine, may be prescribed for eye lesions. Other prescription medications can help ease the discomfort of herpes 2 and prevent infection of open sores.

Outlook: Once you are infected with these viruses, recurrences can happen at any time. Wash your hands after touching the sores to avoid spreading the infection to other parts of your body. Herpes 1 that affects the eye can threaten your vision if not treated promptly. Women infected with herpes 2 may have a slightly increased risk for cervical cancer and should have regular PAP TESTS. If you have active herpes 2 during labor, a cesarean section may be recommended to prevent the baby from being exposed to the virus during vaginal birth.

Tips: If you have recurrent sores in your vaginal area, see a physician immediately. Herpes 1 attacks may be triggered by stress, sunburn, or other environmental factors. If you experience a prodrome before an outbreak of herpes 1, prompt use of aspirin and ice packs sometimes forestalls recurrence. When lesions appear, cold compresses may ease discomfort. To protect others from infection, avoid kissing anyone or sharing dishes or utensils while you are infected. For herpes 2, warm baths or saltwater compresses sometimes alleviate the inflammation. Do not have sexual intercourse during an attack. Tell any prospective sexual partner that you are infected with herpes 2. Using a latex condom may lower but cannot banish the risk of transmitting the infection.

HYPERTHYROIDISM refers to any condition in which too much thyroxine, the thyroid hormone, is produced in your body. One of the most common conditions is called Graves' disease.

Symptoms: Depending on the severity of the thyroxine excess, you may experience nervousness, irritability, or mood swings; increased sweating; increased hunger and thirst but continuing weight loss (although 30 percent of women with Graves' disease gain weight); fatigue; insomnia; hair loss; rapid heartbeat; trembling; more frequent and loose bowel movements; and muscle weakness. Women may notice a decrease in their menstrual flow and less frequent menstruation. In Graves' disease, your eyes may seem larger or appear to bulge. You may develop a swelling, called a goiter, in the lower front of your neck.

Causes: Different types of hyperthyroidism have different causes. Graves' disease, also known as diffuse toxic goiter, is caused by an autoimmune disorder that triggers overactivity of the entire thyroid. Thyroiditis is an inflammation of the thyroid gland. In other cases, only one or a few thyroid nodules become inflamed, for unknown reasons. Hyperthyroidism also may be caused by overtreatment of HYPOTHYROIDISM.

Diagnosis: Blood tests can assess your thyroxine level and determine whether the problem derives from abnormal activity of the thyroid gland itself or from oversecretion of thyroid-stimulating hormone (TSH) by the pituitary gland. A thyroid scan can help identify the underlying cause.

Treatment: Therapy depends on your age, physical condition, and the cause and severity of the disorder. Beta-blocker medications, such as propranolol, are often prescribed immediately to decrease irritation and palpita-

tions within hours, but such drugs do not treat the underlying problem. For Graves' disease, radioactive iodine therapy is most commonly prescribed. You swallow a capsule or liquid containing radioactive iodine and, because the thyroid needs iodine to make hormones, it absorbs the substance. Over the next few weeks, the radioactive material damages some thyroid cells, causing them to shrink and reduce their hormone output, and then the iodine is eliminated from the body. Sometimes a second dose is needed if the thyroid gland is resistant to treatment.

In other cases, the thyroid gland may be very sensitive to treatment so that too much tissue is destroyed and thyroid hormone replacement is necessary. Because this treatment is not precise, your thyroxine levels must be monitored for the rest of your life. Children, pregnant women, and others with special problems may be unable to take radioactive iodine therapy. They must take antithyroid drugs or have all or part of the thyroid gland surgically removed.

Outlook: If you are alert to subtle bodily changes and get prompt medical care, hyperthyroidism can be easily treated. If not treated, it can lead to a sudden explosion of symptoms, called thyroid storm, that can cause cardiovascular collapse and death.

Tips: If you have hyperthyroidism, get regular medical checkups. Life-style changes may require modification of your medication dosage. Subtle feelings of illness may signal a problem.

HYPOTHYROIDISM, also called myxedema, refers to a deficiency of thyroxine, the thyroid hormone.

Symptoms: Depending on the severity of the hormone deficiency, you may experience a few or many of the following: progressive fatigue and lethargy, muscle aches, constipation, increased sensitivity to cold, decreased appetite but continued weight gain, dry skin and facial puffiness, hair loss, decreased sexual drive, deepened voice, impaired reflexes, numbness or tingling in your feet and hands, heavier than normal menstrual flow, and psychological problems.

Causes: The most common type of hypothyroidism is due to Hashimoto's disease, an autoimmune disorder that leads to inflammation of the thyroid gland. Hypothyroidism may also be caused by congenital problems, pituitary disorders, or iodine deficiency, although the latter is rare in the United States because iodine is added to most table salt. It may also be caused by overtreatment of HYPERTHYROIDISM.

Diagnosis: Blood tests can assess your thyroxine level and help determine the source of the problem. If no underlying disorder is found, Hashimoto's disease will be diagnosed.

Treatment: Therapy requires a daily dose of synthetic thyroxine. Unless a treatable underlying cause is found and corrected, you must take thyroxine for the rest of your life.

Outlook: If you are alert to subtle bodily changes and get prompt medical care, hypothyroidism can be easily treated. Otherwise, it can lead to myxedema coma, in which your body temperature drops markedly, breathing is depressed, circulation to the brain is impaired, and you lose consciousness.

Tips: If you have hypothyroidism, get regular medical checkups. Life-style changes may require modification of your medication dosage. Subtle feelings of illness may signal a problem.

HYSTERECTOMY is the surgical removal of the uterus. It is most often performed to treat UTERINE CANCER, although it may also be used in cases of very large fibroids, severe ENDOMETRIOSIS, and other gynecological problems. Hysterectomy is major surgery, requiring general anesthesia, 3 to 7 days of hospitalization, and 1 to 2 months of recuperation.

Procedure: A vertical or horizontal incision is made in the lower abdomen. In supracervical hysterectomy, the uterus is removed, but not the cervix. In total hysterectomy, both the uterus and the cervix are removed. In total hysterectomy with bilateral salpingo-oophorectomy, the Fallopian tubes and ovaries are also removed. If cancer is present, nearby lymph nodes may be removed as well to determine if cancer has spread beyond the uterus. In some cases of benign disease, hysterectomy may be done through the vagina or with the help of a laparoscope. These methods allow a shorter hospital stay and quicker recovery.

Risks and complications: Bleeding and infection are possible complications. Also, as in any abdominal surgery, adjacent organs (such as the intestines, bladder, or ureters) may become injured. Call your doctor right away if vaginal bleeding soaks more than one sanitary pad in an hour, or if you have increased abdominal swelling, pain, fever, headache, dizziness, or muscle aches.

Results: After hysterectomy, you will no longer menstruate or be able to conceive and bear children. You will not, however, experience menopause unless your ovaries are removed (see OOPHORECTOMY). You may resume normal sexual relations within 4 to 6 weeks.

Outlook: If pain or abnormal bleeding prompted the surgery, you should experience relief after recovery. If cancer necessitated the surgery, the long-term outlook depends on the type of cancer and whether it has spread beyond the uterus. When the cancer has spread, radiation or chemotherapy are usually necessary.

Tips: Always get a second opinion before agreeing to any surgery. For information about new therapies and experts in your community, call the National Cancer Institute at 1-800-4-CANCER.

HYSTEROSALPINGOGRAM, also called uterotubography or uterosalpingography, is a test performed primarily to evaluate the Fallopian tubes, although it also reveals information about the uterus. It is most often performed as part of an infertility workup, but may also be used to find polyps, fibroids, or developmental abnormalities.

Procedure: You recline on an examining table as for a routine pelvic examination, in a darkened room with an X-ray machine suspended over you. The radiologist or gynecologist opens your vagina with a speculum, and grasps your cervix and holds it in place with an instrument called a tenaculum. Then a very thin catheter is inserted through your cervix into your uterus. A radio-opaque dye, injected through the catheter into your uterus, spreads up into your Fallopian tubes. X rays then track the path of the dye as it spreads. The procedure takes about 15 to 30 minutes.

Results: The doctor may be able to read the X rays before you leave.

Risks and complications: The dye causes intense uterine contractions that feel like menstrual cramps but last only 5 to 10 minutes. If your tubes are blocked, you may feel some additional pain and the tubes may go into spasm. A serious, but rare, risk is an allergic reaction to the iodine dye. Notify your doctor beforehand if you are allergic to shellfish or iodine. Some women may develop PELVIC INFLAMMATORY DISEASE after the procedure.

Hysterectomy

uterus

lymph nodes

Fallopian tubes

normal

supracervical

total with bilateral salpingo-oophrectomy

total

lymph node sampling

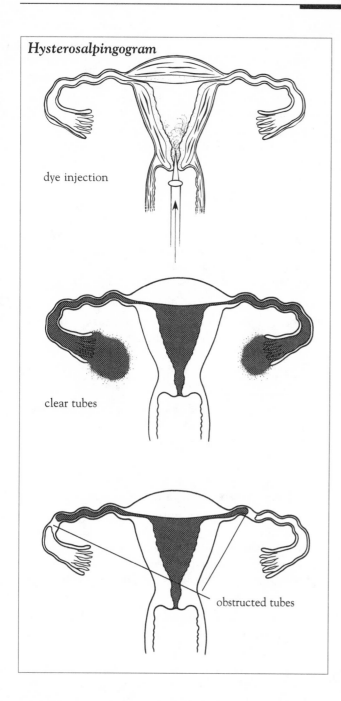

Hysterosalpingogram

dye injection

clear tubes

obstructed tubes

Tips: If your gynecologist recommends several doctors for this procedure, ask previous patients what their experiences were. The doctor's skill and gentleness can make a real difference in your comfort level. Ask if you can take a mild pain-killer or antispasmodic a half hour before the test to lessen cramps. Wear a sanitary napkin for 24 hours after the procedure, and report any excessive bleeding or odor to your doctor right away.

IRRITABLE BOWEL SYNDROME (IBS) is a disorder in which the rhythmic muscle contractions that normally move waste through the intestines are replaced by irregular contractions that cause discomfort as well as diarrhea and/or constipation. Women are affected three times as often as men.

Symptoms: For some people, the primary symptom is painless but urgent diarrhea that usually occurs upon awakening or during or immediately after a meal. For others, constipation is the biggest problem. Still others suffer from alternating bouts of diarrhea and constipation along with abdominal pain, cramps, bloating, and nausea. Other symptoms include fatigue, anxiety, headache, and depression.

Cause: While the cause of IBS is unknown, stress, emotional conflict, or dietary factors may aggravate it.

Diagnosis: There is no single test capable of identifying IBS. It is diagnosed by excluding all other possible causes of your symptoms, such as Crohn's disease, ulcerative colitis, and colorectal cancer. You may require extensive testing. Evaluation often includes blood tests, laboratory examination of your stools, special X rays, and colonoscopy. In the latter procedure, a flexible, hollow tube is inserted into your rectum and passed through the colon, allowing it to be visualized and biopsied if necessary.

Treatment: Dietary modification is the mainstay of treatment. If constipation is more severe than diarrhea, eat a high-fiber diet with plenty of fresh fruits and vegetables and whole grains. If diarrhea is more severe than constipation, or if a high-fiber diet makes your symptoms worse, try eating a bland, low-fiber diet. Your doctor may also prescribe a short-term course of anticholinergic drugs to help alleviate abnormal muscle contractions. Other drugs, such as mild sedatives or antidepressants, may be prescribed if anxiety or depression is severe.

Outlook: Although dietary and life-style changes can reduce your symptoms, IBS is very unpredictable. Symptoms may persist throughout life, disappear permanently, or come and go without warning.

Tips: Keep a diary of the foods you eat and other life-style factors to help you identify and avoid foods or situations that exacerbate IBS. Learn relaxation techniques to lower your stress levels.

LAPAROSCOPY, also known as pelvic endoscopy, is a diagnostic procedure that enables the doctor to see your internal abdominal and pelvic area without major surgery. It may be ordered to evaluate chronic pelvic pain, ENDOMETRIOSIS, or ovarian cysts or tumors. Tiny surgical tools are used to take tissue samples for biopsy and perform some therapeutic procedures, such as tubal ligation for sterilization, removing an ECTOPIC PREGNANCY, or aspirating fluid from a cyst.

Procedure: Laparoscopy is usually performed under general anesthesia in a hospital ambulatory surgery department; in some cases, you may stay overnight. You have nothing to eat or drink after midnight the night before. Once the anesthesia takes effect, the table is tilted so that your head is lower than your pelvis, and a small incision

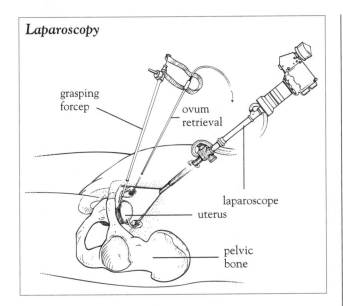

Laparoscopy

grasping
forcep

ovum
retrieval

laparoscope

uterus

pelvic
bone

resides. Other terms used for this surgery, such as "segmental" or "partial mastectomy," are less descriptive of exactly how much tissue is being removed. Breast conservation surgery is always followed by radiation therapy to the remaining breast tissue. The treatments are generally given 5 days a week for 6 to 7 weeks.

If the cancer is an invasive type (see BREAST CANCER), lymph nodes under the arm are also removed to check the possibility of metastasis (spread). This procedure, done in

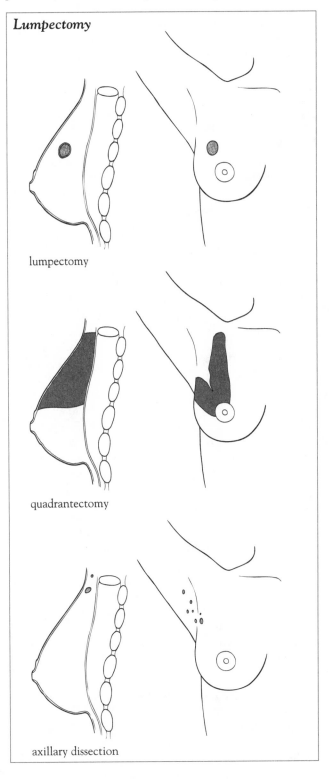

Lumpectomy

lumpectomy

quadrantectomy

axillary dissection

is made just below your navel. Carbon dioxide gas is pumped into your abdomen to provide the doctor with a better view, and the small, rigid laparoscope is inserted through the incision. Other small incisions in the lower abdomen may be made to insert tiny surgical tools. If necessary, tissue samples are taken for laboratory examination. Once the procedure is performed, the gas is allowed to escape and the incision is closed with a few stitches. The procedure lasts about 30 to 60 minutes, depending on what is done. When you awaken, expect some abdominal soreness, cramps, and the lightheadedness and discomfort generally felt after having general anesthesia.

Risks and complications: Any carbon dioxide left in the abdomen may cause so-called referred pain, which is felt in one or both shoulders, but the gas should be absorbed within a day or two. There is a very small risk of excessive bleeding and infection.

Results: Your doctor can tell you about what was visually observed as soon as you are awake. Laboratory analysis of any tissue samples taken should be available within a few days.

Tips: Laparoscopy is also known as "Band-Aid" surgery for the dressing that covers the tiny incision afterward. Do not wet the incision or remove the bandage for a day or two. Take aspirin or ibuprofen for cramps.

LUMPECTOMY, the most common type of breast conservation treatment, is the surgical removal of a cancerous mass in the breast and a margin of tissue surrounding it. It is generally used to treat breast cancer when the tumor is small.

Procedure: There are several approaches to breast conservation therapy. Lumpectomy is the removal of only the cancerous mass and a small margin of healthy tissue around it; quadrantectomy is a more aggressive approach that removes the tumor and the quarter of the breast in which it conjunction with the breast surgery, is known as axillary dissection. Although lumpectomy or quadrantectomy alone may be performed as an outpatient procedure under local anesthesia, the axillary dissection requires general anesthesia and is considered major surgery. Breast conservation surgery requires 1½ to 2 hours in the operating room and 2 to 3 weeks' recuperation.

When the excised lymph nodes are positive, indicating that the cancer has spread beyond the breast, or if the nodes are negative but features of the tumor indicate a high risk of spread, systemic treatment is necessary. Systemic treatment is either chemotherapy, administered orally or by intravenous injections, or hormone therapy. Because the growth of some types of breast cancer cells is stimulated by the hormone estrogen, antiestrogens such as tamoxifen are used to inhibit the proliferation of these cells.

Risks and complications: Complications following breast conservation surgery are unusual. Dissection of the lymph nodes can interrupt lymph drainage and may result in arm swelling if there is injury to the arm at any time after the operation. Consequently, care must be taken to avoid injury if the lymph nodes have been removed.

Results: When the tumor is small and localized, long-term survival rates are excellent. There is no difference in survival between those who have a lumpectomy or quadrantectomy followed by radiation and those who have a MASTECTOMY. In a small percentage of patients, radiation therapy will not kill all of the cancer cells and there may be a recurrence of the tumor in the original site. Although mastectomy will then be necessary, this recurrence does not affect survival rates.

Lumpectomy with radiation is appropriate treatment for most breast cancers, but the tumor must be small enough to be removed with a good cosmetic result. The size of an appropriate tumor will depend on the size of the breast: A large tumor in a small breast is not appropriate. Other exceptions include multiple tumors within a breast or a very diffuse tumor that cannot be removed with a clear margin of healthy tissue.

Tips: Always get a second opinion before agreeing to any surgery. For information about new therapies and experts in your community, call the National Cancer Institute at 1-800-4-CANCER. If you are being treated for breast cancer, you can ask your surgeon for a referral to Reach to Recovery, a program of the American Cancer Society, through which volunteers arrange hospital visits for moral support and give practical tips on dealing with breast cancer surgery.

LUPUS refers to systemic lupus erythematosus (SLE) and discoid lupus erythematosus (DLE), both of which are chronic rheumatic diseases. Lupus strikes women about ten times as often as men. It is most likely to occur in young adults in their twenties and thirties, although it can develop at any time from infancy through old age. Although both types of lupus are mild diseases for many people, SLE can be serious and even life-threatening.

Symptoms: Lupus is a highly variable disease. While the most common symptoms of SLE are fatigue and joint pain, there are many different patterns. You also may have a skin rash, a low-grade fever, hair loss, weakness, weight loss, dry mouth, muscle aches, swollen glands, loss of appetite, nausea, and mouth ulcers. DLE primarily affects the skin. About half of all people with systemic lupus develop a butterfly-shaped rash over the nose and cheeks. It may range from a blush to mild scaliness to a blistery eruption. Symptoms may worsen after exposure to the sun. SLE also may cause severe headaches, anemia, inflammation in the lining of the heart or lungs, and kidney problems.

Causes: The precise causes of lupus remain unknown. However, it is believed that there may be a genetic predisposition to the disorder, which is then triggered by a virus or some other environmental factor. Lupus is an autoimmune disease in which your immune system runs amok. Connective tissue throughout your body is attacked as if it were a foreign invader.

Diagnosis: See a rheumatologist for diagnosis of any problem involving joint pain and stiffness. Lupus can be difficult to spot because of its highly variable symptoms. An important part of a diagnostic evaluation are blood tests to determine whether your body is producing antibodies to your own tissue.

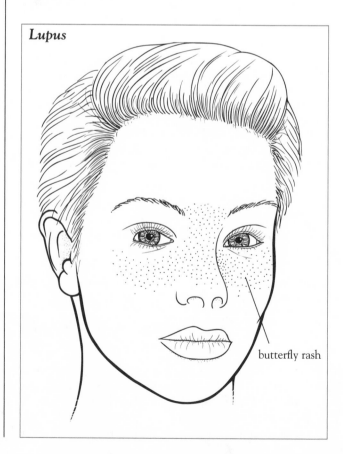

Lupus

butterfly rash

Treatment: You and your doctor may have to experiment with several drug regimens over a period of months to find the right one for you. A relatively mild case of lupus may be controlled with aspirin or other nonsteroidal antiinflammatory drugs (NSAIDs) to suppress inflammation. Antimalarial drugs can increase your resistance to sun exposure and help prevent rashes and joint pain. For more severe problems, your doctor may prescribe prednisone, a potent antiinflammatory medication, or drugs used in transplant medicine to suppress the action of the immune system. Because these drugs have potentially severe side effects, you must be frequently monitored.

Outlook: Although lupus cannot be cured, most patients can lead normal lives with proper treatment tailored to their symptoms. Symptoms may come and go without any clear reason. After some years, the disease may vanish in some people or become severe or even life-threatening in others.

Tips: To lessen fatigue, get enough sleep at night and balance your day with one or more half-hour breaks between periods of activity. To lessen stress, which can trigger flareups, learn relaxation techniques. If your symptoms are worsened by the sun, avoid exposure in midday and always use sunscreens and brimmed hats when you go out. Aspirin and NSAIDs must be taken with meals to help prevent stomach irritation. Because dry mouth increases your risk of caries and gum disease, practice scrupulous dental care.

MASTECTOMY is the surgical removal of the entire breast and sometimes the lymph tissue under the arm and is the most common treatment for BREAST CANCER.

Procedure: In all forms of mastectomy, all of the breast tissue, including the nipple skin, is removed. If the cancer is a noninvasive type, lymph nodes need not be removed, in which case the procedure is called a simple, or total, mastectomy. If the cancer is invasive and the lymph nodes must be removed, the operation is called a modified radical mastectomy. The outdated radical mastectomy (sometimes called a Halsted procedure) removes the breast, all adjacent armpit lymph nodes, and the pectoral muscle on the chest wall. This operation is more disfiguring and is now thought to be unnecessary, since it does not improve survival. Mastectomies require general anesthesia, 2 to 3 hours in the operating room, and about a month of recuperation.

Breast reconstruction can be done at the same time as mastectomy or at any time later on. (See Chapter 14, "Breast Care.") If reconstruction is not done, the skin is closed in a way that will produce a straight-line, horizontal scar on the chest wall, resembling the flat chest of a child without a nipple.

Risks and complications: Complications following a mastectomy are unusual. Dissection of the lymph nodes can interrupt lymph drainage and may result in arm swelling

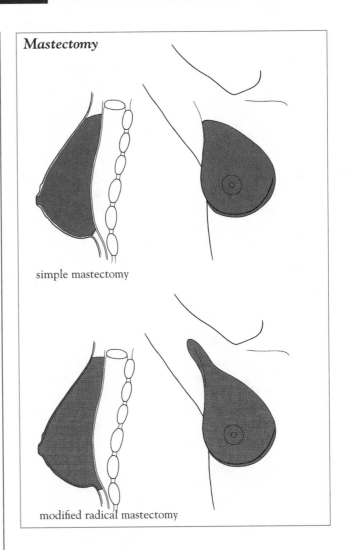

Mastectomy

simple mastectomy

modified radical mastectomy

if there is injury to the arm at any time after the operation. Consequently, care must be taken to avoid injury if the lymph nodes have been removed.

Results: Long-term outlook depends on the type of cancer and whether it has metastasized (spread). If the excised lymph nodes are positive, indicating that the cancer has spread beyond the breast, or if the nodes are negative but features of the tumor indicate a high risk of spread, systemic treatment is necessary. Systemic treatment is either chemotherapy, administered orally or by intravenous injections, or hormone therapy. Because the growth of some types of breast cancer cells is stimulated by the hormone estrogen, antiestrogens such as tamoxifen are used to inhibit the proliferation of these cells.

Tips: Always get a second opinion before agreeing to any surgery. For information about new therapies and experts in your community, call the National Cancer Institute at 1-800-4-CANCER. If you are being treated for breast cancer, you can ask your surgeon for a referral to Reach to Recovery, a program of the American Cancer Society, through which volunteers arrange hospital visits for moral support and give practical tips on dealing with mastectomy.

MIGRAINES are severe and debilitating vascular headaches that afflict women two to three times as often as men. Of the 20 million Americans who suffer with migraines, about 60 percent have a family history of the condition and more than 60 percent are women of childbearing age who usually get these headaches before, during, and just after they menstruate.

Symptoms: Migraines cause excruciating, throbbing pain that usually affects only one side of the head. They may be accompanied by nausea and vomiting, dizziness, tremor, pallor, perspiration, cold hands, and sensitivity to light or sound. In common migraines, the pain hits with no warning. In 20 to 30 percent of cases, called classic migraines, an "aura" starts 5 to 30 minutes before pain occurs. The aura may include visual symptoms, such as flickering lights, jagged lines, or obstructions in the field of vision; tingling or numbness in the face, hands, or feet; speech impairment; and a sense of confusion.

Causes: Although the cause of migraines is not fully understood, the neurochemical serotonin seems to play a pivotal role. When serotonin is released into blood vessels, they narrow. When it is excreted by the kidneys, the vessels widen. When serotonin goes into overdrive, it leads to a rhythmic cycle of constriction and dilation in the blood vessels of the scalp, which produces throbbing pain.

Diagnosis: Your doctor may conduct a number of tests, possibly including special X rays or magnetic resonance imaging of your brain, to rule out other possible causes of your headaches. You may be referred to a neurologist or headache specialist.

Treatment: Therapy may include prophylactic drugs taken daily to prevent attacks completely or decrease their frequency, abortive therapy drugs taken at the beginning of an aura or headache to cut short the attack, and symptomatic drugs that treat migraine symptoms. Among the prophylactic drugs prescribed are beta-blockers, calcium channel blockers, antidepressants, ergot preparations, anticonvulsants, aspirin and other nonsteroidal antiinflammatory agents (NSAIDs). Abortive therapy drugs include ergot preparations, NSAIDs, and sumitriptin. Symptomatic drugs include some of those used for abortive therapy as well as antinauseants and narcotic pain-killers.

Outlook: Although experimentation is necessary to find which therapy is best for you, you can expect treatment at least to decrease the frequency and severity of migraine attacks. Many women have no headaches during pregnancy. Menopause may bring a cessation or a worsening of headaches. Oral contraceptives and postmenopausal estrogen replacement therapy may make headaches worse— or may make them better.

Tips: Chart your headaches to determine what provokes them and then eliminate those factors from your life. Certain known migraine triggers are stress; low blood sugar, which may result from irregular meal schedules; inadequate sleep or frequent changes in sleep habits; smoking or exposure to secondary smoke; exposure to certain chemicals and odors, such as insecticides and perfumes; travel to high altitudes; drugs containing amines, such as nitroglycerine, lithium, certain bronchodilating, antiinflammatory, and high blood pressure medications; and some over-the-counter sinus and cold formulas.

Potential food triggers are ripe cheeses; citrus fruits; chocolate; red wine and other forms of alcohol; caffeinated beverages; processed meats, such as salami, bologna, and frankfurters; snow peas, lima and navy beans, lentils, onions, and avocados; and food additives such as nitrates, nitrites, meat tenderizers, and monosodium glutamate (MSG). Sometimes you can ward off an oncoming migraine by drinking a cup of strong coffee or tea, taking an aspirin or ibuprofen, and lying down in a darkened room.

MISCARRIAGE, also called spontaneous abortion, is the natural termination of a pregnancy before the fetus is able to live independently outside the uterus. About one pregnancy in five ends in a miscarriage, usually during the first trimester.

Symptoms: Bleeding or a brownish discharge from the vagina, sometimes accompanied by cramps or pain in the lower abdomen or back, is the main sign of a threatened miscarriage.

Causes: Miscarriage is usually prompted by a problem in fetal development. If fertilization occurred toward the end of the 24-hour period after ovulation, the egg may have been "stale," which can lead to improper development. Improper early development of the embryo is probably the major cause of miscarriage. Other causes include faulty attachment of the placenta to the uterus, uterine structural defects, maternal hormone imbalance, maternal infection, and complications of other diseases, such as DIABETES. Often, the cause of a miscarriage is never identified.

Diagnosis: When bleeding is heavy and solid, it is presumed that a miscarriage has occurred. ULTRASOUND may be used to confirm it.

Treatment: When minor bleeding occurs in the absence of pain, you may merely have to restrict your activity, go to bed and avoid sexual intercourse and strenuous exercise, for the threatened miscarriage to abate. However, when a true miscarriage has begun, little can be done to prevent it. A miscarriage is often nature's way of preventing a baby with serious health problems from being born. If the miscarriage is not complete, the uterus may have to be suctioned to remove remaining fetal and placental material.

Outlook: If the bleeding is no heavier than your normal menstrual flow and if there is no pain, the fetus may yet develop properly. If the uterus continues to grow normally, it means the baby is probably developing normally. One miscarriage does not mean that your next pregnancy will be threatened. In most cases, a miscarriage happens only once. If you miscarry more than once, you should get a complete evaluation from a specialist before considering another pregnancy. If a treatable cause is diagnosed, steps may be taken to prevent future miscarriages.

Tips: Vaginal bleeding during the early months of pregnancy does not always signal the onset of miscarriage, but you should always report it to your doctor immediately.

MITRAL VALVE PROLAPSE is a disorder caused by the abnormal structure and function of one of the four valves that control blood flow through the heart. The mitral valve controls the passage of freshly oxygenated blood from the lungs as it passes from the left atrium (an upper heart chamber) into the left ventricle (a lower heart chamber). When the valve is prolapsed, one or both of the flaps that open and close to control the flow bulge backward

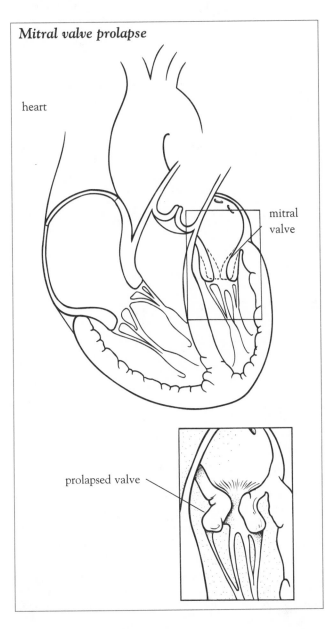

Mitral valve prolapse

heart

mitral valve

prolapsed valve

into the atrium with each heartbeat. As a result, a small amount of blood heading for the ventricle regurgitates, or leaks backward. Depending on the extent of the regurgitation, the heart may have to work harder to pump out enough blood to the body.

Symptoms: Most people have no symptoms. Others experience palpitations, shortness of breath, and chest pains.

Causes: Although the cause is unknown, it is usually present at birth. It occurs more often in women and is particularly common in those who have Marfan's syndrome, scoliosis, and other skeletal abnormalities.

Diagnosis: By listening to your heart with a stethoscope, your doctor can often hear a characteristic clicking sound and, possibly, a heart murmur. To evaluate the sounds and any symptoms, a chest X ray, an electrocardiogram, and an echocardiogram may be required.

Treatment: If you have no symptoms, no treatment is needed. If symptoms occur, your doctor may prescribe beta-blocking drugs to slow your heart rate. If prolapse is severe, you may be advised to avoid strenuous competitive sports.

Outlook: Serious complications are rare. However, you may have a greater risk of bacterial endocarditis (an infection of the heart lining), blood clot formation leading to a stroke, and an irregular heart arrhythmia called ventricular tachycardia. It is unclear whether the risk of other types of stroke is increased.

Tips: If you have severe mitral valve prolapse, ask your doctor about taking antibiotics before any dental extractions or surgery to help protect you from endocarditis. If you are over 45, ask your doctor about taking aspirin every other day to help prevent blood clots.

MULTIPLE SCLEROSIS (MS) is a nervous system disorder in which myelin, a protective coating that surrounds nerves, is destroyed, thus short-circuiting messages traveling to and from the brain. Movement, sensation, vision, balance, speech, and other bodily functions can be impaired as a result. MS usually starts between the ages of 20 and 40, but it can occur at any age. Six out of every ten victims are women.

Symptoms: These vary widely and may come and go. Symptoms commonly include partial or complete paralysis of parts of the body; numbness or prickling "pins and needles" sensations in the arms and legs; noticeable dragging of one or both feet; loss of bladder or bowel control; loss of balance; extreme weakness or fatigue; hand tremors; blurred or double vision; blindness or pain in one or both eyes; dizziness; facial pain; difficulty speaking; and psychological changes, such as mood swings, apathy, and poor judgment.

Causes: The cause of MS is not clearly understood. An immunological abnormality or viral infection may be involved. Environmental factors may also play a role, because MS is far more common in temperate climates than in the tropics.

Diagnosis: Diagnosis is hampered by the variability of symptoms. It can be made only after all other possible causes of your symptoms have been ruled out. Evaluation may include blood tests, a spinal tap, and brain scans. Special tests measuring the speed at which nerve impulses travel can also be helpful.

Treatment: MS cannot be cured, but drugs that suppress inflammation (such as steroids) may reduce the severity of attacks. Immunosuppressive drugs are sometimes used and may help prevent relapses. Treatment to help you maintain your strength for withstanding attacks may include getting extra rest, eating a well-balanced diet, and preserving muscle function through physical therapy.

Outlook: The course of MS can vary dramatically. MS is often associated with dramatic exacerbations and remissions. You may have symptom-free periods lasting weeks or months between flareups, especially in the early years of the disease. Although MS may be a chronic and slowly progressive disease in some people, it can be rapidly debilitating in others.

Tips: Get plenty of rest. Avoid physical and emotional stress, which can provoke flareups.

OBSESSIVE-COMPULSIVE DISORDER (OCD) is an anxiety disorder that is characterized by excessively repetitive thinking or behavior. About 4 million Americans are believed to suffer from OCD.

Symptoms: People who have compulsions repeat certain behaviors according to irrational inner rules. Some compulsives wash their hands dozens of times a day, or constantly check to make sure they have turned off the stove. The behavior is designed to prevent some dreaded situation, but the actions and fears are not realistic and the response is excessive. Affected people may or may not recognize the unreasonableness of their compulsions.

People who have obsessions have recurrent and persistent thoughts, impulses, or images that seem senseless. Some may think about killing a loved family member. Or an otherwise religious person is possessed by blasphemous thoughts. These people are unable to ignore or suppress what they feel. Obsessions or compulsions may be linked to chaotic feelings about sex, anger, or death, but they become all-consuming. Less severe forms of compulsive behavior that do not meet the criteria for OCD are reflected in the workaholic who never relaxes, the inflexible individual who believes his or her ideas are always right, or the timid soul who tends to avoid new situations because of fear of making mistakes.

Causes: Like most psychological illnesses, the causes of OCD are unknown. The disorder most likely stems from childhood, when learning to perform simple tasks repeatedly provides a sense of safety. If stress becomes overwhelming, some people seek emotional security by retreating to the same types of repetitiveness. Biological factors may also play a role.

Diagnosis: There are no special tests to identify OCD, but it can usually be assessed by a psychiatrist based on a short discussion. Among the key elements of diagnosis are that the obsessions or compulsions are upsetting to the person, that they take up more than an hour a day, and that they interfere with work or social relationships.

Treatment: Both therapy and medication are helpful, and are sometimes used in combination. In psychotherapy the patient talks about feelings and experiences so that the therapist can help him or her understand the obsessions or compulsions, their possible causes, and how to control them. In behavioral therapy, the counselor can help modify the rituals without necessarily dealing with the underlying causes; this type of therapy may include oral or written "contracts" between therapist and client to reduce specific behaviors gradually. In severe cases, psychoactive medications, such as fluoxetine or clomipramine, may be prescribed.

Outlook: OCD can take all the joy out of life by filling up so much time with ritualistic thoughts or behaviors. Early therapy may improve the outcome because all behavior patterns tend to become more rigid with age.

Tips: You may be able to reduce the likelihood of a child's developing this disorder if you encourage flexibility, praise creative efforts, and avoid drawing undue attention to life's dangers.

OOPHORECTOMY is the surgical removal of one or both ovaries. When the Fallopian tubes are removed as well, the procedure is called salpingo-oophorectomy. It may be performed to treat benign ovarian tumors or OVARIAN CANCER. When ovarian cancer is present, the procedure is usually performed in conjunction with HYSTERECTOMY. Oophorectomy is major surgery, requiring general anesthesia, 3 to 7 days of hospitalization, and 1 to 2 months of recuperation. In cases where the ovary or ovaries are removed by a laparoscope, hospitalization may be as little as one day and the recovery period is much shorter.

Procedure: A vertical or horizontal incision is made in the lower abdomen. The organs to be removed are cut free from surrounding tissue. If there is any question about the extent of the cancer or whether a tumor is benign or cancerous, tissue samples are sent to the pathology laboratory for analysis and the surgeon receives a report before proceeding. In many cases, nearby lymph nodes are often removed, too, in order to assess whether cancer has spread

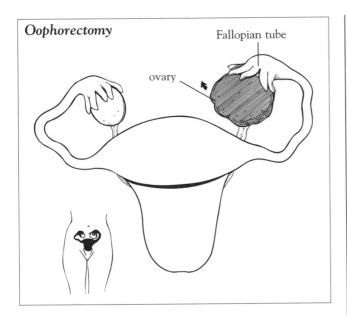

Oophorectomy

Fallopian tube

ovary

---

beyond the reproductive organs. The incision is closed with sutures that dissolve or with staples or sutures that must be removed 4 to 7 days after surgery.

Risks and complications: Abnormal bleeding and infection at the incision site are possible complications. Call your doctor right away if you experience anything more than minor vaginal bleeding, any increased abdominal swelling or pain, fever, headache, dizziness, or muscle aches.

Results: If both ovaries are removed, you will enter menopause immediately. This may precipitate a wide array of intense symptoms, including hot flashes and insomnia. Whether you are a candidate for estrogen replacement therapy to ease such symptoms may depend on why you had to have the surgery.

Outlook: If cancer was the reason for your surgery, the long-term outlook depends on the type of cancer and whether it has spread beyond the uterus. When the cancer has spread, radiation or chemotherapy are usually necessary.

Tips: Always get a second opinion before any elective surgery. For information about new therapies and experts in your community, call the National Cancer Institute at 1-800-4-CANCER.

OSTEOARTHRITIS, also called degenerative joint disease, is a rheumatic disorder that afflicts more than half of American adults over 30, about 16 million of whom have symptoms serious enough to have sought medical care. Most often it afflicts those over 60, but younger people whose occupations or leisure activities involve excess joint wear and tear are also at risk.

Symptoms: Although osteoarthritis can be so mild that symptoms never develop, many people have joint pain,

ranging from mild aches to severe discomfort. There may be loss of mobility due to joint stiffness and pain. Among older people, osteoarthritis usually afflicts the weight-bearing joints, such as the hips and knees. It may also affect the spine and finger joints. In younger people, osteoarthritis may occur at sites of prior joint injury—for example, the elbow joints of tennis players and pneumatic drill workers, the ankles of ballerinas, the knees of football players and runners, and even the hands of knitters.

Causes: Doctors are not sure what causes osteoarthritis, but damage to cartilage, the rubbery shock absorber that surrounds and protects bone ends, is commonly seen in those who suffer from it. Pain occurs when the smooth cartilage surfaces that enable the joints to move freely are worn away. What starts the destructive cycle is still unknown, although some people may inherit a predisposition to it. The damage may be exacerbated by the weight-bearing stress of obesity, the wear and tear of a lifetime of movement, or trauma.

Diagnosis: Many cases can be diagnosed solely by a physical examination and your report of symptoms. Sometimes X rays and blood tests are needed to rule out other possible causes of joint pain.

Treatment: Aspirin is one of the most commonly taken drugs for osteoarthritis. If it does not help, your doctor may prescribe a nonsteroidal antiinflammatory drug (NSAID), such as ibuprofen or naproxen. You may have to learn how to protect the affected joints by doing daily tasks in new ways and doing special exercises to strengthen your mus-

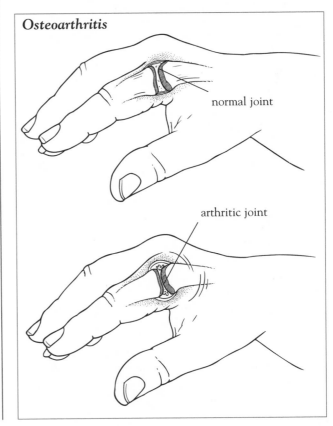

Osteoarthritis

normal joint

arthritic joint

cles and maintain joint mobility. If a knee or hip becomes badly damaged, surgical replacement may be needed.

Outlook: Although osteoarthritis is a progressive disease that cannot be cured, much can be done to prevent pain and disability.

Tips: To ease morning stiffness, take a hot bath or shower upon arising. A nonprescription analgesic cream containing capsaicin, the same chemical in chili peppers, has been shown to relieve pain in some arthritis patients. It appears to work by depleting the chemical that transmits pain impulses through the nerves. Like aspirin, this cream (marketed as Zostrix) must be used regularly. To help prevent stomach irritation, aspirin and NSAIDs should always be taken with meals. If you are overweight, reduce to ease the burden on your joints. Avoid jogging and other exercises that place excessive stress on the joints. Better choices are walking or swimming.

OSTEOPOROSIS causes the bones to become fragile and break easily due to loss of calcium and protein. Osteoporosis afflicts more than 20 million American women, and it occurs most often after menopause. Men are not as likely to develop osteoporosis, and when they do, it occurs much later in life.

Symptoms: The earliest symptom may be back pain. As the bones lose calcium and become less dense, they are vulnerable to spontaneous fracture. Microfractures in the vertebrae cause these spinal bones to compress, ultimately leading to decreased height and what is called "dowager's hump." Or the first signal may be a fractured rib or hip, which can occur with only minimal stress or injury.

Causes: In women, low levels of estrogen after menopause are believed to be the primary cause of osteoporosis. Demineralization of bone can also be caused by Cushing's disease, liver disease, or long-term use of corticosteroid drugs such as prednisone.

Diagnosis: Special scans similar to X rays can measure bone density. Some doctors recommend that women have a baseline scan at menopause, then repeat it at some time later, to help determine whether or not to use estrogen replacement therapy.

Treatment: Therapy includes increasing your calcium intake through diet and supplements, as well as supplements of vitamin D. Estrogen replacement therapy in postmenopausal women may be able to prevent or halt osteoporosis. Other medications such as calcitonin and etidronate can favorably affect bone metabolism.

Outlook: If left untreated, osteoporosis can lead to serious fractures of the spine and hip, which may lead to permanent disability. Treatment may stop the progression of osteoporosis, but it usually cannot repair damage that has already occurred.

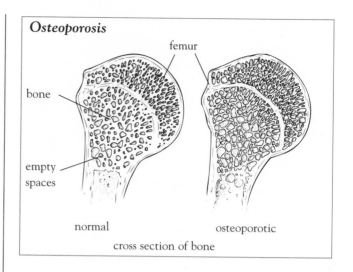

Osteoporosis

femur
bone
empty spaces

normal   osteoporotic

cross section of bone

Tips: To help prevent osteoporosis, start building bone density in youth and middle age. Establish a regular regimen of weight-bearing exercise and consume adequate amounts of calcium. Calcium-rich foods include milk and milk products, green leafy vegetables, and canned salmon and sardines with bones.

OVARIAN CANCER is a malignancy of the ovaries. Although it can occur at any age, it is more frequent after menopause.

Symptoms: Ovarian cancer causes no symptoms in its early stages. With time, there may be recurrent abdominal

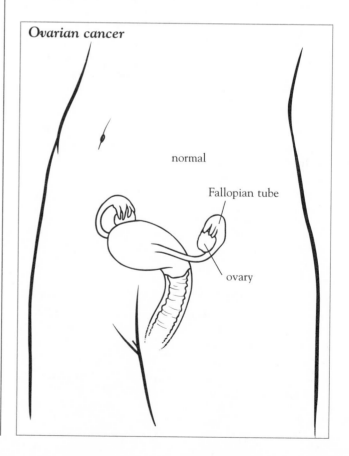

Ovarian cancer

normal

Fallopian tube

ovary

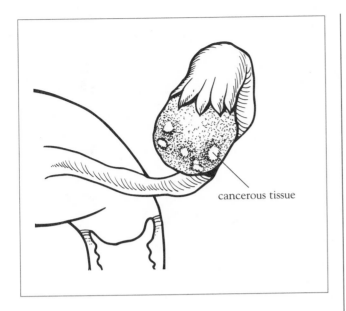

cancerous tissue

discomfort, such as aching or gas pains. Rarely does ovarian cancer cause vaginal bleeding. When the disease is more advanced, abdominal swelling, pain, and weight loss occur.

Causes: Doctors suspect that hereditary factors may be involved because ovarian cancer occurs most often in women in North America and northern Europe. It also is more common in women who have never had children and in those who have previously had cancers of the breast, uterus, colon, or rectum.

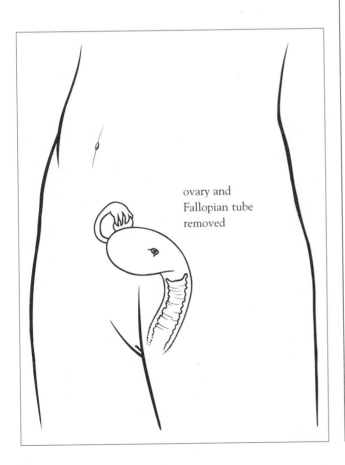

ovary and
Fallopian tube
removed

Diagnosis: Ovarian cancer is difficult to detect. In many cases, the only clue is a slight enlargement of the ovary found during a pelvic examination. If a problem is suspected, a sonogram can detect structural changes in the ovary. Often, the diagnosis is not confirmed until surgery is performed.

Treatment: If only one ovary is involved and the cancer is still localized, young women who hope to have children may in some cases have only the single ovary removed. However, because the cancer has often spread by the time of diagnosis, both ovaries, as well as the uterus, Fallopian tubes, and a sampling of lymph glands, are generally removed. After surgery, radiation and/or chemotherapy can help destroy any remaining cancer cells or slow the progression of the disease.

Outlook: Although ovarian cancer accounts for less than 20 percent of all malignancies in women's reproductive organs, it contributes to a much larger share of fatalities because it can rarely be detected in its early stages.

Tips: To assist early detection, you should have a thorough pelvic examination every year if you are over 40 or more often if you have ovarian cysts. If your mother or sister has had ovarian cancer, discuss the possibility of additional screening tests with your doctor.

PANIC DISORDER is a psychological problem that causes episodes of intense fear and terror that arise seemingly without provocation. It is a type of anxiety disorder. Women are twice as likely as men to have panic attacks associated with agoraphobia—the inability to leave home alone or travel without great mental anguish.

Symptoms: Intense fear characterizes a panic attack. You may feel detached from yourself or your environment and fear that you are going crazy or losing control of yourself, or that you are about to die. You may also experience one or more of the following physical symptoms: rapid heart rate or palpitations; shortness of breath; choking or smothering sensations; chest pain or tightness; dizziness, unsteadiness, or faintness; sudden sweating or chills; nausea, abdominal pain, or other stomach problems; trembling or shaking; and numbness or tingling, particularly in the hands. Panic attacks may last from a few minutes to as long as an hour.

Causes: Both biological and psychological factors can make you vulnerable to panic attacks. Some doctors believe the tendency is inherited, and others think abnormalities in brain blood flow may be involved. About 50 percent of people with panic disorder have a heart valve abnormality called MITRAL VALVE PROLAPSE. Some studies link the onset of panic attacks to female hormones because episodes are more frequent just before monthly periods and during early childbearing years when levels of progesterone are high. Separation anxiety in childhood or sudden loss of important relationships may predispose a person to panic disorder.

Diagnosis: Psychiatrists diagnose panic disorder if you have at least four attacks a month, or only one attack a month—if you live in constant fear of having another.

Treatment: Both medications and psychotherapy have proved to be effective treatments. Some antidepressants can help prevent attacks, while tranquilizers can reduce the anxiety that may contribute to their development. However, some people have problems with the side effects of these drugs, and attacks may recur when the drugs are stopped. Psychotherapy may produce longer-lasting benefits, especially cognitive therapy, which helps you correct distorted ways of thinking that can intensify fear. You can also learn techniques, such as controlled breathing, to help manage your physical symptoms. Sometimes the combination of medication and psychotherapy works best.

Outlook: The initial attacks may be infrequent. However, when you develop a fear of the fear itself, this will more likely cause frequent panic attacks. They occur most commonly in young adults and usually become less severe in middle age. While attacks may disappear spontaneously, therapy can hasten recovery.

Tips: Do not drink coffee, tea, and colas. These beverages contain caffeine, which can make you jumpy and help predispose you to a panic attack. During a panic episode, try to face your feelings rather than fight them, which only worsens the fear. If you can remember that fear cannot hurt you, that you will survive the panic attack, the episode will probably pass quickly.

PAP TEST, short for Papanicolaou smear, detects abnormal cells that may indicate CERVICAL CANCER or precancerous changes of the cervix. All adult women should have this screening test every 1 to 3 years, depending on age, sexual history, and personal and family medical history.

Procedure: The test is done as part of your regular gynecological checkup while you are reclining on the examining table. Do not douche or tub bathe for 24 hours beforehand. In the test, your doctor opens your vagina with a speculum, and with a tiny brush and a small spatula he or she scrapes samples of cervical cells. The secretions are then transferred to a glass slide and sent to a laboratory for examination.

Risks and complications: This is a no-risk procedure. You may experience a slight twinge while the sample is taken.

Results: Depending on the laboratory used and your doctor's procedures, you may be notified of findings by phone or mail within 1 to 3 weeks. Results are often divided into five cell categories: class 1—no abnormal cells; class 2—atypical cells but no evidence of cancer; class 3—cells suggestive of precancerous changes requiring more extensive evaluation; class 4—cells strongly suggestive of cancer requiring more evaluation; class 5—cancer present and treatment required.

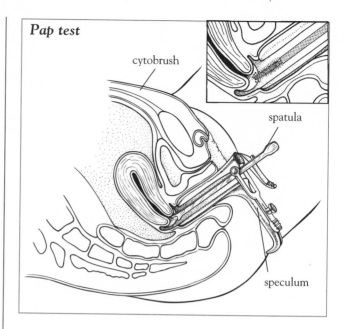

Pap test

cytobrush

spatula

speculum

Tips: Do not be overly concerned about a class 2 result. It is most frequently caused by simple inflammation and will be gone by the time you have a follow-up check a few months later. Although a class 3 result indicates you need further testing, it will frequently be caused by mild abnormalities that may be revealed and removed by office procedures. Never ignore an abnormal Pap test result, however. Follow-up is always essential.

PELVIC INFLAMMATORY DISEASE (PID) refers to any major infection in the pelvis, but it typically affects the Fallopian tubes, uterus, or ovaries. It is most common among young women of reproductive age who are sexually active, and more than half of all cases are sexually transmitted.

Symptoms: There may be few early symptoms. Later ones vary from woman to woman, depending on the site and severity of the infection. Most common are mild to severe pain and tenderness in the lower abdomen or lower back, pain during or after intercourse, heavy vaginal discharge, irregular menstrual periods, irregular bleeding or cramps between periods, and fatigue. Some women experience fever, chills, and other flulike symptoms, painful urination, or nausea and vomiting.

Causes: The most common causes of PID are sexually transmitted infections such as CHLAMYDIA and GONORRHEA. Other bacterial infections may also be involved.

Diagnosis: A pelvic exam, laboratory analysis of cells taken from the cervix, and a blood test to determine white-cell count are necessary for diagnosis. In some cases, the symptoms may be confused with those of appendicitis, a tubal pregnancy, or an ovarian cyst, and the diagnosis may require LAPAROSCOPY for confirmation. About half of all cases are diagnosed retrospectively when evaluation for infertility reveals scar tissue blocking the Fallopian tubes.

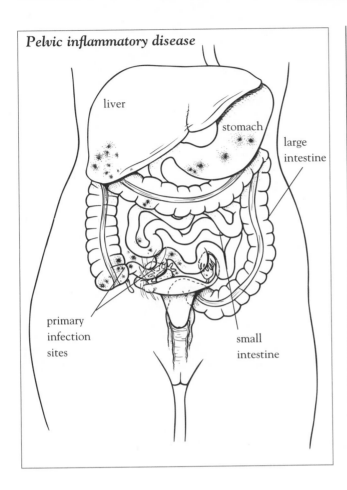

Pelvic inflammatory disease

liver

stomach

large intestine

primary infection sites

small intestine

Sometimes PID is not spotted until rampant infection requires gynecological surgery (see below).

Treatment: If caught early, most cases can be treated with antibiotics, although more than one type of antibiotic may be needed. You also may require analgesics to ease pain. More severe cases may require hospitalization, treatment with intravenous antibiotics and, possibly, surgery to remove the infected organs. Depending upon the causative agent, your sexual partner may have to be treated to eradicate the source of the infection.

Outlook: If not treated promptly, PID can cause permanent damage to the reproductive organs, causing infertility, an increased risk of ECTOPIC PREGNANCY, or life-threatening problems such as rupture of a tubo-ovarian abscess.

Tips: If you are diagnosed with PID, stay in bed for the first week of treatment (or longer if directed by your physician). A heating pad may help ease the pain. Avoid sexual intercourse until both you and your partner have completed treatment. If you are not in a mutually monogamous relationship, use a condom and spermicide to reduce the risk of future infection, and have annual checkups for chlamydia and gonorrhea. Do not douche unless your doctor instructs you to do so, because douching can transfer infectious agents from your vagina to your uterus.

POSTTRAUMATIC STRESS SYNDROME is a psychiatric disorder that may occur after an extraordinarily disturbing experience that threatens your life, physical well-being, home, or those you love. It is a type of anxiety disorder. Although the problem became well known among Vietnam veterans, it can happen to anyone at any age, even in childhood. In acute posttraumatic distress syndrome, symptoms arise within 6 months of the event and last less than 6 months. The chronic form may last for years or may recur periodically.

Symptoms: You may find yourself constantly thinking or dreaming about the traumatic event or, in contrast, totally avoiding thoughts or feelings about it. Secondary symptoms vary widely from one person to another and may include anxiety, depression, insomnia, irritability, difficulty concentrating, feelings of estrangement from those around you or guilt for having survived the experience, decreased interest in your regular activities, an exaggerated response when startled, and impaired memory, possibly including amnesia about the event. Friends or family may find your behavior irrational or impulsive or may be frightened by your violent outbursts.

Causes: Although war is the most common trigger for the syndrome, it has also been seen among survivors of floods, earthquakes, fires, plane crashes and other disasters, as well as among those who have been raped or otherwise assaulted. Why some people who undergo such crises heal uneventfully while others develop emotional problems is unknown. Possibly trauma in early life or other psychiatric problems may increase susceptibility.

Diagnosis: No special tests can identify this disorder. Rather, diagnosis is based on a therapist's discussions with the victim or, possibly, family members and friends. Both emotional and physical disorders that can cause similar symptoms must be ruled out.

Treatment: The type of psychotherapy needed depends on the type and severity of symptoms. When a large number of people have been affected by an event, such as an earthquake, group therapy can be very useful. In some cases, it may be helpful for a spouse or other family members to participate in the therapy. For those with acute problems, counseling can help integrate the trauma into their lives, and medications can do much to alleviate anxiety, depression, or insomnia. If symptoms worsen and/or become chronic, therapy provides long-term emotional support and helps solve specific problems. People who become suicidal may need short-term hospitalization.

Outlook: The outlook for patients who have acute posttraumatic distress syndrome is more favorable than for those with the chronic form of the disorder. In acute cases, symptoms usually lessen gradually and then disappear completely. In chronic cases, symptoms may worsen. Even after apparent healing, symptoms may recur months or years later.

Tips: If you have had a significant traumatic experience, try to confront and discuss the event and your feelings about it with a family member or friend. If you know of others in similar situations, consider joining a support group. If your fears persist, you should seek psychological counseling.

PUNCH BIOPSY, also known as cervical biopsy, is a diagnostic test used to evaluate abnormal cells in the cervix or evaluate an abnormal Pap test. It is likely to be performed if your gynecologist spots any abnormalities suggestive of cancer or precancerous changes during a COLPOSCOPY examination. It is often performed in conjunction with another procedure, known as endocervical curettage.

Procedure: After the colposcopy exam has been performed, your doctor uses a specialized instrument to clip off one or more tiny pieces of tissue, each no larger than 5 millimeters. In order to check the area that cannot be

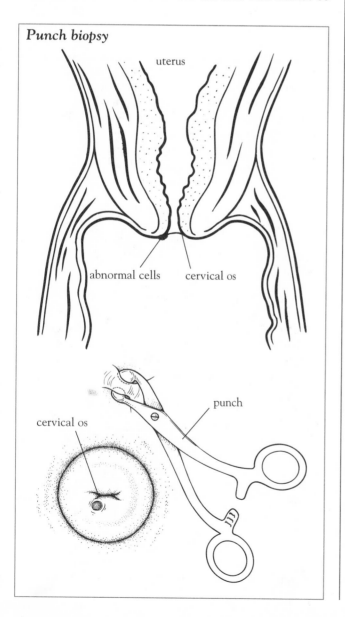

Punch biopsy

uterus

abnormal cells   cervical os

cervical os

punch

fully visualized with the colposcope, an endocervical curettage may be performed as well. Your doctor inserts a tiny instrument called a curette just inside the cervical canal, but not up into the uterus. He or she scrapes the canal for a few seconds to get a sample of the tissue. All tissue samples are sent to a pathology laboratory for examination.

Risks and complications: The punch biopsy may cause an intense but brief pain, lasting only a few seconds. Endocervical curettage may cause cramping. You also may experience mild to moderate cramps afterward. Any biopsy procedure carries a very small risk of excessive bleeding and infection.

Results: The tissue samples are sent to a laboratory for staining and microscopic examination. Results are usually available within a week. When findings fully explain your abnormalities, treatment may be instituted immediately.

Tips: Ask your doctor if you can take a mild pain-killer, such as aspirin or ibuprofen, a half hour before the procedure to lessen the intensity of postbiopsy cramps. Wear a sanitary napkin for 24 hours after the procedure, and report any excessive bleeding to your doctor right away. Avoid sexual intercourse for at least 24 hours.

RAYNAUD'S DISEASE is a condition in which impaired blood circulation in the hands causes the skin over the fingers to turn very pale or even blue in response to cold. Sometimes other parts of the body, such as the nose or tongue, may be affected.

Symptoms: The hypersensitivity to cold first prompts tingling and numb sensations in the fingers. The skin then pales and turns blue, returning to its normal color only when the hands warm up, which may take minutes or hours. Over time, small sores develop on the fingertips and the overlying skin becomes smooth and shiny.

Causes: The impaired circulation is caused by spasms in tiny arteries in the fingers. In most cases, the cause of Raynaud's disease is unknown, although it is more common in young women. In some cases, called simply Raynaud's phenomenon, decreased circulation is caused by RHEUMATOID ARTHRITIS, scleroderma, LUPUS, thyroid disorders, or drug reactions, or by working in a cold, damp atmosphere or long-term use of vibrating equipment.

Diagnosis: Raynaud's disease is diagnosed based on your symptoms. Blood tests are performed to determine whether an underlying condition is present that needs treatment.

Treatment: Therapy for any underlying disease, together with self-care measures, usually helps lessen Raynaud's symptoms. If such efforts do not work, vasodilator drugs may be prescribed to relax and dilate the blood vessels. In the worst cases, an operation that cuts part of the nerves in the hand can sometimes provide relief by preventing the arterial spasms.

Outlook: Raynaud's episodes tend to come and go, and are likely to be less frequent during warm weather. The condition rarely leads to serious complications.

Tips: Protect your hands from the cold by wearing gloves even in only moderately cool circumstances. Use tongs or pot holder mitts to handle items from your freezer or refrigerator. Use thermal glasses for cold beverages to avoid an episode when you handle them. Do not smoke, because nicotine constricts the blood vessels.

RECTOCELE is a prolapse of the rectal wall that causes it to push against the outer wall of the vagina and protrude into the space occupied by the vaginal canal.

Symptoms: Unlike other pelvic prolapse problems, rectocele usually causes few if any difficulties unless you are chronically constipated. In such cases, feces may collect and harden in the pouch of rectal wall that protrudes into the vagina. As they continue to accumulate there, it can become progressively more difficult to move your bowels.

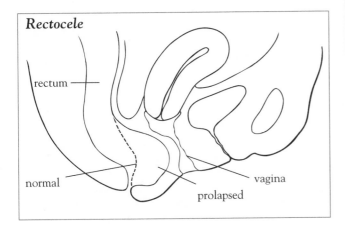

Rectocele

rectum

normal

prolapsed

vagina

Causes: Rectocele is caused by weak ligaments that support pelvic organs, and by a weakness in the vaginal wall that allows the protrusion. Most prolapse problems stem from damage caused by childbirth. You also may be at greater risk if you are obese or have chronic constipation, which strains the pelvic support system, or if you cough excessively from a lung disease. The decrease in hormones after menopause can worsen a previously mild prolapse.

Diagnosis: Your gynecologist can usually diagnose rectocele simply by observing and feeling the bulge in the vagina and the pouch in the rectum.

Treatment: If the rectocele is causing significant problems, a surgical procedure, performed through the vagina, can repair the weaknesses in the vaginal and rectal walls.

Outlook: You can help prevent rectocele from getting worse by keeping your stools soft and developing regular bowel habits.

Tips: You can often ease bowel movements by putting a finger in your vagina and pushing against the bulging rectal wall. Eat plenty of fresh fruits and vegetables and whole grains, and drink six to eight glasses of fluid daily, to ensure soft, moist stools. If these measures are not sufficient, ask your doctor for a stool softener. Do not delay going to the toilet when you feel the urge. Try to relax and move your bowels at about the same time each day.

RHEUMATOID ARTHRITIS (RA), one of the most severe forms of arthritis, is an inflammatory disorder that can be extremely painful and crippling. RA usually strikes people between their mid-twenties and mid-forties, although it can even begin in childhood. Women are afflicted three times as often as men.

Symptoms: Joint pain, stiffness, and deformity are the major symptoms. Joints are affected symmetrically; that is, the same joint—the wrist or the knee—is affected on both sides of the body. In some people, widespread joint involvement may cause aching all over the body. They may also experience weight loss and fatigue. RA can also damage the lungs, skin, blood vessels, muscles, heart, and eyes.

Causes: The precise causes remain unknown. However, it is believed that some people are born with a genetic predisposition to the disorder, which is then triggered by a virus or some other environmental factor. RA is an autoimmune disease in which your immune system runs amok and attacks healthy tissue as if it were a foreign invader. The attack starts with the synovial membrane that surrounds the joint, extends to the rubbery cartilage that protects bone ends, and even affects the underlying bone.

Diagnosis: See a rheumatologist for any problem involving widespread joint pain and stiffness. Diagnosis is based on a complete history and physical examination, as well as blood tests and sometimes X rays.

Treatment: Aspirin is most commonly used for rheumatoid arthritis, but it must be taken in high doses on a regular schedule (not just when you have pain) to have long-term beneficial effects.

If aspirin does not help, your doctor may prescribe a nonsteroidal antiinflammatory drug (NSAID), such as ibuprofen or naproxen. For severe RA, more potent drugs may be used, such as methotrexate, gold compounds, penicillamine, hydroxychloroquine, sulfasalazine, corticosteroids, and other immunosuppressives used in transplant medicine. These drugs all have potentially serious side effects, so you will need frequent blood and urine tests.

Hot or cold compresses and other physical therapy techniques may help relieve pain. Complete treatment of RA also requires learning how to protect affected joints by doing daily tasks in new ways and doing special exercises to strengthen your muscles and maintain joint mobility. If a joint becomes badly damaged, surgery may be required to remove the damaged tissue, stabilize the joint, or replace it completely with an artificial one.

Outlook: RA cannot be cured, but effective treatment can help you lead a relatively normal life. The course of the disease is variable: It may sometimes flare up or it may go into remission for unknown reasons.

Self-care: To ease joint stiffness, take a hot bath or shower upon arising. To help prevent stomach irritation, always take aspirin and NSAIDs with meals. A nonprescription analgesic cream containing capsaicin, the ingredient that makes chili peppers hot, may be helpful in treating arthritis pain by depleting the chemical that transmits pain impulses through the nerves. Like aspirin, this cream (marketed as Zostrix) must be used regularly. To cope with fatigue, get sufficient sleep at night and balance your day with one or more half-hour rest breaks between periods of activity. To help lower stress, which can trigger flareups, learn relaxation techniques. If you are overweight, reduce to ease the burden on your joints.

STROKES are the result of a disruption of the blood supply to the brain. Deprived of oxygen, the nerve cells in the brain die. Cerebral thromboses and cerebral embolisms are caused by blood clots that interfere with the delivery of oxygen to the brain. In a transient ischemic attack, also known as a TIA or ministroke, such a clot causes only temporary obstruction. Less common are cerebral and subarachnoid hemorrhages, which occur when a blood vessel in the brain bursts.

Causes: Cerebral thromboses tend to occur in older people who have atherosclerosis that has narrowed cranial arteries. Cerebral embolisms are more frequent in people who have atrial fibrillation, a heart rhythm disorder. Hemorrhagic strokes can be caused by a ruptured blood vessel (more common in smokers and people with high blood pressure) or by a head injury.

Symptoms: Stroke may cause a sudden weakness and/or numbness of the face, arm, and leg on one side of the body; difficulty speaking or understanding others; dimness or impaired vision in one eye; or dizziness and unsteadiness. TIA symptoms are similar but milder: a temporary weakness or loss of feeling on one side of the body, or other symptoms that last only a few minutes.

Diagnosis: A complete physical and neurological examination, blood tests, an electroencephalogram, a brain scan, and evaluations of neck and cerebral artery blood flow by sonogram may be needed to identify a TIA or stroke and assess its cause and severity.

Treatment: Stroke treatment during the acute phase centers on maintaining body fluids and blood electrolytes (such as sodium and potassium). Anticoagulant drugs, to prevent clotting, may be administered in certain kinds of stroke. Long-term therapy involves rehabilitation and certain steps, such as surgical removal of atherosclerotic plaque in a neck artery or aggressive treatment of heart disease, to prevent the stroke from recurring.

Outlook: Prompt use of anticoagulants may help minimize damage. However, when areas of the brain are deprived of normal blood flow and oxygen, local nerve cells die quickly. Then, the body parts that are controlled by those nerves can no longer function. Depending on the extent of the stroke, this may mean temporary or permanent impairment of movement, sensation, speech, memory, vision, behavior, and other functions. The extensive bleeding caused by hemorrhagic strokes can cause severe and potentially life-threatening pressure within the brain.

Tips: TIAs are a significant warning sign that a stroke is likely to occur within the next month to year. Aggressive efforts should be made to treat any risk factors, such as hypertension, DIABETES, high blood cholesterol, and obesity, as well as to quit smoking. Aspirin therapy or anticoagulant drugs may be effective in reducing the risk of progression to a stroke.

SYPHILIS is a serious sexually transmitted disease.

Symptoms: The first stage of syphilis, which usually occurs within a month after infection, is usually a painless open sore called a chancre. It may appear in the vagina, rectum, or mouth. In some women, the sore may occur inside the vagina, where it is never observed. Even if not treated, this sore soon disappears, but the infection continues to spread inside the body.

Within a few weeks to a few months later, the second stage of syphilis may cause new symptoms: swollen lymph glands, headaches, fever, and a rash that may spread all over your body or appear only on the palms of your hands and soles of your feet. Because these symptoms may be confused with other illnesses they may be missed. With time they will also disappear without treatment, but damage continues inside the body. The third stage of syphilis occurs years later and may cause serious harm to the heart and nervous system, blindness, or death.

Causes: Syphilis is caused by a spirochete that is almost invariably spread through direct sexual contact. It is infectious throughout the first and second stages. A pregnant woman can also pass the disease to her unborn baby through the placenta.

Diagnosis: Syphilis can be diagnosed by laboratory examination of cells from the chancre in the first stage, of a blood sample in the second stage, or of a sample of cerebrospinal fluid in the third stage.

Treatment: In the first and second stages, syphilis can usually be cured by injections of large doses of penicillin or, if you are allergic to it, other antibiotics. Avoid sexual intercourse for at least 2 months after treatment begins. In the third stage, hospitalization for intravenous antibiotics usually is necessary.

Outlook: In about 10 percent of cases, the disease recurs within a year and needs to be treated again. For this reason, many doctors recommend having regular blood tests for 6 months to 2 years after the initial treatment to make sure that the infection has been completely eradicated.

Tips: If there is even the slightest possibility that you have been exposed to syphilis, seek medical diagnosis and treatment immediately. If you or your partner are not monogamous, consider having annual tests for syphilis and other venereal diseases.

TRICHOMONAS (often called trich) is one of the three most common causes of VAGINITIS (see also YEAST INFECTION and GARDNERELLA).

Symptoms: Trichomonas causes a thin, foamy discharge that is yellowish green or gray and has a foul odor. Vaginal irritation causes an inflammation, which may produce mild to severe vaginal or vulvar itching, burning, redness or swelling, and pain or stinging during intercourse.

Causes: The parasite *Trichomonas vaginalis* is usually sexually transmitted, but occasionally may live normally in the vagina in small numbers without causing any problem. The vagina normally cleanses itself continuously with secretions that bathe its mucous membrane lining. Trich may overgrow if this normal self-cleansing process breaks down, such as through excessive douching. Stress, poor blood sugar control by people with DIABETES, and the use of oral contraceptives also increase susceptibility to trich.

Diagnosis: Your doctor can usually diagnose trich by examining a sample of your vaginal discharge under a microscope. In other cases, a smear of the discharge is taken for laboratory evaluation.

Treatment: Trich is usually treated with metronidazole (Flagyl), given orally or as a vaginal gel. For women who cannot take this drug because they are pregnant, are nursing, or have a peptic ulcer, certain blood diseases, or a central nervous system disorder, an alternative but less effective treatment may be used.

Outlook: If you are sexually active, your partner must be treated at the same time you are. During treatment, genital contact should be avoided to prevent reinfection.

Tips: If your doctor prescribes a therapeutic vaginal cream or suppository, use it just before getting into bed to help keep the medicine in place as long as possible.

ULTRASOUND is a diagnostic test that uses inaudible sound waves to produce images of internal organs. It is also called sonography, and the resulting "pictures" are known as sonograms. While ultrasound may be used to examine many parts of the body, it is most often used to evaluate the pelvis, especially during pregnancy, or if you have pelvic pain, or fertility or menstrual problems. Ultrasound can spot cysts and other masses, help diagnose ENDOMETRIOSIS, identify an ECTOPIC PREGNANCY, and evaluate a fetus.

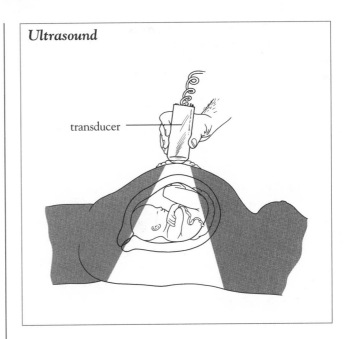

Ultrasound

transducer

Procedure: Prior to a pelvic ultrasound, you will be asked to drink at least a quart of water to fill your bladder, which pushes the bowel away from the uterus and ovaries and ensures better images. During the test, you recline on an examining table in a semidarkened room, and a technician rubs your abdomen with gel or mineral oil so that the ultrasound probe (called a transducer) slides more easily over your skin. The transducer is moved over your skin to deliver the sound waves and receive image information.

In a newer technique, called transvaginal ultrasonography, the probe is inserted in your vagina. This procedure provides superior images and eliminates the need to fill your bladder. The transvaginal technique may be used in early pregnancy or when a mass or cyst is small. When there is a large pelvic mass or an advanced pregnancy, the pelvic approach must be used. In some situations, both techniques are used.

Risks and complications: This is a safe, noninvasive procedure that involves no radiation.

Results: You may be able to watch the sonogram on a monitor as the test is being performed, although the interpretation may come from your doctor later. The technician may point out what you are seeing and provide a snapshot of the image. Since ultrasonography is often done to monitor pregnancy, this photograph of the fetus is often appreciated.

Tips: Maintaining a full bladder can be difficult while traveling to the doctor's office. Try drinking only half the recommended amount of fluid at home. Then get to the appointment at least a half hour early and drink the rest. If you're having a transvaginal ultrasonography exam, some technicians allow you to insert the probe yourself.

URETHROCELE is a ballooning of the walls of the urethra, the tube that carries urine from the bladder to the outside of the body. Instead of being tucked against the pubic bone, the urethra sags downward and pushes against the outer wall of the vagina, protruding into the space occupied by the vaginal canal.

Symptoms: Minor urethroceles exhibit no symptoms. Larger ones may cause a lump or bulge inside the vaginal opening.

Causes: The prolapse is caused by a weakness in the ligaments that support the pelvic organs, and a weakness in the vaginal wall that allows the protrusion. Most prolapse problems stem from damage caused by childbirth. You also may be at greater risk if you are obese or are chronically constipated, which strains the pelvic support system, or if you cough excessively from a lung disease. The decrease in hormones after menopause can worsen a previously mild prolapse.

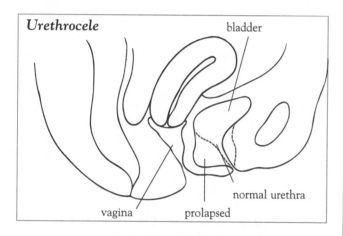

Urethrocele — bladder, normal urethra, prolapsed, vagina

Diagnosis: Your gynecologist can usually diagnose urethrocele simply by observing and feeling the bulge.

Treatment: If the urethrocele is causing symptoms, the weakness in the vaginal wall and bulging urethra can be repaired by surgery, which is performed through the vagina.

Outlook: A severe urethrocele can lead to URINARY INCONTINENCE.

URINARY INCONTINENCE is the inability to control urine flow, which can be very embarrassing and uncomfortable.

Symptoms: Incontinence can range from leakage of a few drops on occasion, to sudden bursts of flow (urge incontinence), to a constant dripping from the urethra. Among women, the most common type is stress incontinence, in which small amounts of urine leak when you sneeze, cough, or laugh.

Causes: Urinary incontinence can be caused by injury to the bladder support muscles during childbirth; systemic diseases that damage nerves, such as MULTIPLE SCLEROSIS, DIABETES, Parkinson's, and Alzheimer's; and spinal cord injury, brain damage, or stroke. Taking diuretics, tranquilizers, antidepressants, and alcohol can also cause urinary incontinence. If you have a URINARY TRACT INFECTION, the frequent, urgent need to urinate may cause mild incontinence. Rarely, as a result of injury incurred during surgery, an accident, or childbirth, some women have a urinary fistula—a duct connecting the ureter, bladder or urethra to the vagina—that causes urine to leak from the vagina.

Diagnosis: A thorough history of the type of incontinence and the situations in which it occurs is very important in determining its cause. A physical examination and tests to evaluate bladder function are also helpful. Occasionally, X rays or cystoscopy (looking into the bladder with a scope) may be necessary.

Treatment: In systemic diseases, therapy for the underlying problem may reduce or eliminate incontinence. Urinary tract infections can be treated with antibiotics. In cases of urge incontinence, drug therapy may help. Bladder relaxants can decrease bladder contractions and thus prevent urine leakage. In other situations, medications that strengthen bladder contractions can facilitate complete bladder emptying and limit later leakage. Postmenopausal women may be helped by estrogen replacement therapy. For others, behavioral training or surgery may be necessary.

Outlook: Women too often put up with the embarrassment of incontinence and do not seek medical help. However, with proper treatment from a gynecologist or urologist, many of these problems can be reduced or eliminated.

Tips: If you have stress incontinence, doing Kegel exercises, which strengthen the muscles involved in urination, may help you regain better bladder control. Learn to isolate the muscles involved by starting and stopping your urinary stream. Then practice slowly tightening and releasing these muscles several times a day while sitting or standing. As you become skilled, you should be able to do 20 to 30 repetitions three or four times a day. (See box, Chapter 2, "Sexual Health.")

URINARY TRACT INFECTIONS, also known as UTIs, affect the bladder, kidneys, or urethra (the tube that carries urine from the bladder out of the body). Infections of the bladder are called cystitis; those of the urethra, urethritis; and those of the kidneys, pyelonephritis. Bladder infections are particularly common in women.

Symptoms: The most common problem is frequent urination, which may come on suddenly and be severe, especially at night. This condition is usually caused by inflammation of the bladder. Urination may be accompanied by pain or a burning sensation. If the infection is very severe, only small amounts of urine may pass and it may be bloody. If you also have fever, chills, vomiting, or pain in the abdomen or back, the infection is more likely to be in your kidneys.

Causes: UTIs are usually caused by bacteria, which enter the body through the urethra. Because a woman's urethra is much shorter than a man's and is located so near to the vagina and anus, where unfriendly bacteria may flourish, women are much more susceptible to UTIs than men. Women who have a CYSTOCELE or who are past menopause may also be at greater risk of these infections.

Diagnosis: A sample of your urine is given to a laboratory to confirm an infection and identify the bacteria causing it so that the proper drug can be prescribed.

Treatment: A 5- to 14-day course of antibiotics usually cures UTIs, although longer regimens may be necessary for recurring infections. Take the full course, even though your symptoms disappear within a few days. However, if the infection is severe, especially if it has spread into the kidneys, hospitalization may be necessary.

Outlook: If UTIs are left untreated, the symptoms sometimes last only a few days and then disappear, but the bacteria may continue to do permanent damage inside your body. Due to an abnormality in the urethra, bladder, or kidneys, some people get repeated infections. If you have recurrent UTIs, see a urologist for evaluation. Your doctor may recommend that you take a low-dose antibiotic on a continuing basis as a preventive measure.

Tips: After moving your bowels, make sure to wipe yourself from front to back to avoid fecal contamination of the urethra and vagina. If you have or are prone to UTIs, drink six to eight glasses of fluid daily to help flush out bacteria in the bladder. Always empty your bladder completely when you urinate and be sure to urinate immediately after intercourse. Do not use vaginal deodorants, bubble baths, or other potentially irritating substances. If you use a diaphragm, be sure that it fits properly to avoid irritation and infection.

UTERINE CANCER most often develops in the endometrium, the membrane lining the uterus, where it is called ENDOMETRIAL CANCER. A small percentage of uterine cancers arise in the myometrium, the muscular tissue that forms the walls of the uterus.

Symptoms: Uterine cancer usually causes no symptoms in its early stages. Abnormal vaginal discharge or bleeding, pain or pressure in the pelvic area, or abdominal swelling may occur as the cancer grows.

Causes: As with most malignancies, the cause of uterine cancer is unknown. However, hormonal factors are believed to be involved because this cancer occurs more frequently after menopause. Women who have not had children and those who entered puberty late and went through menopause early may be at higher risk.

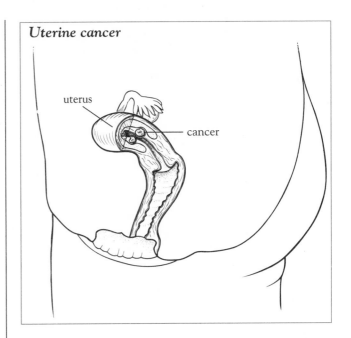

Uterine cancer

uterus

cancer

Diagnosis: Although the PAP TEST is excellent for detecting cervical cancer, it is not very good for diagnosing uterine cancer. If such a malignancy is suspected, you may need ULTRASOUND or some other imaging procedure. Definitive diagnosis requires a tissue sample, which may be obtained by ENDOMETRIAL BIOPSY or a D&C. If cancer is diagnosed, further studies will be done to determine whether it has spread to other parts of the body.

Treatment: Removal of the uterus and cervix by HYSTERECTOMY is the standard treatment for uterine cancer. The Fallopian tubes and ovaries are also removed, a procedure known as bilateral salpingo-oophorectomy. Following surgery, radiation or chemotherapy is often recommended to destroy any remaining cancer cells.

Outlook: When uterine cancer is diagnosed early, the outlook is very favorable—a 5-year survival rate of 80 percent. Unfortunately, most cases that are advanced by the time of diagnosis have a 5-year survival rate of only 20 to 30 percent.

Tips: Report any abnormal bleeding, especially bleeding that occurs after menopause, to your gynecologist. A D&C or endometrial biopsy can be done to rule out endometrial cancer.

UTERINE PROLAPSE is a condition in which the uterus becomes displaced, protruding downward into the vagina and, in some extreme cases, out of the vagina. Uterine prolapse should not be confused with a retroverted or tipped uterus, a benign variation of the normal position that occurs in about 20 percent of women.

Symptoms: If the prolapse is mild, you may not experience any symptoms. If your uterus descends further into the vaginal canal, you may have pain during sexual intercourse if penetration is deep, or low back pain, especially

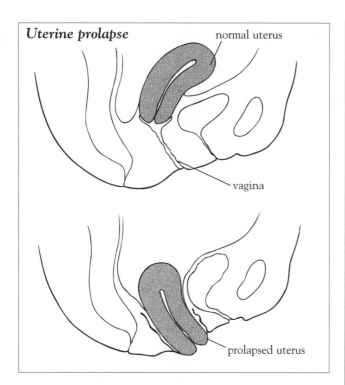

Uterine prolapse   normal uterus

vagina

prolapsed uterus

during menstruation or when standing for long periods. If the prolapse is severe, you may feel the lower part of the uterus protruding through the labia.

Causes: The muscles and ligaments that support the uterus sometimes become weakened by childbirth. This may be more pronounced in women who have had long or difficult labors, large babies, or many pregnancies. There is also a genetic component, meaning that women in some families are more likely than others to develop prolapse after childbirth. As the hormone levels drop in a woman's forties and fifties, the prolapse may worsen. Occasionally prolapse occurs in a woman who has not had children and is thought to be due to a congenital weakness.

Diagnosis: Your gynecologist can feel even a mild prolapsed uterus during a routine pelvic examination.

Treatment: A mild prolapse does not require treatment. If the prolapse is severe, surgery may be recommended to reposition the uterus by reconstructing the ligaments and supporting muscles. There are several different surgical procedures, some of which involve the partial or total removal of the uterus as well. For a woman who is not a candidate for surgery, a pessary (a rubber ring or donut) may be inserted to keep the uterus in place. This is not an ideal solution because it frequently causes vaginal irritation, requires scrupulous cleaning, and in most cases makes it impossible for the wearer to have sexual intercourse.

Outlook: Many cases of prolapse require no treatment; if the prolapse is severe or produces symptoms, surgery is usually successful in relieving them.

Tips: If you experience pain during intercourse, use positions that avoid deep penetration.

VAGINAL CANCER is the growth of abnormal, malignant cells in the vagina. It is the least common cancer of the female reproductive tract. When such growths do occur, most are squamous cell carcinomas similar to a type of skin cancer. Other types of cancer are rare in the vagina.

Symptoms: There are no symptoms in the early stages. Later, you may develop an abnormal vaginal discharge or bleeding, especially after sexual intercourse, or pain during intercourse. If the cancer has spread to the bladder, frequent urination may occur; bowel movements may be painful if the cancer has spread to the rectum.

Causes: As with most types of cancer, the cause is unknown. Vaginal cancer occurs slightly more often in women who have had GENITAL WARTS or HERPES 2, and in those aged 45 to 65. Women whose mothers took DES are at greater risk of clear cell carcinoma, a very rare type of vaginal cancer.

Diagnosis: Long before symptoms occur, vaginal cancer can be detected at its earliest and most curable stage by a PAP TEST during a normal pelvic examination. If the Pap test is abnormal, the vagina may be examined more closely by COLPOSCOPY, after which a tissue sample of any abnormal cells can be taken for laboratory examination. If cancer is diagnosed, further tests can assess whether it has spread to other areas of the body.

Treatment: If you want to have children and the cancer has not progressed much, it may be possible to have only the diseased area surgically removed, with follow-up radiation therapy. However, in most cases, all or part of the vagina must be removed along with nearby lymph nodes; in many cases, the uterus and ovaries are also removed. If the cancer has spread to the bladder or rectum, more extensive surgery will be needed. If it has spread to other parts of the body, radiation or chemotherapy may be required after surgery.

Outlook: Because vaginal cancer is usually not diagnosed until it has reached an advanced stage, only 30 percent of women with this malignancy survive for 5 years without a recurrence.

Tips: If you are over 19—or younger if you are sexually active—you should have regular Pap tests as recommended by your gynecologist.

VAGINAL CYSTS are benign growths, filled with fluid or white material, that develop in the vagina.

Symptoms: Most cysts, especially small ones, do not cause symptoms. Larger or multiple cysts may cause abnormal bleeding or vaginal discharge or painful intercourse.

Causes: When they occur, inclusional cysts generally develop at the site of an episiotomy or a vaginal tear resulting from childbirth or trauma. Gartner duct cysts are remnants of embrionic ducts that disappear in most women but re-

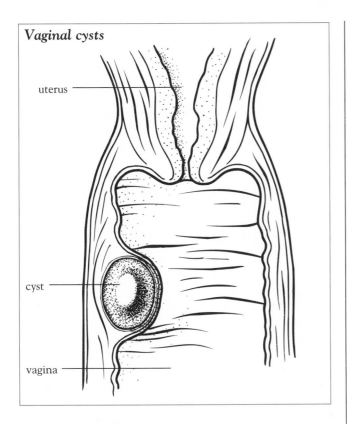

Vaginal cysts

uterus

cyst

vagina

main in a few. An abnormal overgrowth of epithelial tissue in the vagina, called adenosis, sometimes forms cysts. This condition is most often seen among women whose mothers took DES during pregnancy. ENDOMETRIOSIS also can occasionally cause vaginal cysts.

Diagnosis: The fluid in a cyst can usually be withdrawn easily by needle aspiration for laboratory evaluation. Samples of other cysts can be taken for analysis, or the entire cyst can be surgically removed and sent to the laboratory.

Treatment: Large or inflamed inclusional cysts may need to be drained. Cysts due to endometriosis diminish along with other areas of overgrowth when the disorder is treated. Most other cysts require no treatment.

Outlook: Most cysts cause no problems. Endometrial cysts are often mistaken for cancer, a confusion easily cleared up with a biopsy. However, cysts due to adenosis can sometimes lead to a rare type of vaginal cancer and require not only a biopsy but close monitoring by your gynecologist.

VAGINITIS, or inflammation of the vagina, is the condition most frequently reported by women to their gynecologists. Most women have one or more attacks of vaginitis during their lives, and they are easily cured with medication. For others, vaginitis is a recurrent problem that requires more extensive examination and life-style changes to alleviate.

Symptoms: You may experience a discharge from the vagina, accompanied by mild to severe vaginal or vulvar itch-ing, burning, redness or swelling, or pain or stinging during intercourse. A certain amount of clear, odorless vaginal discharge is normal; the discharge caused by vaginitis may change in color, consistency, odor, and amount.

Cause: If the inflammation is not due to simple irritation, the three most common causes are YEAST INFECTIONS, TRICHOMONAS, and GARDNERELLA (also called nonspecific or bacterial vaginitis). Yeast and gardnerella may be present in the vagina in small amounts and cause no symptoms. At other times, they may overgrow and produce symptoms. Trichomonas is usually sexually transmitted and usually symptomatic, although occasionally it may exist without symptoms. Other causes are such sexually transmitted diseases as GONORRHEA, SYPHILIS, CHLAMYDIA, and HERPES—all of which require treatment with antibiotics or antiviral drugs. In rare cases, a vaginal discharge, usually bloody, may be an early sign of VAGINAL, CERVICAL, or ENDOMETRIAL CANCER.

Diagnosis: Your doctor may be able to diagnose the cause by the appearance and odor of your vaginal discharge. In other cases, a smear of the discharge is taken for laboratory evaluation. To rule out cancer, a Pap test may also be taken.

Treatment: Often what is thought to be vaginitis is only a simple irritation that can be eliminated by avoiding excessive douching, vaginal sprays, perfumed soaps, strong detergents, tampons (especially scented ones), pantyhose, and noncotton underwear. An over-the-counter hydrocortisone product can ease vulvar itching temporarily. Some repeat yeast infections can be treated with nonprescription medication (see separate entry). If these measures do not yield prompt improvement, call your doctor. Never self-treat vaginitis if you also have a fever, pain anywhere in your body (especially the abdomen), or a foul-smelling vaginal discharge. These symptoms may indicate a more serious problem that requires medical diagnosis and therapy.

Outlook: Simple irritation should respond to self-care within a week. Yeast infections should respond to a week of over-the-counter vaginal medication. If you are entering or are past menopause and have frequent vaginitis due to dryness and irritation, ask your doctor about estrogen replacement therapy. Applying an estrogen cream directly to the vagina or taking oral estrogen replacement can restore normal lubrication to the vaginal tissues and help prevent future vaginitis episodes.

Tips: If your vagina does not produce adequate lubrication during intercourse, it may become irritated or abraded, which can lead to vaginitis. K-Y jelly or another sterile, water-soluble vaginal lubricant (not Vaseline) applied before intercourse can help avoid irritation.

VARICOSE VEINS, or varicosities, are abnormally enlarged and twisted blood vessels. These veins, which can be uncomfortable and unsightly, usually occur in the legs. Varicose veins result from a malfunction of vein valves that normally control the flow of blood back to the heart and prevent its backup in the legs. When a series of valves degenerates, the vein becomes distended by the blood that pools inside it.

Symptoms: Varicosities look like twisting blue bulges just below the skin. In addition to, or instead of, these bulges, you may experience heaviness or dull stabbing pain, itching around the ankles, tenderness and soreness along the veins, or leg cramps. Sitting down and raising your legs usually alleviates discomfort. Symptoms often worsen during pregnancy and may vary with the menstrual cycle.

Causes: Doctors suspect that some inherent weakness in the blood vessel walls or valves initiates the problem, and the disorder is known to run in families. Hypertension, heavy lifting, pregnancy, and abdominal tumors can result in an increase in internal blood pressure, which also can strain the valves.

Diagnosis: Visible varicosities may require no special testing. If the veins are not evident but are suspected, wrapping an elastic tourniquet around your legs may cause them to stand out. In some cases, though, special studies that measure the flow of blood through the veins of the legs are necessary to determine the severity and locations of the weak valves. Blood tests and other studies may be performed to rule out other possible causes of painful symptoms.

Treatment: Therapy depends on the severity and site of the varicosities. If commercial support stockings do not alleviate your discomfort, you can obtain specially fitted elastic hose. If your problem is more severe, sclerosing therapy may be recommended. This method of treatment involves injecting chemicals into the veins that cause them to become inflamed and then close up, eliminating them as blood-carrying vessels. In some cases, a surgical procedure called vein stripping can be performed to eliminate the distended veins.

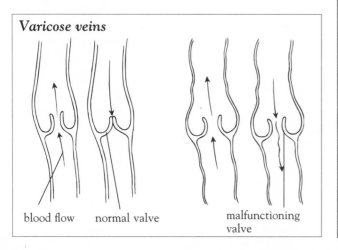

Varicose veins

blood flow   normal valve   malfunctioning valve

Outlook: Untreated varicosities may worsen and can cause leg ulcers that are difficult to heal. Even if the varicosities are removed or destroyed, in many cases new ones are likely to develop.

Tips: If you are overweight, reduce. Because standing can aggravate varicose veins, if your job requires you to be on your feet for long periods, sit down from time to time and elevate your legs, preferably above the level of your chest. If you must sit for long periods, do not cross your legs. Take regular breaks to stand up and stretch. Exercise regularly to improve your circulation. If you are pregnant, discuss the use of support stockings with your physician. Never wear round garters because they impair circulation.

VULVAR CANCER is the growth of abnormal, malignant cells in the vulva, the tissue surrounding the vagina, including the labia minora and labia majora and the clitoris. It is a rare malignancy, accounting for less than 5 percent of cancers of the female reproductive tract.

Symptoms: The first signs are usually thick white patches of skin, called leukoplakia, or a lump or sore that does not heal. These sores most commonly appear on the labia, although they may occur anywhere in the area. Such abnormalities, and others that are not visible to the naked eye, may cause itching, tenderness, pain, slight bleeding, or a burning sensation when you urinate.

Causes: As with most types of cancer, the cause in usually unknown. However, vulvar cancer occurs more frequently in women who have had certain venereal diseases, especially GENITAL WARTS; in those whose estrogen levels are low because of menopause or ovarian dysfunction.

Diagnosis: Your gynecologist can observe abnormalities in vulvar skin during a normal pelvic examination. A sample of the lesion must be taken for laboratory examination to confirm the diagnosis. If cancer is detected, other tests may be necessary to determine whether the malignancy has spread to other areas of the body.

Treatment: If the cancer has been diagnosed early and has not spread below the skin, a condition called carcinoma *in situ*, it can usually be treated by removing the affected area and a surrounding margin of seemingly healthy tissue. If the malignancy has already penetrated the skin, called invasive cancer, vulvectomy must be performed to remove the entire vulva and nearby lymph nodes in the groin. Skin grafting is often necessary to close the wound, and surgery may be preceded or followed by radiation treatments.

Outlook: As with most cancers, early diagnosis and treatment mean that your chances of cure are excellent.

Tips: Sexually active women who have undergone vulvectomy may find it helpful to consult a sex therapist who specializes in treating cancer patients who have had this surgery. In some cases, reconstructive surgery is necessary to restore sexual functioning.

YEAST INFECTION, also called fungus, *Monilia*, and *Candida albicans*, is the most common cause of VAGINITIS. More than 20 million cases of vaginal yeast infection are diagnosed in the United States each year. Yeast infections outnumber TRICHOMONAS, another common cause of vaginitis, by seven to one among women who are not pregnant and by fifteen to one among pregnant women.

Symptoms: An overgrowth of yeast causes a thick, white discharge that may look like cottage cheese and smell like baking bread. The vaginal irritation causes an inflammation that may give you mild to severe vaginal or vulvar itching, burning, redness or swelling, and pain or stinging during intercourse.

Causes: The vagina normally cleans itself constantly, using secretions that bathe its mucous membrane lining. Yeast is among the many microorganisms that live naturally in the vagina, and are kept in check by secretions from lactobacilli that help maintain the normal vaginal acidity. A yeast overgrowth may occur when the normal self-cleansing process breaks down, such as may happen with excessive douching.

Stress, poor blood sugar control by diabetics, and the use of oral contraceptives also make you more susceptible. Powerful antibiotics taken to treat an infection elsewhere in your body also can destroy the vaginal bacteria that control the yeast fungi. Some couples use saliva to lubricate a condom prior to intercourse, which may also contribute to a yeast infection.

Diagnosis: Your doctor is usually able to diagnose the cause by the appearance and odor of your vaginal discharge. In other cases, a smear of the discharge is taken for laboratory evaluation.

Treatment: If you catch a yeast infection early, unpasteurized plain yogurt that contains live lactobacilli cultures can help restore a healthy flora balance. The yogurt may be dissolved in water and applied as a douche or inserted directly into the vagina with an applicator such as those used to insert contraceptive spermicides. Or a vinegar and water douche may halt the attack. However, in most cases, vaginal applications of a cream or suppository containing clotrimazole, miconazole nitrate, or nystatin are necessary to cure it.

Outlook: For recurrent vaginal yeast infections, your doctor may recommend that you douche once a week with a mild acidic solution of 1 to 2 tablespoons of vinegar to a quart of warm water. This added acidity can help promote

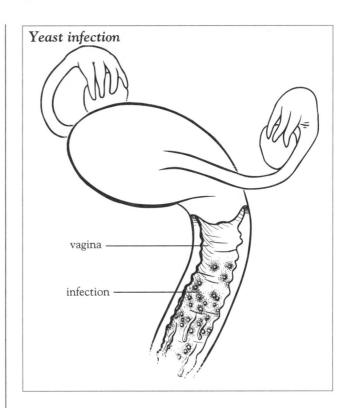

Yeast infection

vagina

infection

the growth of normal vaginal bacteria. If you are prone to yeast infections when taking antibiotics, ask your doctor to prescribe a countervailing medication to keep the condition under control.

Tips: Creams and suppositories for yeast infections are now available over the counter. Because women who have had these infections can spot the symptoms, such at-home treatment helps assure faster relief and saves the cost of a doctor's visit. Look for products containing clotrimazole (Gyne-Lotrimin, Fem Care, or Mycelex-7) or miconazole nitrate (Monistat 7) and follow package directions carefully. Never self-treat vaginitis if you also have a fever, pain anywhere in your body (especially the abdomen), or a foul-smelling vaginal discharge. You probably have a more serious problem that requires medical diagnosis and therapy.

Glossary

Absorptiometry: a scanning technique used to detect osteoporosis, or brittle bones

Adrenaline: one of the catecholamines, substances released by the adrenal glands to help the body mobilize its resources in response to extreme conditions or perceived danger

Aldosterone: a hormone that helps maintain the body's balance of fluids

Amenorrhea: absence of menstruation, or monthly periods

Amniocentesis: a test done during pregnancy to detect certain genetic defects and other fetal abnormalities

Amniotic fluid: the fluid that surrounds and protects the fetus as it grows in the uterus

Androgens: male sex hormones, also present in women in smaller amounts

Androsterone: one of the male sex hormones

Areola: the circle of darker-colored skin that surrounds the nipple on the breast

Arteriosclerosis: a condition in which the walls of arteries thicken and lose elasticity

Aura: a vision of light or feeling of temperature change that may precede a migraine headache or hot flash

Basal (body) temperature: a person's body temperature at rest, usually taken before rising from bed in the morning

Beta-blocker: a class of drugs that slow the heart rate, used in the treatment of certain heart conditions and high blood pressure

Biopsy: the surgical removal of skin or other tissue for diagnosis or for tracking the progress of certain diseases, including cancer

Breech presentation: the presentation of a baby's buttocks or feet first, rather than head first, at delivery

Calcitonin: a hormone produced by the thyroid gland to control the levels of calcium and phosphorus in the blood and inhibit the breakdown of bone tissue

Capsular contracture: the formation of scar tissue around a breast implant, causing the implant and the breast to feel unnaturally hard

Carcinoma in situ: a cancerous tumor that has not yet spread to other tissue

Catecholamines: a class of chemicals produced by the body in response to perceived danger or stress. Examples include adrenaline and noradrenaline

Cesarean section: a surgical procedure in which a baby is delivered via incisions in the abdomen and uterus

Chlamydia: a microorganism responsible for some sexually transmitted diseases, including pelvic inflammatory disease

Chorionic villus sampling: a test performed during pregnancy in order to detect genetic abnormalities in the fetus

Climacteric: the time before menopause in which a variety of hormonal and other body changes take place

Coitus: sexual intercourse between two people of opposite sex

Corpus luteum: the shell left behind in an ovary when an egg is released. It secretes progesterone, which helps the endometrium prepare to receive a fertilized egg

Corticosterone: a hormone released by the adrenal gland to assist in metabolism of carbohydrates

Cortisol: a hormone released by the adrenal gland in response to stress or injury; a synthesized form may be used to reduce swelling. Also called hydrocortisone

Creatinine: one of the waste products of metabolism that is excreted in urine

Cystocele: a condition in which the bladder protrudes into the vaginal wall, resulting in frequent urination and other symptoms

DES (diethylstilbestrol): a synthetic hormone similar to estrogen that was given to some pregnant women in the 1950s and 1960s to prevent miscarriage. Use of the drug has been linked to reproductive abnormalities in offspring, primarily in daughters

Dilation and curettage (D&C): a procedure in which the cervical opening is widened and the lining of the uterus (endometrium) is scraped out

Diuretic: any substance that increases urination

Dysmenorrhea: painful menstruation or cramping during the menstrual period

Ectopic pregnancy: a fertilized egg that develops outside the uterus, usually in the Fallopian tubes

Electronic fetal monitoring: a method of monitoring the fetal heart rate during labor and delivery

Endocrine glands: glands that secrete substances, such as hormones, directly into the bloodstream

Endometrial tissue (endometrium): the lining of the uterus, which grows in order to receive a fertilized egg; if pregnancy does not occur, the tissue is shed during menstruation

Endorphins: chemicals released by the pituitary gland that influence perceptions of pain and pleasure

Epidemiology: the study of disease and its occurrence in a community or population

Episiotomy: a surgical incision in the perineum (the area between the vagina and the rectum) made to enlarge the birth opening during delivery

Estradiol: a potent form of estrogen, the female sex hormone

Estrogen: the female sex hormone, which promotes the development of female attributes and cycles, such as menstruation and pregnancy. Also present in males in smaller amounts

Estrogen replacement therapy: a regimen of synthetic estrogen and other hormones used in some menopausal women to treat symptoms such as hot flashes and to prevent osteoporosis

Exocrine glands: glands that produce substances that are released onto the skin or outside the body, such as sweat or saliva

Fetoscope: a specially designed stethoscope for listening to a fetal heartbeat through the mother's abdomen

Fibromyalgia: a condition of unknown origin characterized by increased sensitivity to temperature changes, pain, and stress as well as by headaches, depression, chronic fatigue, and other symptoms

FSH (follicle-stimulating hormone): a hormone that stimulates the ovarian follicles to release an egg in women. In men, FSH stimulates the testes to release androgens

Galactorrhea: flow of milk from the breasts not associated with breast-feeding or pregnancy

Glandular tissue: tissue containing an organ that releases substances, such as hormones, that affect other bodily functions, cycles, or organs

Gonadotropins: hormones that stimulate the ovaries in women or the testes in men

Growth-stimulating hormone (somatotropin): stimulates the growth of muscle and bone in children and adolescents

Hernia: protrusion of an organ through the muscle that surrounds it

Hydrocortisone: a hormone released by the adrenal gland in response to stress or injury; a synthesized form may be used to reduce swelling. Also called cortisol.

Hypercalcemia: an excessive amount of calcium in the blood, a symptom of several conditions, including osteoporosis

Hyperthyroidism: a condition in which the thyroid gland releases increased amounts of thyroid hormones, accelerating the body functions and causing an array of symptoms

Hypothyroidism: a condition in which the thyroid gland secretes greatly reduced amounts of thyroid hormones, causing metabolism to slow down and leading to weight gain, poor appetite, depression, and other symptoms

Hysterogram: an X ray of the uterus used to detect abnormalities, including those sometimes seen in daughters of women who used DES during pregnancy

Hysterosalpingogram: a test that is performed primarily to evaluate the Fallopian tubes, most often as part of an infertility workup, but which may be used to find polyps, fibroids, or developmental abnormalities. Also called uterotubography or uterosalpingography.

Immunology: the study of the body's reaction to infection or other foreign bodies, such as in an allergic reaction

Induction: the use of a stimulant (usually a drug called pitocin) to start labor contractions and encourage the delivery of a baby

Intrauterine device (IUD): a device placed in the uterus in order to prevent pregnancy

Kegel exercises: a series of exercises designed to strengthen the pelvic muscles to enhance sexual satisfaction and to prevent or reduce bladder control problems after pregnancy or menopause

Laparoscopy: a surgical procedure for examining the ovaries and Fallopian tubes

Lumpectomy: a surgical procedure used to treat breast cancer by removing only the tumor and some surrounding tissue rather than the entire breast

LH (luteinizing hormone): a hormone produced by the pituitary gland that helps regulate the reproductive and menstrual cycles in women

Macrophage: a type of cell that plays an important role in the immune system by digesting foreign substances, such as bacteria

Malignancy: a cancerous tumor that grows, spreads, or involves more than one organ

Mammaplasty: a surgical procedure that changes the shape of the breasts. The procedure may be done to reconstruct breasts after mastectomy or to enlarge or reduce breasts for cosmetic reasons

Mastectomy: the surgical removal of one or both breasts, usually performed to treat cancer of the breast

Mastodynia: breast pain, especially the swelling and tenderness sometimes experienced by women before their menstrual period

Mastopexy: a surgical procedure by which sagging breasts are lifted

Meconium: the greenish-black or brown feces excreted by an infant in the first 36 hours or so after birth

Melatonin: a hormone that helps regulate the sleep-wake cycle and suppress the secretion of other hormones, including the sex hormones in men and women, during sleep

Menarche: a girl's first menstrual period, usually occurring between the ages of 9 and 17

Menorrhagia: menstrual periods characterized by particularly heavy or long bleeding

Metastasize: to spread, as in a cancerous tumor that spreads to other organs

Metrorrhagia: bleeding from the uterus that occurs apart from the menstrual cycle

Micturition: urination, or the act of emptying the bladder through the urethra

Mitral valve prolapse: a heart condition in which the valve between the upper and lower chambers does not close properly, allowing blood to flow back into the atrium. Symptoms may include irregular heartbeat, chest pain, and difficulty breathing.

Montgomery's glands: glands in the areola of the breast that get larger and secrete an oily material that protects the breast during breast-feeding

MSH (melanocyte-stimulating hormone): a hormone that regulates the amount of pigment in the skin

Neural tube defects: abnormalities of the central nervous system caused by faulty formation of the spinal column in the fetus

Neurotransmitter: a chemical that carries messages to the brain and the nervous system

Noradrenaline: hormones that increase the heart rate and blood pressure during times of stress or danger

Oligomenorrhea: lack of, or unusually light, bleeding during menstrual periods

Oophorectomy: a surgical procedure in which one or both of the ovaries is removed

Osteoarthritis: a form of arthritis (joint disease) in which the tissue of one or more joints breaks down, causing pain, swelling, and reduced mobility

Osteoporosis: a condition characterized by a loss of bone density, causing brittle bones that fracture easily

Ovulation: the time in the reproductive cycle when an egg is released into the Fallopian tube

Oxytocin: a hormone that induces labor and promotes milk production and release in pregnant women

Pap smear: a test in which cervical cells are examined to detect cancer of the cervix in the early stages of the disease

Pelvic inflammatory disease: an inflammation of the female pelvic organs, usually caused by a bacterial infection

Phenylketonuria: a condition characterized by the lack of an enzyme essential to the breakdown of the amino acid phenylalanine in the body

Pheromones: substances that are sensed by and elicit a response from another member of the same species, often of the opposite sex. Pheromones have not been positively identified in humans

Pitocin: a synthetic form of oxytocin, the naturally occurring hormone that regulates labor contractions. Pitocin is used to induce labor in some pregnant women

Pituitary gland: a small gland located in the base of the brain that regulates many bodily functions, including menstruation and the reproductive system

Placenta: the tissue that forms on the uterine wall about the third month of pregnancy in order to transfer nourishment and oxygen from a pregnant woman to the fetus

Posterior presentation: the position of the fetus in the birth canal when the back of its head is to the spine instead of the more usual face-to-spine position

Primigravida: a woman pregnant for the first time

Progesterone: the female sex hormone that regulates the preparation of the uterus for possible pregnancy

Prolactin: a hormone that stimulates the breasts to produce milk in a woman who is about to deliver or who has just had a baby

Prolapsed uterus: a condition in which the uterus sags into the vagina

Prostaglandin: a hormonelike fatty acid that is instrumental in a number of hormone-mediated functions in the body, such as stimulating uterine contractions during labor and birth

Puberty: the age at which secondary sex characteristics, such as breasts in females, develop and the reproductive system becomes functional

Rectocele: a condition in which the rectum protrudes into the vagina

Relaxin: a hormone present in pregnant women that relaxes the joints in preparation for pelvic expansion during labor

Serotonin: a chemical in the body that constricts the blood vessels

Sonogram: (See Ultrasound.)

Thyroxine: the primary hormone secreted by the thyroid gland that affects metabolism, body temperature, and other bodily functions

Toxic Shock Syndrome (TSS): a form of blood poisoning associated with superabsorbent tampons, contraceptive sponges, diaphragms, and other devices left in the vagina for longer than recommended

Toxoplasmosis: a parasitic disease spread by cat feces or the ingestion of raw meat that can cause blindness if the fetus is exposed to it during the first twelve weeks of pregnancy

Trichomonas: an inflammation, usually of the vagina, caused by a parasite, *Trichomonas vaginalis*

Triglyceride: a compound of fatty acid and glycerol found in fatty tissue. High triglyceride levels are thought to be a risk factor for coronary heart disease when found in combination with other risk factors

Tropins: hormones that stimulate the production of other hormones

Ultrasound: a scan using high-frequency sound waves to create a picture of internal organs or of the fetus during pregnancy. The picture is called a sonogram.

Vaginitis: swelling or inflammation of the vagina, usually due to infection

Vasoconstriction: tightening or narrowing of blood vessels

Vasomotor: the nerves and muscles that regulate the constriction or dilation of blood vessels

Vasopressin: a hormone that regulates the body's fluid balance and constricts small blood vessels

Resources

The sources listed offer information, free or low-cost brochures, or referrals to physicians and other health care providers or self-help groups. Those resources listed without a phone number prefer to be contacted by mail. When writing them, however, be as specific as possible with your questions and make sure to enclose a self-addressed stamped envelope.

General Health Information and Organizations

American Red Cross
17th and D Streets, NW
Washington, DC 20006
(908) 737-8300

Centers for Disease Control and Prevention
1600 Clifton Road, NE
Building 1 SSB249, MS A 34
Atlanta, GA 30333
(404) 332-4555

National Self-Help Clearinghouse
33 West 42nd Street
New York, NY 10036

Office of Disease Prevention and Health Promotion
National Health Information Center
P.O. Box 1133
Washington, DC 20013-1133
(800) 336-4797

Specific Health Concerns

AGING/NURSING HOMES
American Association of Homes and Services
  for the Aging
901 E Street, NW, Suite 500
Washington, DC 20004
(202) 783-2242

American Health Care Association
1201 L Street, NW
Washington, DC 20005
(202) 842-4444

National Council on Aging
409 Third Street, SW
Washington, DC 20024
(202) 479-1200

National Institute on Aging
Building 21, Room 5C27
Bethesda, MD 20892
(301) 496-1752
(800) 222-2225

U.S. Administration on Aging
Eldercare Locator
(800) 677-1116

ALCOHOLISM AND SUBSTANCE ABUSE
Ad Care Hospital
(800) 252-6465

Al-Anon Family Group Headquarters
1372 Broadway
New York, NY 10018
(212) 302-7240
(800) 356-9996

Alcoholics Anonymous
475 Riverside Drive
New York, NY 10015
(212) 870-3400

Children of Alcoholics Foundation
Grand Central Station, P.O. Box 4185
New York, NY 10163-4185
(800) 359-2627

Do It Now Foundation
P.O. Box 27568
Tempe, AZ 85285-7568
(602) 257-0797

Drug Abuse and Narcotic Addiction
Cocaine Abuse Hotline
(800) COCAINE
(201) 522-7055 (in Alaska or Hawaii)

Drug Abuse Clearinghouse
Room 10A53
5600 Fishers Lane
Rockville, MD 20857
(301) 443-6500

Narcotics Anonymous
(212) 874-0700

National Association of Alcohol and Drug
    Counselors
3717 Columbia Pike, Suite 300
Arlington, VA 22204
(703) 920-4644

National Association of Children of Alcoholics,
    Inc.
11426 Rockville Pike, Suite 100
Rockville, MD 20852
(301) 468-0985

National Clearinghouse for Alcohol
    and Drug Information
P.O. Box 2345
Rockville, MD 29847
(301) 468-2600
(800) 729-6686

National Council on Alcoholism and Drug
    Dependence, Inc.
12 West 21st Street
New York, NY 10010
(212) 206-6770

National Drug Abuse and Treatment Hotline
(800) 662-4357
(800) 662-9832 (Spanish speakers)

National Institute on Alcohol Abuse and
    Alcoholism
Willco Building, Suite 400
6000 Executive Boulevard
Rockville, MD 20892
(301) 443-3885

National Institute on Drug Abuse
(800) 638-2045
(301) 443-2450 (in Alaska, Hawaii, or Maryland)

Rational Recovery
P.O. Box 800
Lotus, CA 95651
(916) 621-2667

Women for Sobriety, Inc.
109 West Broad Street
P.O. Box 618
Quakertown, PA 18951
(215) 536-8026

ARTHRITIS
Arthritis Foundation
1314 Spring Street, NW
Atlanta, GA 30309
(404) 872-7100

National Institute of Arthritis and Musculoskeletal
    and Skin Diseases
Box AMS
Bethesda, MD 20814
(301) 495-4484

ASTHMA AND ALLERGIES
American Lung Association
1740 Broadway
New York, NY 10019
(800) 586-4872

Asthma and Allergy Foundation of America
1125 15th Street, NW, Suite 502
Washington, DC 20005
(202) 466-7643

National Jewish Center for Immunology and
    Respiratory Medicine
1400 Jackson Street
Denver, CO 80206
(800) 222-5864

National Asthma Education Program
4733 Bethesda Avenue, Suite 350
Bethesda, MD 20814
(301) 495-4484

National Institute of Allergy and Infectious
   Diseases
Building 31, Room 7A32
Bethesda, MD 20892
(301) 496-5717

BREAST-FEEDING
Breastfeeding National Network
P.O. Box
McHenry, IL 60051
(800) 835-5968

La Leche League International
Box 1209, 9616 Minneapolis Avenue
Franklin Park, IL 60131
(800) 525-3243
(708) 455-7730

CANCER
American Cancer Society, Inc.
National Headquarters
1599 Clifton Road, NE
Atlanta, GA 30329

Cancer Counseling and Research Center
P.O. Box 7237
Little Rock, AR 72217
(501) 224-1933

Cancer Response System
(800) ACS-2345

Leukemia Society of America, Inc.
600 Third Avenue
New York, NY 10016
(212) 573-8484

Living with Cancer, Inc.
P.O. Box 3060
Long Island City, NY 11101

National Cancer Institute
Cancer Information Clearinghouse
Office of Cancer Communications
Memorial Sloan-Kettering Cancer Center
1275 York Avenue, P.O. Box 166
New York, NY 10021
(800) 4-CANCER

Rose Kushner Breast Cancer Advisory Center
P.O. Box 224
Kensington, MD 20895

Y-ME
National Organization for Breast Cancer
   Information and Support
18220 Harwood Avenue
Harwood, IL 60430
(800) 221-2141
(708) 799-8228 (Illinois only)

YWCA
ENCORE
726 Broadway
New York, NY 10003
(212) 614-2827

CAREGIVING
CAPS (Children of Aging Parents)
1609 Woodbourne Road
Levittown, PA 19057
(215) 945-6900

National Association for Home Care
519 C Street, NE
Washington, DC 20002
(202) 547-7424

CHRONIC FATIGUE SYNDROME AND
   FIBROMYALGIA
Chronic Fatigue and Immune Dysfunction
   Syndrome Association of America
P.O. Box 220398
Charlotte, NC 28222-0398

National Chronic Fatigue Syndrome and
   Fibromyalgia Association
3521 Broadway, Suite 222
Kansas City, MO 64111
(816) 931-4777

COLITIS
Crohn's & Colitis Foundation
386 Park Avenue South
New York, NY 10016
(800) 343-3637

DEATH AND DYING
Choice in Dying (Living Wills)
200 Varick Street, Suite 1001
New York, NY 10107
(212) 366-5540

Hospice Education Institute
Hospicelink
P.O. Box 713
5 Essex Square, Suite 3-B
Essex, CT 06426
(800) 331-1620
(203) 767-1620

National Hospice Organization
1901 North Moore Street, Suite 901
Arlington, VA 22209
(800) 658-8898
(703) 243-5900

DIABETES
American Diabetes Association, Inc.
149 Madison Avenue
New York, NY 10016
(212) 725-4925

Juvenile Diabetes Foundation International
432 Park Avenue South
New York, NY 10016
(212) 889-7575

National Diabetes Information Clearinghouse
9000 Rockville Pike, Box NDIC
Bethesda, MD 20892

DIGESTIVE DISEASES
Crohn's and Colitis Foundation of America, Inc.
386 Park Avenue South
New York, NY 10016
(800) 343-3637

National Digestive Disease Education and
    Information Clearinghouse
1555 Wilson Boulevard, Suite 600
Rosslyn, VA 22209

National Foundation for Ileitis and Colitis, Inc.
386 Park Avenue South
New York, NY 10016
(212) 685-3400
(800) 343-3637

EATING DISORDERS
American Anorexia Nervosa Association, Inc.
133 Cedar Lane
Teaneck, NJ 07666
(201) 836-1800

Anorexia Nervosa and Associated Disorders
Box 7
Highland Park, IL 60035
(708) 831-3438

Bulimia Anorexia Self-Help
(800) 227-4785
(800) 762-3334

Help Anorexia, Inc.
P.O. Box 2992
Culver City, CA 90231
(213) 558-0444

Overeaters Anonymous
4025 Spencer Street, Suite 203
Torrance, CA 90503
(310) 618-8835

Take Off Pounds Sensibly
(800) 932-8677

EXERCISE AND FITNESS
Aerobics and Fitness Foundation
15250 Ventura Boulevard, Suite 310
Sherman Oaks, CA 91403
(800) BE-FIT-80

American College of Sports Medicine
P.O. Box 1440
Indianapolis, IN 46206-1440

President's Council on Physical Fitness and Sports
707 Pennsylvania Avenue, NW, Suite 250
Washington, DC 20004
(202) 272-3430

FAMILY PLANNING/SEX EDUCATION
Alan Guttmacher Institute
120 Wall Street, 21st Floor
New York, NY 10005
(212) 248-1111

Association for Voluntary Surgical
    Contraception, Inc.
79 Madison Avenue
New York, NY 10016
(212) 561-8000

Family Life Information Exchange
P.O. Box 37299
Washington, DC 20013
(301) 585-6636

Natural Family Planning Program
Center for Life
O'Conner Hospital
2105 Forest Avenue
San Jose, CA 95128

Ovulation Method Teachers Association
P.O. Box 101780
Anchorage, AK 99510

Planned Parenthood Federation of America, Inc.
810 Seventh Avenue
New York, NY 10019
(212) 541-7800
(800) 223-3303

San Francisco Sex Information
(415) 621-7300

Sex Information and Educational Council
    of the United States
130 West 42nd Street, Suite 2500
New York, NY 10036
(212) 819-9770

FAMILY VIOLENCE/CHILD ABUSE
American Humane Association
63 Inverness Drive East
Inglewood, CA 80112
(303) 792-9900

CALM (Child Abuse Listening Mediation, Inc.)
1236 Chapala Street
Santa Barbara, CA 93101
(805) 965-2376

National Child Abuse Hotline
Childhelp USA
1345 El Centro Avenue
P.O. Box 630
Hollywood, CA 90028
(800) 422-4453

National Clearinghouse on Child Abuse
    and Neglect
P.O. Box 1182
Washington, DC 20013
(800) 394-3366

National Coalition Against Domestic Violence
P.O. Box 18749
Denver, CO 80218
(303) 839-1852

National Council on Child Abuse and
    Family Violence
1155 Connecticut Avenue NW, Suite 20036
Washington, DC 20036
(202) 429-6695

Parents Anonymous
6733 South Sepulveda Boulevard
Los Angeles, CA 90045
(800) 421-0353

VOICES in Action, Inc. (Victims of Incest Can
    Emerge Survivors in Action, Inc.)
P.O. Box 148309
Chicago, IL 60614
(312) 327-1500

GENERAL REHABILITATION
National Rehabilitation Association
633 South Washington Street
Alexandria, VA 22314
(703) 836-0850

GENETIC DISEASES AND BIRTH DEFECTS
American Genetic Association
P.O. Box 39
Buckeystown, MD 21717
(301) 695-9292

March of Dimes/Birth Defects Foundation
1275 Mamaroneck Avenue
White Plains, NY 10605
(914) 428-7100

National Hemophilia Foundation
110 Greene Street, Suite 303
New York, NY 10012
(212) 219-8180

National Institute of Child Health and
    Human Development
Building 31, Room 2A32
Bethesda, MD 20892
(301) 496-5133

National Sickle Cell Disease Branch
Division of Blood Diseases and Resources
National Heart, Lung, and Blood Institute
Room 504, Federal Building
7550 Wisconsin Avenue
Bethesda, MD 20892
(301) 496-6931

National Tay-Sachs and Allied Disease
   Association, Inc.
92 Washington Avenue
Cedarhurst, NY 11516
(516) 569-4300
or
2001 Beacon Street
Brookline, MA 02146
(617) 277-4463

Spina Bifida Association of America
4590 McArthur Boulevard, NW, Suite 250
Washington, DC 20007
(800) 621-3141
(202) 944-3285

HEART DISEASE
American Heart Association
7272 Greenville Avenue
Dallas, TX 75231
(800) 242-8721

Arizona Heart Institute and Foundation
(800) 345-4278

Coronary Club, Inc.
9500 Euclid Avenue, Room E4-15
Cleveland, OH 44195
(216) 444-3690

National Heart, Lung, and Blood Institute
Building 31, Room 4A21
Bethesda, MD 20892
(301) 496-4236

National High Blood Pressure Education Program
Information Center
National Institutes of Health
7200 Wisconsin Avenue, Suite 500
Bethesda, MD 20814
(301) 951-3620

HIV/AIDS
AIDS Hot Line
(800) 342-AIDS
(202) 245-6867 (Call collect if in Alaska
   or Hawaii)

National AIDS Information Clearinghouse
P.O. Box 6003
Rockville, MD 20850
(800) 458-5231
(800) 342-2437
(800) 334-7492 (Spanish speakers)
(800) 243-7889 (TTY-Deaf access)

Women's AIDS Network
(415) 864-4376
(800) 367-2437

INFERTILITY
American Fertility Society
1209 Montgomery Highway
Birmingham, AL 35216
(205) 978-5000

RESOLVE, Inc.
1310 Broadway
Somerville, MA 02114
(617) 623-0744

IRRITABLE BOWEL SYNDROME
International Foundation for
   Bowel Dysfunction
P.B. Box 17864
Milwaukee, WI 53217
(414) 964-1799

LEARNING DISABILITIES
Association for Children with Learning Disabilities
4156 Library Road
Pittsburgh, PA 15234
(412) 341-1515

National Center for Learning Disabilities
381 Park Avenue South, Suite 1420
New York, NY 10016
(212) 545-9665

LUPUS (SLE)
American Lupus Society
23751 Madison Street
Torrance, CA 90505
(213) 373-1335

Lupus Foundation of America
(800) 558-0121

National Institute of Arthritis, Musculoskeletal,
    and Skin Diseases
Box AMS
Bethesda, MD 20892
(301) 495-4484

MENTAL HEALTH

American Association of Pastoral Counselors
9504-A Lee Highway
Fairfax, VA 22031
(703) 385-6967

American Board of Examiners in
    Clinical Social Work
8484 Georgia Avenue, Suite 800
Silver Spring, MD 20910
(301) 587-8783

American Family Therapy Association
2020 Pennsylvania Avenue NW, Suite 273
Washington, DC 20006
(202) 994-2776

American Mental Health Counselors Association
5999 Stevenson Avenue
Alexandria, VA 22304
(703) 823-9800

American Mental Health Foundation
2 East 86th Street
New York, NY 10028
(212) 737-9027

American Nurses' Association
600 Maryland Avenue, Suite 100
Washington, DC 20024-2571

American Psychiatric Association
1400 K Street, NW
Washington, DC 20005
(202) 682-6000

American Psychological Association
750 First Street, NE
Washington, DC 20002
(202) 336-5500

Anxiety Disorders Association of America
6000 Executive Boulevard, Suite 200
Rockville, MD 20852
(301) 231-8368

Association of Humanistic Psychology
1772 Vallejo Street
San Francisco, CA 94123
(415) 346-7929

National Association for Mental Health
66 Canal Center Plaza, Suite 302
Alexandria, VA 22314
(703) 139-9333

National Association of Social Workers, Inc.
750 First Street, NE, Suite 700
Washington, DC 20002
(202) 408-8600
(800) 638-8799

National Foundation for Depressive Illness
P.O. Box 2257
New York, NY 10016
(800) 248-4344

National Institute of Mental Health
Public Inquiries Section
Room 15 C-05
5600 Fishers Lane
Rockville, MD 20857
(301) 443-4513

National Register of Health Service Providers
    in Psychology
1120 G Street, NW
Washington, DC 20005
(202) 783-7663

MENTAL RETARDATION

American Association on Mental Deficiency
(800) 424-3638
(202) 387-1968 (in District of Columbia)

American Association on Mental Retardation
1719 Kalorama Road, NW
Washington, DC 20009
(202) 387-1968

Association for Retarded Citizens
500 East Border Street, Suite 300
Arlington, TX 76010
(817) 261-6003

Kennedy Child Study Center
151 East 67th Street
New York, NY 10021
(212) 988-9500

National Down Syndrome Society
(800) 221-4602
(212) 460-9330 (in New York)

MINORITY HEALTH ISSUES
National Black Women's Health Project
1237 Ralph Davis Abernathy Boulevard, NW
Atlanta, GA 30310
(404) 758-9590

Office of Minority Health Resource Center
P.O. Box 37337
Washington, DC 20013
(800) 444-6472

NERVE AND MUSCLE DISORDERS
Multiple Sclerosis Association of America
(800) 833-4672

National Multiple Sclerosis Society
733 Third Avenue
New York, NY 10017
(212) 986-3240

**OCCUPATIONAL HEALTH AND
    SEXUAL HARASSMENT**
Department of Health and Human Services
200 Independence Avenue, SW
Washington, DC 20201
(202) 619-0257

9to5, National Association of Working Women
(800) 522-0925

Office of Federal Contract Compliance Programs
Department of Labor
200 Constitution Avenue, NW
Washington, DC 20210
(202) 401-8818

ORGAN DONATION
The Living Bank
P.O. Box 6725
Houston, TX 77265
(800) 528-2971
(713) 528-2971

United Network for Organ Sharing
P.O. Box 13770
1100 Boulders Parkway, Suite 500
Richmond, VA 23225-8770
(800) 24-DONOR

OSTEOPOROSIS
National Osteoporosis Foundation
1150 17th Street, NW, Suite 500
Washington, DC 20036
(202) 223-2226
(800) 223-9994

PAIN DISORDERS
American Chronic Pain Association, Inc.
P.O. Box 850
Rocklin, CA 95677
(916) 632-0922

American Council for Headache Education
875 Kings Highway, Suite 200
West Deptford, NJ 08096
(800) 255-ACHE
(609) 845-0322

American Pain Society
5700 Old Orchard Road
Skokie, IL 60077
(708) 966-5595

Chronic Pain Support Group
P.O. Box 148
Peninsula, OH 44264
(216) 657-2948

National Chronic Pain Outreach Association
7979 Old Georgetown Road
Bethesda, MD 20814
(301) 652-4948

National Headache Foundation
5252 North Western Avenue
Chicago, IL 60625
(800) 843-2256
(312) 878-7715

PARKINSON'S DISEASE
American Parkinson's Disease Association
116 John Street
New York, NY 10038
(212) 685-2741

National Institute of Neurological Disorders
    and Stroke
(800) 352-9424

National Parkinson's Foundation
(800) 327-4545
(800) 433-7022 (in Florida)
(305) 547-6666 (in Miami)

Parkinson's Disease Foundation
650 West 168th Street
New York, NY 10032
(212) 923-4700

Parkinson Support Group of America
11376 Cherry Hill Road, Suite 204
Beltsville, MD 20705
(301) 937-1545

United Parkinson's Foundation
800 West Washington Boulevard
Chicago, IL 60607
(312) 733-1893

PREGNANCY AND CHILDBIRTH
American College of Nurse-Midwives
1522 K Street, NW, Suite 1000
Washington, DC 20005

Compassionate Friends, Inc.
101 Shelter Road, Suite B-103
Lincolnshire, IL 60069
(708) 990-0010

Depression After Delivery
P.O. Box 1282
Morrisville, PA 19067
(215) 295-3994

International Childbirth Education Association,
    Inc.
P.O. Box 20048
Minneapolis, MN 55420
(612) 854-8660

National Association of Childbearing Centers
3123 Gottschall Road
Perkiomenville, PA 18074-9546
(215) 234-8068

PSORIASIS
American Academy of Dermatology
Box 681069
Schaumburg, IL 60168

National Psoriasis Foundation
6600 South West 92nd Avenue, Suite 300
Portland, OR 97223
(503) 244-7404

SEX THERAPY
American Association of Sex Educators,
    Counselors, and Therapists
435 North Michigan Avenue, Suite 1717
Chicago, IL 60611-4067
(312) 664-0828

Center for Human Sexuality
Department of Psychiatry, Box 1203
Downstate Medical Center
450 Clarkson Avenue
Brooklyn, NY 11203
(718) 270-2576

Impotence Foundation
(800) 221-5517

Sexual Behaviors Consultation Unit
550 North Broadway, Suite 114
Baltimore, MD 21205
(410) 955-6318

SEXUALLY TRANSMITTED DISEASES
Centers for Disease Control
National Sexually Transmitted Disease Hotline
P.O. Box 13827
Research Triangle Park, NC 27709
(800) 227-8922

National Herpes Hotline
(919) 361-8488

VD National Hotline
(800) 227-8922
(800) 982-5883 (in California)

SLEEP DISORDERS
American Narcolepsy Association
425 California Street, Suite 201
San Francisco, CA 94104-6230
(800) 222-6085
(415) 788-4793

American Sleep Disorders Association
1610 Fourteenth Street, NW, Suite 300
Rochester, MN 55901
(507) 287-6006

National Sleep Foundation
122 South Robertson Boulevard,
3rd Floor, Department FC
Los Angeles, CA 90048

SMOKING
Centers for Disease Control Office on
    Smoking and Health
Public Information Branch
Mail Stop K-50
1600 Clifton Road, NE
Atlanta, GA 30333
(404) 488-5705

National Center for Health Promotion
Smoke Stoppers Program
3920 Varsity Drive
Ann Arbor, MI 48108
(313) 971-6077

Office on Smoking and Health
U.S. Department of Health and Human Services
Centers for Disease Control
1600 Clifton Road, NE
Mail Stop K50
Atlanta, GA 30333
(404) 488-5705

Seventh-day Adventists
Community Health Services
P.O. Box 1029
Manhasset, NY 11030
(Ask for "How to Stop Smoking" pamphlet.)

Smokenders
1430 East Indian School Road, Suite 102
Phoenix, AZ 85014
(800) 828-4357

48 East 92nd Street
New York, NY 10128
(212) 369-7300

STROKE
American Paralysis Association
P.O. Box 187
Short Hills, NJ 07078
(800) 255-0292
(201) 379-2690

National Aphasia Association
P.O. Box 1887, Murray Hill Station
New York, NY 10156-0611
(800) 922-4622

National Stroke Association
8480 East Orchard Road, Suite 1000
Inglewood, CO 80111
(303) 839-1992

Stroke Connection
7272 Greenville Avenue
Dallas, TX 75231
(800) 242-8721

Stroke Foundation
898 Park Avenue
New York, NY 10021
(212) 134-3434

SUDDEN INFANT DEATH SYNDROME (SIDS)
New York City Program for Sudden Infant Death
520 First Avenue
New York, NY 10016
(212) 686-8854

Pregnancy and Infant Loss Center
1421 East Wayzata Boulevard
Wayzata, MN 55391
(612) 473-9372

Sudden Infant Death Syndrome (SIDS)
    Clearinghouse
8201 Greensboro Drive, Suite 600
McLean, VA 22102
(703) 821-8955

SURGERY
American College of Surgeons
Office of Public Information
55 East Erie Street
Chicago, IL 60611
(312) 644-4030

American Society for Aesthetic Plastic Surgery
444 East Algonquin Road
Arlington Heights, IL 60005
(708) 228-9131

American Society of Plastic and Reconstructive
    Surgeons
444 East Algonquin Road
Arlington Heights, IL 60005
(708) 228-9900

Non-Emergency Surgery Hotline
(800) 638-6833
(800) 492-6603 (in Maryland)

URINARY TRACT DISORDERS
Bladder Health Council
1120 North Charles Street
Baltimore, MD 21201
(410) 727-2896

Continence Restored, Inc.
785 Park Avenue
New York, NY 10021
(212) 879-3131

Help for Incontinent People
P.O. Box 544
Union, SC 29373
(800) 252-3337
(803) 579-7900

National Kidney Foundation
30 East 33rd Street
New York, NY 10016
(800) 622-9010

WOMEN'S HEALTH
American College of Obstetricians and
    Gynecologists
409 Twelfth Street, SW
Washington, DC 20024

HERS (Hysterectomy Educational Resources
    and Services)
422 Bryn Mawr Avenue
Bala Cynwyd, PA 19004
(215) 667-7757

Melpomene Institute
1010 University Avenue
St. Paul, MN 55104

National Women's Health Center (NWHC)
2440 M Street, NW, Suite 201
Washington, DC 20037
(202) 293-6045

National Women's Health Network
1325 G Street, NW
Washington, DC 20005
(202) 347-1140

PMS and Menopause Self-Help Center
101 First Street, Suite 441
Los Altos, CA 94022
(415) 964-7268

Index

Page numbers in *italics* refer to illustrations.